DNA Repair and Mutagenesis in Eukaryotes

BASIC LIFE SCIENCES
Alexander Hollaender, General Editor
Associated Universities, Inc.
Washington, D.C.

A Continuation Order Plan is available for this series. A continuation order will bring
delivery of each new volume immediately upon publication. Volumes are billed only upon
actual shipment. For further information please contact the publisher.

DNA Repair and Mutagenesis in Eukaryotes

EDITED BY

W. M. GENEROSO

Oak Ridge National Laboratories
Oak Ridge, Tennessee

M. D. SHELBY

AND

F. J. DE SERRES

National Institute of Environmental Health Sciences
Research Triangle Park, North Carolina

PLENUM PRESS · NEW YORK AND LONDON

Library of Congress Cataloging in Publication Data VFDUCat

Symposium on DNA Repair and Mutagenesis in Eukaryotes, Atlanta, 1979.
  DNA repair and mutagenesis in eukaryotes.

  (Basic life sciences; v. 15)
  "Proceedings of the Symposium on DNA Repair and Mutagenesis in Eukaryotes,
sponsored by the National Institute of Environmental Health Sciences, and held in
Atlanta, Georgia, June 25–29, 1979."
  Includes index.
  1. Deoxyribonucleic acid repair—Congresses. 2. Mutagenesis—Congresses. I. Generoso,
W. M. II. Shelby, Michael D. III. De Serres, Frederick J. IV. National Institute of En-
vironmental Health Sciences. V. Title. [DNLM: 1. DNA repair—Congresses. 2. Muta-
tion—Congresses. 3. Cells—Congresses. W3 BA255 v. 15 1979/QH467 S989d 1979]
QH467.S95 1979   574.87'3282   80-18743
  ISBN 0-306-40552-0

Proceedings of the Symposium on DNA Repair and Mutagenesis in Eukaryotes,
sponsored by the National Institute of Environmental Health Sciences,
and held in Atlanta, Georgia, June 25–29, 1979.

© 1980 Plenum Press, New York
A Division of Plenum Publishing Corporation
227 West 17th Street, New York, N.Y. 10011

Printed in the United States of America

FOREWORD

Not many years ago most discussion of mutation induction by physical and chemical agents concentrated on the initial lesions induced in the DNA with the implicit assumption that once the lesions were made they were converted almost automatically to mutations by relatively simple processes associated with DNA replication. The discovery of a variety of enzymatic processes that can repair these lesions, the great increase in our understanding of the molecular steps involved in repair, replication, and recombination, and the increasing availability of cells with genetic defects in these processes have led to the realization that mutation induction is a far more complex process than we originally thought. Repair systems can remove lesions before they can be converted to mutation, they can also convert initial lesions to secondary ones that are themselves mutagenic, and they can remove potentially lethal lesions at the expense of making mutations. The error-avoiding systems associated with replication are themselves complex and may be caused to make mistakes in various ways.

These different pathways for mutation production and mutation avoidance are still being worked out in prokaryotes and are less well understood in eukaryotes. This symposium shows, however, that very encouraging progress has been made in the last several years, and the progress is now accelerating. Among eukaryotes, the repair systems are probably best understood in mammals but, as shown by a number of papers in this symposium considerable progress has been made in working them out for those favorite organisms for studying mutation, yeast, Neurospora, and Drosophila. The analysis of the relations between repair and mutagenesis is probably furthest along in yeast but very encouraging progress has been made with the other systems, including mammalian germ cells.

These developments are of fundamental importance for understanding the basic mechanisms that cells have developed to protect the integrity of the genome. They are also of great practical interest for our attempts to evaluate the risks to human health and well being of the various physical and chemical agents which are the result of the activities of modern society. Various prokaryotic and

v

eukaryotic systems, including especially those discussed in this
symposium, are now in widespread use for the identification and
evaluation of such risks. The confidence with which we extrapolate
from such laboratory test systems to humans depends on how similar
we believe the mutagenic mechanisms to be. It is becoming clear
that the simple assumption that mutagenic mechanisms are the same
in all cells and organisms is incorrect. Only by becoming much more
familiar with the mutagenic processes in our various test systems
can we judge with confidence how serious the variations between test
systems may be and know which features they share with the human
cells of interest. The hope of advancing from the largely empirical
procedures of today to a science firmly based on molecular and
cellular principles depends upon developments in the enzymology of
mutagenesis. This symposium by bringing together workers in this
field should accelerate our progress in this direction.

R. F. KIMBALL

PREFACE

The role of DNA repair processes in modifying radiation-induced genetic damage in eukaryotic organisms was the major subject of a conference held in Leiden, The Netherlands in 1962. The proceedings of that conference were published a year later (Repair from Genetic Radiation Damage and Differential Radiosensitivity in Germ Cells, F. H. Sobels, Ed., The MacMillan Company, New York, 1963) and became an important source of information on the subject. There has been much progress since 1962, particularly in the understanding of the molecular nature of repair processes and their role in mutation induction. Although many are aware of this progress, there has been no comprehensive compilation of information on the relationship between repair and mutation induction in eukaryotes in recent years. Because progress in repair biochemistry and basic mutagenesis are closely linked, it seemed essential not only to convene many of the active researchers in this field in a forum for the review and exchange of research results in eukaryotic organisms from fungi to man but also to produce a publication based on such a meeting. Thus, a conference, supported through funds from the National Institute of Environmental Health Sciences, was organized and held in Atlanta, Georgia on June 25-28, 1979.

The conference was attended by 64 researchers from Argentina, England, Italy, Japan, The Netherlands, Switzerland, and the USA. The success of this meeting is attributable to the enthusiasm of the participants and the high quality of their research and presentations. We believe that this book, which contains the proceedings of the conference, truly reflects on the many exciting new developments in repair and mutagenesis and will provide an important reference in this rapidly advancing field of biology.

W. M. Generoso
M. D. Shelby
F. J. de Serres

CONTENTS

CHAPTER 1

RELATIONSHIP BETWEEN REPAIR PROCESSES AND MUTATION INDUCTION
IN BACTERIA*

R. F. KIMBALL

Biology Division, Oak Ridge National Laboratory
Oak Ridge, TN 37830 (U.S.A.)

SUMMARY

A summary is given of the main repair and replication-
associated processes that can influence the induction of mutations
by various mutagens in bacteria. These include both constitutive
and induced, error-free and error-prone systems. The mutation
yield from a treatment with a mutagen can be markedly affected by
which of these systems is operating in a given bacterial species
or strain. The effect of these systems on mutation induction by
ultraviolet light, monofunctional alkylating agents, base analogues,
and frameshift mutagens is discussed in some detail. The bearing
of these studies on the practical problems of estimating hazards
is briefly considered.

INTRODUCTION

In recent years it has become increasingly evident that to
understand how physical and chemical agents produce mutations we
have to understand both how they interact with DNA and how these
interaction products are handled by the various enzymes that repair
and replicate DNA. These enzymes may remove much of the damage
from the DNA, but they may also make mutations while rescuing the
cell from potentially lethal damage. Both constitutive and induced
enzymes are involved. Cells can differ in the complement of such
enzymes, and such differences can have major effects on the action
of potential mutagens. Thus mutagens such as UV light, that are
strong mutagens for many cells, are almost nonmutagenic for some
cells.

This situation raises important questions about such practical matters as dose-rate effects, the form of the dose-response curve, and the applicability of test results from one species to another and even from one cell type to another in the same species. If mutagenesis testing and hazards evaluation is to advance from the empiricism that dominates it today to a science based on strong theory, then we must be just as concerned with the enzymatic mechanisms that handle damaged DNA as with the molecular mechanisms by which the damage is produced in the first place.

In a preceding paper Setlow [72] has covered the major features of DNA repair. I will concentrate on the role of repair in mutation induction. However, I cannot discuss this subject without also talking about replication and to a lesser extent recombination. I shall confine myself to bacteria since the work with them is further along than that with other organisms and since I know this work better.

A previous review [38] covered much of the same material as the present paper in more detail and with a more complete set of references. Other recent reviews on mutagenesis in bacteria have been published by Bridges [4, 5, 7], Doudney [14], Kondo [44], and Witkin [82]. More detailed information on repair processes, together with some of the relations to mutagenesis, can be found in the published proceedings of two workshops [23, 24].

MAIN ENZYMATIC PROCESSES

Table 1 lists the main enzymatic processes that can influence mutation yields. Some of these occur prior to replication and some occur during or after replication. Two prereplication processes, photomonomerization of pyrimidine dimers and the rejoining of strand breaks with 3'-hydroxy and 5'-phosphoryl ends, restore the initial state of the DNA directly and thus should prevent mutation as has been clearly demonstrated for photomonomerization (photoreactivation).

The prereplication process that has been most studied is excision repair. References to the many papers on this subject may be found in the reviews and workshop proceedings mentioned above. As will be brought out in subsequent discussions, several different excision processes with different substrates and combinations of enzymes exist. In all cases, excision repair is a multistep process requiring an endonuclease for the initial incision and an exonuclease, polymerase, and ligase to excise a series of bases, resynthesize the excised region, and join the strand ends back together again. There are reasons to believe that, in some instances at least, resynthesis is subject to error and thus can be a source of mutation. Recently Linn et al. [49] reported some evidence from human fibroblasts that altered bases can be removed from the DNA and replaced

TABLE 1

MAIN ENZYMATIC PROCESSES IN MUTATION INDUCTION

Process	Error
Prereplication processes	
Photomonomerization of dimers	Error-free
Strand-break rejoining	Error-free
Excision repair	Errors possible
Base removal and replacement ?	Error-free ?
Recombination	Errors possible
Replication-associated processes	
Replication with proofreading	Errors possible
Gap formation with postreplication repair	Errors possible
Mismatch repair	Errors ?

by normal bases without excision. Presumably this process is error-free. Finally, recombination between strands may, on the one hand, allow the reconstruction of a normal genome from several damaged ones or, alternatively, when recombination is between different regions in the same strand, it can cause deletions and inversions. In eukaryotes, translocations can arise by recombination between different chromosomes.

Prereplication processes may remove many lesions, but some lesions will usually remain at the time of DNA replication. In Escherichia coli each of the three known DNA polymerases has associated with it a $3' \rightarrow 5'$ exonucleolytic activity that can remove newly inserted bases that are detected by the systems as pairing improperly [10]. This "proofreading" activity prevents many errors but cannot avoid the insertion of some "wrong" bases opposite bases that have been altered by a mutagen. It can also "stall" replication at a noncoding lesion, such as a pyrimidine dimer. Synthesis apparently starts up again further along the strand so that gaps are left in the new DNA. These gaps can be filled by postreplication repair. There are probably several forms of this process and some of them are subject to error. Finally, mismatched bases left in the DNA at replication can be removed shortly after replication by a process known as mismatch repair which will eliminate some potentially mutagenic mismatched base combinations. Discussions of these processes are to be found in the reviews and workshop proceedings referred to earlier. Information on mismatch repair in relation to spontaneous mutation can be found in a review by Cox [13].

TABLE 2

EFFECT OF BLOCK IN DIMER EXCISION REPAIR (Uvr⁻ STRAINS)

Induced mutation	Agent	Conclusions
Increased	UV 4-Nitroquinoline 1-oxide Hycanthone, Others[a]	Replication errors predominate
Unaffected	Monofunctional alkylating agents Ionizing radiation Hydroxylamine Others[a]	Dimer excision not active on these lesions
None	Mitomycin C, Cis-platinum dichlorodiamine	Lesions lethal at replication; Prereplication repair required for viable mutants

[a]See Kimball [38] for a more complete list and for references to the data for those listed.

THE PYRIMIDINE DIMER EXCISION REPAIR SYSTEM

UV-induced pyrimidine dimers can be removed before replication by the dimer excision system. The first step is an incision (strand break) introduced into the DNA by a UV endonuclease. This endonuclease can also incise the DNA near other bulky lesions, such as large adducts and crosslinks, but apparently does not act on slightly altered bases. The section on "Nucleotide Excision Repair in Bacteria" in a recent workshop [23] can be consulted for more information on this subject.

Mutants of E. coli at the uvrA and uvrB loci lack the incision step and do not remove dimers. UV and several other agents that produce bulky lesions in DNA produce a much higher frequency of mutations in such strains than in wild type (Table 2). This suggests that such lesions produce mutations most effectively if, because of the repair deficiency, they persist to replication. It does not exclude the possibility that some mutations are formed during the

excision process though with a lower probability than if the same
lesions had persisted to replication. Indeed there is evidence
that errors can happen during excision [9, 57, 58].

The absence of the dimer incision enzyme has little, if any,
effect on mutation induction by ionizing radiation, monofunctional
alkylating agents, and several other mutagens. No mutations are
induced by mitomycin C or the platinum compound in an excision-
negative strain. Apparently the crosslinks produced by mitomycin C
and lesions produced by the platinum compound are lethal if they
persist to replication but can be converted to a mutagenic but
nonlethal lesion by excision repair.

AN INDUCED ERROR-PRONE SYSTEM (SOS SYSTEM)

Much work has been done in recent years on an error-prone
system induced by UV light. This work has been reviewed extensively
by Witkin [82] and a section in a recent workshop [23] was devoted
to it. It was given the name "SOS repair" by Radman [61], and this
is a convenient term for referring to this system.

The initial evidence for an error-prone system under gene
control was the observation by Witkin [80] that exr⁻ (now usually
called lexA⁻) mutants of E. coli were not mutable by UV (Table 3)
whether or not the excision system was present. The exr⁻ strains
with excision repair survived better than those without it (uvrA⁻,
uvrB⁻). Therefore, it was concluded that excision repair was
probably error free and that the error prone step was in postreplication repair, the only other known repair process at that time.
It was at first suggested that recombination was error-prone, since
postreplication repair in E. coli involved recombination, and this
suggestion was given support by the finding that recA⁻ strains, in
which recombination is lacking, were not mutated by UV [81].
However, more recent studies on various combinations of recB or
recC and recF strains suggest that recombination is not involved in
the error-prone reaction. The single mutants recB⁻, recC⁻, and
recF⁻ are mutable by UV as is the double mutant recB⁻recF⁻, but
recombination is blocked almost as completely in the double mutant
as it is in recA⁻ [36]. Moreover, the recA locus appears to have
more than one complementing unit, only one of which is involved in
recombination [18]. The lexB mutant, which is probably an allele
of recA, is not mutable by UV but is not blocked in recombination.
Mutants of lexC [34, 37] and the combination of recB and uvrD [73]
can block UV mutagenesis, but too little work has been done to
determine how they act.

Other work has shown that UV induced a whole series of
different events that also require the lexA and recA functions.
These are phage induction, reactivation of irradiated phage by

TABLE 3

MUTANT LOCI E. coli THAT PREVENT UV-INDUCED MUTATION

Locus	Action	UV-induced mutation when locus mutant
lexA (= exr)	SOS system	None
recA	All recombination, SOS system, protein X	None
Alleles of recA ?		
lexB	SOS system	None
tif-1	Temperature-sensitive induction of SOS system	Increased at 42°C
lexC (= umuC)	Not known	None
recB uvrD	See below	None
recB	RECBC recombination pathway, exonuclease V	Nearly normal
uvrD	Mutator, proofreading(?), Mismatch repair(?)	High spontaneous, Nearly normal induced

irradiated hosts (Weigle reactivation), filament formation, and mutations induced in unirradiated phage by irradiated hosts [82]. These same phenomena are induced by high temperature (42°C) in a temperature-sensitive mutant, tif-1, which is probably an allele of recA. At 42°C the tif-1 mutant has an elevated spontaneous mutation frequency and is also more mutable by low doses of UV than is wild type.

This set of properties and other considerations led to the formulation of the hypothesis that all these effects, including an error-prone replication or repair system, were coinduced by UV, and Witkin [82] has discussed in some detail the induction system and the role of the lexA and recA loci in induction. There is some evidence, however, that at low doses of UV not all these functions are coinduced in the same cell [84]. Radman and his colleagues [3, 62, 63] have developed the view that one of the major consequences of the induced system is a modification of, or block to, the proofreading (3'→5' exonuclease) function of one or more of the polymerases. An alternative suggestion has been made by Lark [47] that the replication complex has been modified in such a way that it can synthesize past a dimer. A discussion of some of these same observations from a somewhat different perspective is given by Clark and Volkert [12]. The paper by Strauss in this volume [74] should be consulted for an alternative view of the block to synthesis caused by certain lesions.

The consequences of the hypothesis that the proofreading system is modified or blocked are diagramed in Fig. 1. The proofreading activity normally prevents synthesis past such noncoding lesions as pyrimidine dimers. Synthesis appears to start up again further along the strand, perhaps at the initiation site for the next Okazaki fragment. The gaps left in the newly synthesized DNA are usually repaired in E. coli by recombination repair, as diagramed at the top of Fig. 1. From the studies with the rec mutants, it would appear that this process is probably error free. The alternatives to recombination repair are either gap-filling synthesis past the dimer or replication past the dimer. Both would probably require some sort of block to the proofreading activity.

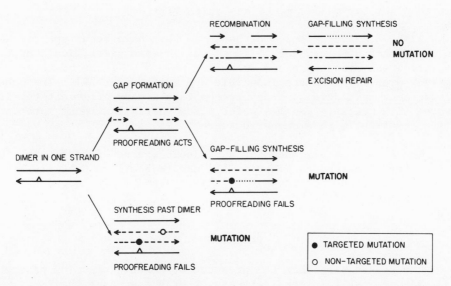

Fig. 1.   Diagram of replication and postreplication repair in DNA that contains pyrimidine dimers: (——) old DNA;   (---) newly replicated DNA; (···) gap-filling or excision-repair synthesis.

Sedgwick [71] has suggested that synthesis past the dimer is the only way in which synthesis could be completed when there are two dimers closely spaced in opposite strands and suggests that such double lesions are a major source of UV-induced mutations at the higher doses at which the SOS system is fully induced.

Once the proofreading system is blocked or modified, errors could also occur even in synthesis on sections of DNA without lesions. There is evidence that such "nontargeted" mutations do occur [6, 30, 32, 82]. However, it seems likely that at higher doses the bulk of the mutations are "targeted," perhaps many of them being initiated by Sedgwick's double lesions.

Bridges [8] has concluded that those mutations fixed prior to replication result from a constitutive error-prone process that is different from the induced error-prone process responsible for fixation during and after replication. If so, the two processes must have important common components since the functions of the lexA and recA loci are required for both.

A number of other agents also require the functions of the lexA and recA loci to produce mutations and so may act primarily through the SOS-induced system (Table 4). The monofunctional alkylating agents produce some mutations through this system, but, with the exception of methyl methanesulfonate (MMS) many of the mutations they produce are induced by other mechanisms. A number of other agents seem to have no dependence at all on this system, but the data for these agents are quite limited.

There are four species of bacteria that have been reported not to be mutated by ultraviolet light and, in some cases, ionizing radiation and other mutagens as well (Table 5). Three of these species probably lack the inducible SOS system [38, 39]. The other, Micrococcus radiodurans, probably combines a very efficient repair system with multiple genomes which allow survival without mutation after treatment with a number of agents [25, 54].

There is some evidence for an inducible error-free repair system for UV damage to E. coli [55] and to Bacillus subtilis [16], but too little has been done with this system, if it indeed exists, to discuss it further here.

PLASMIDS

The observation that the presence of certain plasmids protect bacteria against the lethal effects of UV but enhance their susceptibility to mutation induction by a variety of agents led to the incorporation of one such plasmid (pKM101) in stocks of Salmonella typhimurium used in the Ames assay [52]. In general

TABLE 4

MUTAGENS ACTING THROUGH THE SOS SYSTEM[a]

Dependence	Mutagen
Major or total dependence on system (lexA, recA dependence)	Ultraviolet light Ionizing radiation 4-Nitroquinoline oxide Mitomycin C Methyl methanesulfonate Cis-platinum dichlorodiamine
Some mutations by system, many by other system(s)	Nitrous acid Monofunctional alkylating agents other than MMS
No dependence on system?	Hydroxylamine ICR 191 Others?

[a]See Kimball [38].

TABLE 5

BACTERIA SPECIES NOT MUTATED BY UV

Species	
Proteus mirabilis Haemophilus influenzae Haemophilus parainfluenzae	SOS system absent?
Micrococcus radiodurans	Very efficient repair, recombination between multiple genomes

(Table 6), the plasmid enhances the activity of a large number of agents [38, 51, 52], including those that depend on the SOS system in E. coli. The plasmid enhances the activity of mutagens producing base-substitution mutations more frequently than it enhances the activity of mutagens producing frameshift mutations. However, it does increase the frequency with which some of the mutagens produce frameshifts, and in addition causes them to produce some base

TABLE 6

EFFECTS OF THE pKM101 PLASMID ON
CHEMICAL MUTAGENESIS IN SALMONELLA[a]

Mutagen	Effect of plasmid
4-Nitroquinoline oxide Methyl methanesulfonate N-Methyl-N'-nitro-N-nitrosoguanidine Benzyl chloride Aflatoxin B_1	Base-subtitution mutations increased
Ethyl methanesulfonate Bis(2-chloroethyl)amine Dimethylcarbamyl	Base-substitution mutations unaffected
Benzo[a]pyrene 7-12-Dimethylbenz[a]anthracene Aflatoxin B_1	Frameshift mutations increased
ICR 191 2-Aminoanthracene 2-Nitrosofluorene	Frameshift mutations unaffected

[a]Sample list only. Much more information available [33].

substitutions as well. Therefore, the system seems to be involved
in producing both base-substitution and frameshift mutations,
although it is more effective with the former.

    Some evidence suggests that the plasmid enhances the activity
of the SOS system [77-79]. However, other evidence suggests that it
is not the SOS system that is involved [53]. Some evidence [20]
suggests that the plasmid is responsible for a constitutive error-
prone system distinct from the SOS system. It is possible, but not
certain, that this is a constitutive modification of the proofreading system.

MONOFUNCTIONAL ALKYLATING AGENTS

    The main observable molecular effects of monofunctional
alkylating agents on DNA are the alkylation of specific positions
on certain bases and the production of lesions that may be single-
strand breaks, alkali-labile sites, or both. It seems probable that
minor alkylated species, O^6-methylguanine for example, are the

important ones for mutation [17, 50]. Several different mechanisms
for the elimination (repair) of alkylated bases from DNA have been
proposed (Fig. 2). These include removal of the base by a DNA
glycosylase followed either by direct base replacement without
strand breakage [49] or by incision by an AP (apurinic, apyrimidinic)
endonuclease followed by excision repair [48]. Alternatively, a
number of endonucleolytic activities have been described that appear
to incise directly at the altered base with subsequent excision
repair [44]. Lindahl [48] has reviewed these repair pathways, and
they are also discussed in the section on base excision repair in
Hanawalt et al. [23].

Mutation data have confirmed in various ways that repair of
potentially mutagenic lesions does occur after treatment with
alkylating agents [1, 33, 42, 43, 68]. These data also show that
UV endonuclease is not involved since mutants blocked in dimer
excision are just as mutable by monofunctional alkylating agents as
wild type [38].

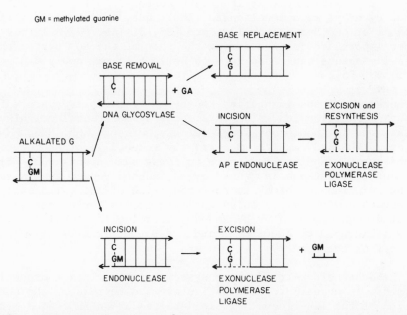

Fig. 2. Diagram of prereplication repair processes for alkylated
bases: (——) old DNA; (---) excision-repair synthesis.

The mechanisms that have been proposed for mutation induction by monofunctional alkylating agents [38] are: (1) mispairing at replication; (2) localized damage to replication complex; (3) induced SOS error-prone system (lexA⁺ required); (4) induced error-free repair (lexA-independent); (5) constitutive error-free repair (lexA⁺ required). The simplest and most obvious hypothesis is that alkylated bases are produced at random in the genome, are subject to removal by one of the repair processes prior to replication, and are converted to mutation by mispairing at replication. Evidence mainly consistent with this hypothesis has been obtained with H. influenzae for MNNG [42, 43] and nitrosocarbaryl [1, 2].

The second mechanism that has been suggested is some special action at the replication fork. Evidence from E. coli treated with nitroso compounds such as N-methyl-N'-nitro-N-nitrosoguanidine (MNNG), N-methyl-N-nitrosourea (MNUA or N-ethyl-N-nitrosourea (ENUA) has been interpreted as favoring such an hypothesis [11, 22, 26-28]. The evidence for the existence of such a component for EMS is equivocal [21, 28]. In H. influenzae, this component, if it exists, is probably less important than it is in E. coli [42].

The role of the SOS system in mutation induction by monofunctional alkylating agents probably varies with the agent. It seems to be the major component of mutation induction by MMS in E. coli [28, 31, 46, 69]. It is also involved, though to a lesser extent, in mutation induction by MNNG and MNUA [27, 28, 31, 46, 69]. There is a possibility that it may be responsible for some mutations induced by ethyl methanesulfonate (EMS), but, if so, it is a minor component at the doses normally used [28, 31, 46, 69]. It may be of some importance in considering the role of the SOS system that alkylating agents can cause gaps to be left in the newly synthesized DNA [1, 42, 75].

Recent work has identified two error-free repair systems for preventing mutation induction in E. coli by monofunctional alkylating agents. One is induced by low-level exposures to MMS, EMS, MNNG, ENNG, and MNUA and results in a greatly reduced level of mutation by subsequent high-level exposure to these same agents [33, 68]. The induced resistance is caused by an induced repair system rather than by some induced block to the production of initial damage, and it disappears with time. This repair system is not effective against damage produced by UV and 4-nitroquinoline 1-oxide (4NQO), nor is it induced by 4NQO. The induced system removes O⁶-methylguanine from the DNA [70].

The other error-free repair system has been less thoroughly analyzed. It appears to be constitutive and to require the normal function of the lexA locus. It is detected by an increased mutation yield at very low doses in lexA⁻ strains as compared to lexA⁺ ones, just the opposite of the result expected with lexA+-dependent error-prone repair [69].

BASE ANALOGS

The main mechanisms that influence mutation induction by base analogs are: (1) misincorporation and misreplication (main or only source); (2) SOS system (probably not a source of mutation); (3) repair and prevention, which, may involve selection against incorporation of analog (occurs), mismatch repair with new strand recognition (occurs: dam locus), or possibly recognition of 5-bromouracil as thymine analog only.

Base analogs probably induce mutations only by mispairing either during incorporation or during subsequent replication. Thus the thymine analog 5-bromouracil might be incorporated in place of cytosine or might be treated as cytosine once it was incorporated for thymine [15]. Some evidence was published by Pietrzykowska and colleagues to show that the SOS system was involved [59, 60]. However, more recent work has failed to repeat some of the results and makes it very improbable that the SOS system is responsible for mutation induction by base analogs [29, 83].

Some of this recent work has shown, however, that there are systems that can reduce or prevent mutagenesis by base analogues. In both E. coli [35] and H. influenzae [40] there is a strong preference for incorporation of thymidine when both thymidine and 5-bromodeoxyuridine are present. In H. influenzae no detectable mutation was produced even when the levels of incorporation of 5-bromodeoxyuridine were quite high. The suggestion was made that the polymerase of this species may always treat 5-bromodeoxyuridine as a thymidine not a cytidine analog [40].

There is a series that can prevent mutation after the analog has been incorporated. This is the mismatch repair system. E. coli DNA is methylated, primarily at the 6 position of adenine, by a deoxyadenosine methylase. This reaction takes time, however, and the newly synthesized DNA is at first undermethylated. This provides a "marker" so that the mismatch repair system can distinguish between old and new strands (Fig. 3). A mutant, dam-3, that fails to methylate the DNA properly is more mutable than wild type by 5-bromouracil [19]. Presumably this is because of the difficulty of distinguishing old and new strands in this mutant. Mismatch repair probably also accounts for the threshold-like dose curve with 5-bromouracil [66, 67]. At low levels of incorporation there is essentially no mutation induced. Once the ratio of newly incorporated bromouracil to newly incorporated thymine reaches about 50%, the frequency of mutation rises rapidly. The suggestion is made that at these higher levels of incorporation the mismatch

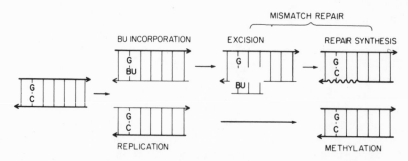

Fig. 3.   Diagram of mismatch repair and the role of strand methylation in removal of a mismatched base: (heavy lines) strand methylated at 6-adenine position;   (wavy line) resynthesized section.

repair system becomes saturated.   It may be that the mismatch repair system in <u>H</u>. <u>influenzae</u> is not as readily saturated as in <u>E</u>. <u>coli</u>.

FRAMESHIFT MUTATION

Earlier work on frameshift mutagenesis in prokaryotes led to a model, proposed by Streisinger et al. [76], that frameshift mutagenesis results from mispairing when there is a strand break in a region of repeated base sequences followed by repair of the break. Because of this mispairing, base additions or deletions could be produced in the repaired strand.   It was suggested that frameshift mutagens acted to stabilize the mispairing by intercalation within the DNA double helix.   The most effective frameshift mutagens have a ring structure which could intercalate.   However, some other mutagens, UV for example, that could not intercalate can produce some frameshift mutations as well as base substitutions.   That mechanisms other than intercalation may be involved is suggested by the finding that the frequency of frameshift mutations produced by some, but not other, frameshift mutagens is higher in stocks of <u>S</u>. <u>typhimurium</u> containing a plasmid (Table 7) (see section on Plasmids).

Some information about repair processes other than that controlled by the pKM101 plasmid comes from work with ICR191 (Table 7).   This compound has an alkylating group that can bind it to DNA, as well as a ring structure that can intercalate in the helix.   Its mutagenic potency is not affected by the presence of the pKM101 plasmid.   Strains of <u>E</u>. <u>coli</u> defective in the incision step of dimer excision (<u>uvrA</u>⁻ and <u>uvrB</u>⁻) are much more mutable than wild type,

TABLE 7

FRAMESHIFT MUTAGENS

Agent	Effect
Plasmid	Increases frameshift mutation by some but not other mutagens Increases base substitution mutations by some frameshift mutagens

ICR 191	Influence of blocked excision
	  E. coli: increased mutation
	  H. influenzae: decreased mutation
	Role of replication
	  E. coli: major role
	  H. influenzae: major role
	Blocked recombination
	  Both species: no effect

suggesting that excision repair can remove the compound from the DNA and that when it is not removed it is much more likely to produce mutations [56]. This is the expected result for an agent that produces mutations most effectively when it persists to replication, and the association with replication has been confirmed with synchronized cultures [56]. However, work in progress with H. influenzae indicates that, if anything, a strain defective in dimer excision is much less mutable than wild type [41]. This strain is much more susceptible to killing by ICR191 than is wild type. It may be that the potentially mutagenic lesions it induces are lethal in H. influenzae unless excision occurs, whereas they are not in E. coli. Recombination is probably unimportant for mutagenesis by ICR191 in either E. coli [56] or H. influenzae [41], since strains defective in recombination are just as mutable as wild type.

PRACTICAL CONSIDERATIONS

It is obvious that the processes by which mutagens produce mutations are multiple and complex. A number of different enzyme systems are involved, and the relative importance of different repair and replication systems is not the same for the different major classes of mutagens. Some of the enzymatic systems are constitutive; others are induced by the mutagens. Mutant strains of bacteria exist in which one or more of these systems are missing.

Such defects can make strains nearly totally nonresponsive to agents such as UV that are strong mutagens in wild type strains or, conversely, make them much more mutable. There is evidence that different species of bacteria may differ very markedly in their response to mutagens, presumably because of differences in the enzymatic systems they possess.

What does all this have to do with the practical problems of assessment of risks for humans and interpreting data from mammalian or other eukaryotic test systems? In the first place, the extreme differences that have been found between strains, and even species, of bacteria in response to common mutagens suggest that it is possible that similar differences may be found between mammalian species and stocks. What is more important, and more likely, is that major differences might exist between different cells in the same body so that even tests with cells from the same stock might not apply to other cells from the same stock. For example, there might be major differences between some somatic cells and germ cells. Indeed, there is some evidence that the germ cells of the mouse may react in an unusual way to alkylating agents [64, 65].

The second point is that both error-prone and error-free systems can be induced by low levels of mutagen. If error-prone systems are induced, then low-level exposures, which do not induce the error-prone system, might be much less mutagenic than would be suggested by high-level acute exposures, which do induce it. If error-free repair systems are induced, then low-level exposure, including low-level chronic exposure, might actually protect the individual against subsequent high levels of exposure by inducing the error-free repair system. It is also possible that people in today's high technology societies are exposed to a sufficient level of a combination of mutagens so that all systems, error-prone and error-free, are permanently induced. All that can be said at present is that extrapolations from acute high-level exposures to chronic low-level ones are suspect.

This applies specifically to the use of the plasmid-containing strains of Salmonella as prescreens for mutagens. The evidence suggests that such strains may have a constitutive error-prone system that has many, if not all, the mutagen specificities of the inducible error-prone SOS system. If an SOS-like system exists in mammals and is inducible not constitutive, then the apparent high correlation between tests for mutagenicity in the plasmid-bearing bacteria and tests for carcinogenicity in mammals may be a conse-quence of the latter being carried out under acute, high-level exposure conditions that induce much the same error-prone system as is present constitutively in bacteria. In that case results with the plasmid-free strain might be more pertinent to chronic exposure situations.

I do not want to imply that any of these speculations should be considered seriously in hazards evaluations at present. I do urge, however, the importance of getting a thorough understanding of the various mutagenic mechanisms in the bacteria that are being so widely used as prescreens, in the mammalian test systems that must be used in the laboratory, and in the human systems, which after all are the real goal of all this work. In my view, it is only in this way that we can hope to advance from today's largely empirical approach to a more sophisticated science based on a strong foundation of theory. Though the system in bacteria may seem complicated, I believe we already have enough information so that fairly broad generalizations are beginning to develop. Examples of such generalizations are the SOS hypothesis, the induction of error-free repair by monofunctional alkylating agents, and the role of the proofreading system in induced, as well as spontaneous, mutations. I am hopeful that out of these initial generalizations will emerge a still broader theoretical framework for induced mutagenesis.

ACKNOWLEDGEMENT

*This research was sponsored by the Office of Health and Environmental Research, U.S. Department of Energy, under contract W-7405-eng-26 with the Union Carbide Corporation.

REFERENCES

1. Beattie, K. L., N-Nitrosocarbaryl-induced mutagenesis in Haemophilus influenzae strains deficient in repair and recombination, Mutat. Res., 27 (1975) 201-217.
2. Beattie, K. L., and R. F. Kimball, Involvement of DNA replication and repair in mutagenesis of Haemophilus influenzae induced by N-nitrosocarbaryl, Mutat. Res., 24 (1974) 105-115.
3. Boiteux, S., G. Villani, S. Spardari, F. Zambrano, and M. Radman, Making and correcting errors in DNA synthesis: in vitro studies of mutagenesis, in: DNA Repair Mechanisms, P. C. Hanawalt, E. C. Friedberg, and C. F. Fox (Eds.), Academic Press, New York, 1978, pp. 73-84.
4. Bridges, B. A., Mutation induction, In: Second International Symposium on the Genetics of Industrial Microorganisms, K. D. Macdonald (Ed.), Academic Press, New York, 1976, pp. 7-14.
5. Bridges, B. A., Bacterial Reaction to Radiation, Patterns in Progress, Meadowfield, Durham, England, 1976.
6. Bridges, B. A., Mutagenic DNA repair in Escherichia coli. VI. Gamma radiation mutagenesis in tif-1 strain, Mol. Gen. Genet., 151 (1977) 115-120.

7. Bridges, B. A., Recent advances in basic mutation research,
    Abh. Akad. Wiss. DDR, Abt. Mathematik, Naturwiss.,
    Technik, N 9 (1977) 9-21.
8. Bridges, B. A., The involvement of E. coli DNA polymerase III
    in constitutive and inducible mutagenic repair, In: DNA
    Repair Mechanisms, P. C. Hanawalt, E. C. Friedberg, and
    C. F. Fox (Eds.), Academic Press, New York, 1978, pp.
    345-348.
9. Bridges, B. A., and R. Mottershead, RecA$^+$-dependent mutagenesis
    occurring before DNA replication in UV and γ-irradiated
    Escherichia coli, Mutat. Res., 13 (1971) 1-18.
10. Brutlage, D., and A. Kornberg, Enzymatic synthesis of deoxy-
    ribonucleic acid. XXXVI. A proofreading function for the
    3'→5' exonuclease activity in deoxyribonucleic acid
    polymerases, J. Biol. Chem., 247 (1972) 241-248.
11. Cerdá-Olmedo, E., P. C. Hanawalt, and N. Guerola, Mutagenesis
    of the replication point by nitrosoguanidine: Map and
    pattern of replication of the Escherichia coli chromosome,
    J. Mol. Biol., 33 (1968) 705-719.
12. Clark, A. J., and M. R. Volkert, A new classification of
    pathways repairing pyrimidine dimer damage, In: DNA Repair
    Mechanisms, P. C. Hanawalt, E. C. Friedberg, and C. F.
    Fox (Eds.), Academic Press, New York, 1978, pp. 57-72.
13. Cox, E. C., Bacterial mutation genes and the control of
    spontaneous mutation, Ann. Rev. Genet., 10 (1976) 135-156.
14. Doudney, C. O., Mutation in ultraviolet light-damaged micro-
    organisms, In: Photochemistry and Photobiology of Nucleic
    Acids, S. Y. Wang (Ed.), Academic Press, New York, 1976,
    pp. 309-374.
15. Drake, J. W., The Molecular Basis of Mutation, Holden-Day,
    San Francisco, 1970.
16. Dubinin, N. P., V. D. Filippov, and E. E. Zagoriuko, Induction
    of antimutagenic activity in Bacillus subtilis cells by
    ultraviolet radiation, Dokl. Biol. Sci., 232 (1977) 32-35.
17. Gerchman, L. L., and D. B. Ludlum, The properties of 0^6-
    methylguanine in templates for RNA polymerase, Biochim.
    Biophys. Acta, 308 (1973) 310-316.
18. Glickman, B. W., N. Guijt, and P. Morand, The genetic charac-
    terization of lexB32, lexB33, and lexB35 mutations of
    Escherichia coli: Location and complementation pattern
    for UV resistance, Mol. Gen. Genet., 157 (1977) 83-89.
19. Glickman, B. W., P. van den Elsen, and M. Radman, Induced
    mutagenesis in dam⁻ mutants of Escherichia coli: A role
    for 6-methyladenine residues in mutation avoidance. Mol.
    Gen. Genet., 163 (1978) 307-312.
20. Gose, A., and R. Devoret, Plasmid pKM101 promoted repair is
    different from SOS repair, Mutat. Res., in press.

21. Guerola, N., and E. Cerdá-Olmedo, Distribution of mutations
     induced by ethyl methanesulphonate and ultraviolet radiation
     in the Escherichia coli chromosome, Mutat. Res., 29 (1975)
     145-147.
22. Guerola, N., J. L. Ingraham, and E. Cerdá-Olmedo, Induction of
     closely linked multiple mutations by nitrosoguanidine,
     Nature New Biol., 230 (1971) 122-125.
23. Hanawalt, P. C., E. C. Friedberg, and C. F. Fox (Eds.), DNA
     Repair Mechanisms, Academic Press, New York, 1978.
24. Hanawalt, P. C., and R. B. Setlow (Eds.), Molecular Mechanisms
     for the Repair of DNA, Plenum Press, New York, 1975.
25. Hansen, M. T., Multiplicity of genome equivalents in the
     radiation-resistant bacterium Micrococcus radiodurans,
     J. Bacteriol., 134 (1978) 71-75.
26. Hince, T. A., and S. Neale, A comparison of the mutagenic action
     of the methyl and ethyl derivatives of nitrosamides and
     nitrosamidines on Escherichia coli, Mutat. Res., 24 (1974)
     383-387.
27. Hince, T. A., and S. Neale, Physiological modification of
     alkylating-agent induced mutagenesis. I. Effect of growth
     rate and repair capacity on nitrosomethyl-urea-induced
     mutation of Escherichia coli, Mutat. Res., 46 (1977) 1-10.
28. Hince, T. A., and S. Neale, Physiological modification of
     alkylating agent induced mutagenesis. II. Influence of
     the numbers of chromosome replicating forks and gene copies
     on the frequency of mutations induced in Escherichia coli,
     Mutat Res., 43 (1977) 11-24.
29. Hutchinson, F., and J. Stein, Mutagenesis of lambda phage:
     5-bromouracil and hydroxylamine, Mol. Gen. Genet., 152
     (1977) 29-36.
30. Ichikawa-Ryo, H., and S. Kondo, Indirect mutagenesis in phage
     lambda by ultraviolet preirradiation of host bacteria,
     J. Mol. Biol., 97 (1975) 77-92.
31. Ishii, Y., and S. Kondo, Comparative analysis of deletion and
     base-change mutabilities of Escherichia coli B strains
     differing in repair capacity (wild type, urvA⁻, polA⁻,
     recA⁻) by various mutagens, Mutat. Res., 27 (1975) 27-44.
32. Jacob, F., Mutation d'un bacteriophage indirite par l'irradia-
     tion des senles bactéries-hôtes avant l'infection, C. R.
     Acad. Sci. (Paris) D, 238 (1954) 732-734.
33. Jeggo, P., M. Defais, L. Samson, and P. Schendel, An adaptive
     response of E. coli to low levels of alkylating agent:
     Comparison with previously characterized DNA repair path-
     ways, Mol. Gen. Genet., 157 (1977) 1-9.
34. Johnson, B. F., Genetic mapping of the lexC-113 mutation,
     Mol. Gen. Genet., 157 (1977) 91-97.
35. Kanner, L., and P. Hanawalt, Efficiency of utilization of
     thymine and 5-bromouracil for normal and repair DNA
     synthesis in bacteria, Biochim. Biophys. Acta, 157 (1968)
     532-545.

36. Kato, T., R. H. Rothman, and A. J. Clark, Analysis of the role
     of recombination and repair in mutagenesis of Escherichia
     coli by UV irradiation, Genetics, 87 (1977) 1-18.
37. Kato, T., and Y. Shinoura, Isolation and characterization of
     mutants of Escherichia coli deficient in induction of
     mutations by ultraviolet light, Mol. Gen. Genet., 156 (1977)
     121-131.
38. Kimball, R. F., The relation of repair phenomena to mutation
     induction in bacteria, Mutat. Res., 55 (1978) 85-120.
39. Kimball, R. F., M. E. Boling, and S. W. Perdue, Evidence that
     UV-inducible error-prone repair is absent in Haemophilus
     influenzae Rd, with a discussion of the relation to error-
     prone repair of alkylating-agent damage, Mutat. Res., 44
     (1977) 183-196.
40. Kimball, R. F., and S. W. Perdue, Attempts to induce mutations
     in Haemophilus influenzae with the base analogues
     5-bromodeoxyuridine and 2-aminopurine, Mutat. Res., 44
     (1977) 197-206.
41. Kimball, R. F., and S. W. Perdue, unpublished data.
42. Kimball, R. F., S. W. Perdue, and M. E. Boling, The role of
     prereplication and postreplication processes in mutation
     induction in Haemophilus influenzae by N-methyl-N'-nitro-
     N-nitrosoguanidine, Mutat. Res., 52 (1978) 57-72.
43. Kimball, R. F., and J. K. Setlow, Mutation fixation in MNNG-
     treated Haemophilus influenzae as determined by trans-
     formation, Mutat. Res., 22 (1974) 1-14.
44. Kirtikar, D. M., J. P. Kuebler, A. Dipple, and D. A. Goldthwaite,
     Enzymes involved in repair of DNA damaged by chemical
     carcinogens and γ-irradiation, Miami Winter Symp., 12 (1976)
     139-155.
45. Kondo, S., Misrepair model for mutagenesis and carcinogenesis,
     In: Fundamentals in Cancer Prevention, P. N. Magee,
     S. Takayama, T. Sugimura and T. Matsushima (Eds.),
     University Park, Baltimore, 1976, pp. 417-429.
46. Kondo, S., H. Ichikawa, K. Iwo, and T. Kato, Base-change
     mutagenesis and prophage induction in strains of Escherichia
     coli with different DNA repair capacities, Genetics, 66
     (1970) 187-217.
47. Lark, K. G., Some aspects of the regulation of DNA replication
     in Escherichia coli, In: Biological Regulation and
     Development, Vol. 1, R. F. Goldberger (Ed.), Plenum Press,
     New York, 1979, pp. 201-217.
48. Lindahl, T., DNA glycosylases, endonucleases for apurinic/
     apyrimidinic sites, and base excision-repair, Progr. Nucleic
     Acid Res. Mol. Biol., 22 (1979) 135-192.
49. Linn, S., U. Kuhnlein, and W. A. Deutsch, Enzymes from human
     fibroblasts for the repair of AP DNA, In: DNA Repair
     Mechanisms, P. C. Hanawalt, E. C. Friedberg, and C. F. Fox
     (Eds.), Academic Press, New York, 1978, pp. 199-203.

50. Loveless, A., Possible relevance of O-6-alkylation of deoxy-
    guanosine to the mutagenicity and carcinogenicity of
    nitrosamines and nitrosamides, Nature, 223 (1969) 206-207.
51. McCann, J., E. Choi, E. Yamasaki, and B. N. Ames, Detection of
    carcinogens in the Salmonella/microsome test: assay of
    300 chemicals, Proc. Natl. Acad. Sci. (U.S.), 72 (1975)
    5135-5139.
52. McCann, J., N. E. Spingarn, J. Kobori, and B. N. Ames,
    Detection of carcinogens as mutagens: bacterial tester
    strains with R factor plasmids, Proc. Natl. Acad. Sci.
    (U.S.), 72 (1975) 979-983.
53. Monti-Bragadin, N. Babudri, and L. Samer, Expression of the
    plasmid pKM101-determined DNA repair system in recA⁻ and
    lex⁻ strains of Escherichia coli, Mol. Gen. Genet., 145
    (1976) 303-306.
54. Moseley, B. E. B., and H. J. R. Copland, Four mutants of
    Micrococcus radiodurans defective in the ability to repair
    DNA damaged by mitomycin-C, two of which have wild type
    resistance to ultraviolet radiation, Mol. Gen. Genet., 160
    (1978) 331-337.
55. Mount, D. W., C. D. Kosel, and A. Walker, Inducible, error-free
    repair in tsl recA mutants of E. coli, Mol. Gen. Genet.,
    146 (1976) 37-41.
56. Newton, A., D. Masys, E. Leonardi, and D. Wygal, Association
    of induced frameshift mutagenesis and DNA replication in
    Escherichia coli, Nature New Biol., 236 (1972) 19-22.
57. Nishioka, H., and C. O. Doudney, Different modes of loss of
    photoreversibility of mutation and lethal damage in
    ultraviolet-light resistant and sensitive bacteria,
    Mutat. Res., 8 (1969) 215-228.
58. Nishioka, H., and C. O. Doudney, Different modes of loss of
    photoreversibility of ultraviolet light-induced true
    and suppressor mutations to tryptophan independence in an
    auxotrophic strain of Escherichia coli, Mutat. Res., 9
    (1970) 349-358.
59. Pietrzykowska, I., On the mechanism of bromouracil-induced
    mutagenesis, Mutat. Res., 19 (1973) 1-9.
60. Pietrzykowska, I., K. Lewandowsky, and D. Shugar, Liquid-
    holding recovery of bromouracil-induced lesions in DNA
    of Escherichia coli CR-34 and its possible relation to
    dark repair mechanisms, Mutat. Res., 30 (1975) 21-32.
61. Radman, M., SOS repair hypothesis: phenomenology of an
    inducible DNA repair which is accompanied by mutagenesis,
    In: Molecular Mechanisms for Repair of DNA, Part A,
    P. C. Hanawalt and R. B. Setlow (Eds.), Plenum Press,
    New York, 1975, pp. 355-367.
62. Radman, M., Inducible pathways in deoxyribonucleic acid repair,
    mutagenesis, and carcinogenesis, Biochem. Soc. Trans., 5
    (1977) 903-921.

63. Radman, M., G. Villani, S. Boiteux, M. Defais, and P.
    Caillet-Facquet, On the mechanism and genetic control of
    mutagenesis induced by carcinogenic mutagens, Cold Spring
    Harbor Conf. Cell Proliferation, 4 (1977) 903-921.
64. Russell, W. L., Radiation and chemical mutagenesis and repair
    in mice, In: Molecular and Cellular Repair Processes,
    R. F. Beers, Jr., R. M. Herriott, and R. C. Tilghman (Eds.),
    Johns Hopkins Press, Baltimore, 1972, pp. 239-247.
65. Russell, W. L., The role of mammals in the future of chemical
    mutagenesis research, Arch. Toxicol., 38 (1977) 141-147.
66. Rydberg, B., Bromouracil mutagenesis in Escherichia coli:
    Evidence for involvement of mismatch repair, Mol. Gen.
    Genet., 152 (1977) 19-28.
67. Rydberg, B., Bromouracil mutagenesis and mismatch repair in
    mutator strains of Escherichia coli, Mutat. Res., 52 (1978)
    11-24.
68. Samson, L., and J. Cairns, A new pathway for DNA repair in
    Escherichia coli, Nature, 267 (1977) 281-282.
69. Schendel, P. F., M. Defais, P. Jeggo, L. Samson and J. Cairns,
    Pathways of mutagenesis and repair in Escherichia coli
    exposed to low levels of simple alkylating agents, J.
    Bact., 135 (1978) 466-475.
70. Schendel, P. F., and P. E. Robins, Repair of 0^6-methylguanine
    in adapted Escherichia coli, Proc. Natl. Acad. Sci. (U.S.),
    75 (1978) 6017-6020.
71. Sedgwick, S. G., Misrepair of overlapping daughter strand gaps
    as a possible mechanism for UV-induced mutagenesis in uvr
    strains of Escherichia coli. A general model for induced
    mutagenesis by misrepair (SOS repair) of closely spaced
    DNA lesions, Mutat. Res., 41 (1976) 185-200.
72. Setlow, R. B., DNA repair pathways, This volume, p. 45.
73. Smith, K. C., D. A. Youngs, E. Van der Scheuren, E. M. Carlson,
    and N. J. Sargenti, Excision repair and mutagenesis are
    complex processes, In: DNA Repair Mechanisms, P. C.
    Hanawalt, E. C. Friedberg and C. F. Fox (Eds.), Academic
    Press, New York, 1978, pp. 247-250.
74. Strauss, B., K. N. Ayers, K. Bose, P. Moore, R. Sklar, and
    K. Tatsumi, Role of cellular systems in modifying the
    response to chemical mutagens, This volume, p. 25.
75. Strauss, B., R. Wahl-Synek, H. Reiter, and T. Searashi, Repair
    of damage induced by a monofunctional alkylating agent in
    Bacillus subtilis: relation to the repair of UV-induced
    damage, In: Symposium on the Mutational Process, Academia,
    Prague, 1965, pp. 39-48.
76. Streisinger, G., Y. Okada, J. Emrich, J. Newton, A. Tsugita,
    E. Terzaghi, and M. Inouye, Frameshift mutations and the
    genetic code, Cold Spring Harbor Symp., 31 (1966) 77-84.

77. Walker, G. C., Plasmid (pKM101)-mediated enhancement of repair
     and mutagenesis: dependence on chromosomal genes in
     Escherichia coli K-12, Mol. Gen. Genet., 152 (1977) 93-103.
78. Walker, G. C., and P. P. Dobson, Mutagenesis and repair
     deficiencies of Escherichia coli mumC mutants are suppressed
     by the plasmid pKM101, Molec. Gen. Genet., 172 (1979) 17-24.
79. Witkin, E. M., Mutation-proof and mutation-prone modes of
     survival in derivatives of Escherichia coli B differing in
     sensitivity to ultraviolet light, Brookhaven Symp. Biol.,
     29 (1967) 17-55.
80. Witkin, E. M., The role of DNA repair and recombination in
     mutagenesis, Proc. XII Int. Congr. Genet., 3 (1969)
     225-245.
81. Witkin, E. M., Ultraviolet mutagenesis and inducible DNA repair
     in Escherichia coli, Bacteriol. Rev., 40 (1976) 869-907.
82. Witkin, E. M., and E. C. Parisi, Bromouracil mutagenesis:
     mispairing or misrepair?, Mutat. Res., 25 (1974) 407-409.
83. Witkin, E. M., and I. E. Wermandsen, Induction of lambda
     prophage and of mutations to streptomycin resistance in
     separate small fractions of a lysogenic derivative of
     Escherichia coli B, or by very low doses of ultraviolet
     light, Mol. Gen. Genet., 156 (1977) 35-39.

CHAPTER 2

ROLE OF CELLULAR SYSTEMS IN MODIFYING THE RESPONSE TO

CHEMICAL MUTAGENS

B. STRAUSS, K. N. AYRES, K. BOSE, P. MOORE,
R. SKLAR, and K. TATSUMI

Department of Microbiology, The University of Chicago
Chicago, Illinois 60637 (U.S.A.)

SUMMARY

Neocarzinostatin (NCS) produces apurinic/apyrimidinic (AP) sites in DNA which are repaired by the AP excision repair system. Survival after NCS treatment is not determined exclusively by this repair system, presumably because of the production of other, lethal, lesions. MNNG also produces multiple lesions which may be handled by cells in different ways. In E. coli, MNNG treatment results in rapid induction of a system which removes O^6-methylguanine. Inhibition of this induction with chloramphenicol results in a large increase in mutation frequency. Induction of an enzyme which removes O_6-methylguanine probably accounts for the enrichment of mutations near DNA growing points. MNNG also induces multiple closely linked mutations. The production of multiple mutations but not of single-site mutations is blocked in rec A and uvr E strains. The exact nucleotide site at which DNA synthesis is blocked in vitro by reaction with mutagens can be observed in a ØX174 system in which the nucleotide sequence is known. DNA polymerase I catalyzed synthesis is blocked one nucleotide before the reacted base on the template strand. In contrast, with some damaged templates, AMV reverse transcriptase can insert a base at the level of the reacted nucleotide on the template.

INTRODUCTION

Although most carcinogens are mutagens and most mutagens are carcinogens [2], the reasons for this correlation remain obscure. The simplest hypothesis is that carcinogenesis results from particular mutations, but there are alternative interpretations, for

25

example, that it is the process leading to mutation which is carcinogenic rather than the mutations produced as an end result. In any
case, the hypothesis that reaction with, or alteration of DNA is
critical for carcinogenesis and certainly for mutagenesis continues
to be the best available. We are therefore interested in the modification of DNA by mutagens and in the response of cells to such
modification. Our recent work falls into three main categories:
(a) study of the DNA excision repair response elicited by the anti-
tumor drug, Neocarzinostatin (NCS); (b) studies on the mechanism
of mutation induced by N-methyl-N'-nitro-N-nitrosoguanidine (MNNG)
in bacteria; and (c) development of in vitro models for the study
of repair and mutation. This manuscript reports on our progress
in these three areas.

RELATION BETWEEN EXCISION REPAIR AND CELL SURVIVAL

The antitumor agent Neocarzinostatin (NCS) is a polypeptide of
molecular weight 10,700 which in the presence of sulfhydryl reagents
produces single- and double-strand breaks in DNA [4]. Recently it
has been demonstrated that the breaks occur at the sites of dT and
dA residues with dT being the preferred substrate [7, 9]. Free
thymine is released in an amount correlated with the number of
strand scissions [19]. D'Andrea and Haseltine [7] suggest that the
double-strand breaks are likely to result from two independent
single-strand break events. The following experiments show that
apurinic/apyrimidinic (AP) endonuclease sensitive sites are intermediates in the breakage pathway.

Col El DNA is a supercoiled double stranded DNA circle of 4.2
$\times 10^6$ molecular weight. Relaxed circles with single-strand breaks
and linear DNA molecules produced by double-strand breaks can be
separated from each other and from the circles by gel electrophoresis
(Fig. 1) [28]. Treatment of col El with NCS and mercaptoethanol
produced both single- and double-strand breaks (Fig. 2). The proportion of molecules with breaks is greatly increased (Fig. 3) when
reaction occurs in the presence of an apurinic endonuclease prepared
from the Daudi line of Burkitt's lymphoma [5]. We conclude that AP
(apurinic plus apyrimidinic) endonuclease-sensitive sites are intermediates in the degradation and that NCS-induced breaks are formed
by the sequence: DNA ⟶ AP sites ⟶ single-strand breaks
⟶ double-strand breaks.

Although deficient in nucleotide excision and unable to repair
damage induced by polynuclear aromatic hydrocarbons, lymphoblastoid
cells from xeroderma pigmentosum patients [3] are competent in their
ability to carry out AP repair [1]. Xeroderma lymphoblastoid cells
are also competent in their ability to respond to NCS treatment with
repair synthesis (Fig. 4). Even when corrected for differences in

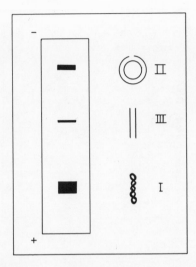

Fig. 1.   Scheme for the separation of supercoiled circles, relaxed
circles, and linear molecules by gel electrophoresis.

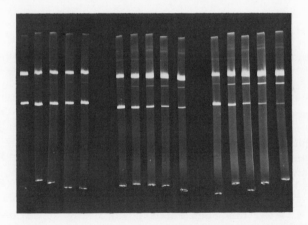

Fig. 2.   Treatment of col E1 with NCS and mercaptoethanol.   Col E1
^{3}H-DNA (126 µg/ml, 6000 cpm/µg) was incubated for 30 min with 0, 1,
2.5, 4, and 5 µg/ml of NCS.   Left to right: (1-5) without mercaptoethanol;   (6-10) plus 5 mM mercaptoethanol;   (11-15) plus 5 mM
mercaptoethanol plus 0.6 µg apurinic endonuclease in a 50 µl reaction
mixture.   Stop solution was added and 10 µl (0.4 µg DNA) was electro-
phoresed (5 hr at 5 ma/gel).   The gels were stained with ethidium
bromide.

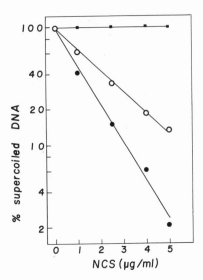

Fig. 3.   Effect of NCS on supercoiled DNA: (■) no mercaptoethanol;
(○) plus mercaptoethanol;   (●) plus mercaptoethanol plus AP endonuclease.   The bands shown in Fig. 2 were cut out, placed in 2 ml
of water, boiled, and 12 ml of Aquasol added.   The radioactivity
was determined and the percentage remaining supercoiled calculated.

pyrimidine metabolism [26], the xeroderma cells are more active in
their repair response than the lymphoblastoid line L33-6-1 (Fig. 4).
NCS-induced repair is similar in its kinetics to the repair of damage
induced by MMS [31] and is complete within a few hours, so that
repair measured in the first hour is likely to reflect the overall
repair capability.   Determination of the concentration of NCS required to inhibit [3H]dThd uptake by 50% gave values of less than
0.1 µg/ml for the Raji lymphoma line and 1-2 µg/ml for XPA-3 and
L33-6-1.   These data indicate that Raji is, if anything, more re-
active to NCS than are the other two strains.

Strain L33-6-1 has been reported as being sensitive to methyl
methanesulfonate (MMS)-induced killing, low in repair activity
for damage induced by MMS [10] and sensitive to ethyl methanesulfonate [24].   The dose reduction factor for MMS-killing of L33-6-1
as compared to the lymphoma line Raji was 2.5 over the whole range
[10].   Although the dose reduction factor for L33-6-1 compared to
Raji after treatment with NCS is about 2 at lower doses, the killing
curves for the two strains approach each other so that at higher
dose there is no difference in survival (Fig. 5).   Furthermore, not-
withstanding the difference in repair activity, L33-6-1 is not more
sensitive to NCS than is the xeroderma line (Fig. 5).

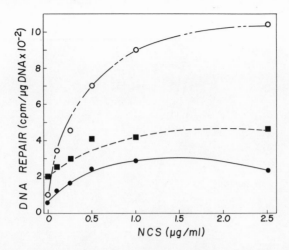

Fig. 4.   Repair synthesis as a function of NCS dose for (●) Raji,
(○) XPA-3, and (■) L33-6-1 lymphoblast lines. Rapidly growing
cells were preincubated with 10 mM hydroxyurea for 30 min and then
incubated for 60 min with NCS. 10 mM hydroxyurea, and [³H]dThd
(10 μCi/ml; 19 Ci/mmole). Cells were harvested and lysed and
repair synthesis was determined by the BND cellulose method [11].
The maximum values for repair (cpm/μg DNA) corrected for pool size
(determined at 10 μg/ml NCS) were: Raji, 1583; L33-6-1, 632;
XPA-3, 3843. The relative pool sizes at 10 μg/ml NCS were Raji,
4.4; L33-6-1, 0.65; XPA-3, 2.7.

        The observed lack of consistency in repair synthesis, DNA syn-
thesis inhibition and cell survival means that AP excision repair
activity as measured by the BND cellulose methodology is not the
sole determinant of survival from NCS-induced damage. NCS induces
double-strand breaks [4] as well as AP sites and single-strand
breaks. Production of a double-strand break may well be the lesion
leading to cell death, and such lesions may accumulate in both AP
repair-proficient and -deficient strains at higher NCS doses at
which double-strand breaks can be formed because of the accumulation
of apurinic sites on opposite strands. Since AP endonuclease is not
the limiting step in repair [15], such apurinic sites would lead to
a lethal double strand break in both repair competent and incompetent
cells. If this is so, excision repair would not determine cell
survival because of the nature of the lesions produced by NCS. Indeed because NCS can induce AP sites at the same nucleotide level
on opposite strands of the DNA [7], the first step in the repair
sequence may actually contribute to the lethality by producing
double-strand breaks.

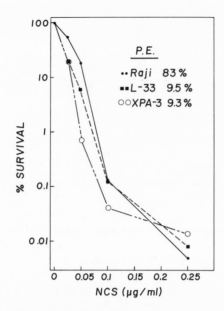

Fig. 5.   Inactivation of (●) Raji, (■) L33-6-1, and (○) XPA-3
lymphoblastoid lines by incubation with NCS. Rapidly growing cells
were suspended in RPMI 1640 (without serum) and incubated for 1 hr
at 37°C with NCS. The cells were then diluted and plated at three
concentrations in soft agar [24] without a feeder layer. Cells
were fed at one day and then weekly. Counts were made after one
month.

MULTIPLE RESPONSE TO COMPLEX MUTAGENS

That single mutagenic agents can produce multiple effects is
particularly evident in the action of N-methyl-N'-nitro-N-nitroso-
guanidine (MNNG) on the bacterium <u>Escherichia</u> <u>coli</u>. Treatment of
<u>E</u>. <u>coli</u> with MNNG induces a system which removes O^6-methylguanine
residues from DNA and thereby serves to protect the organism from
MNNG mutagenesis and killing [4, 21, 25]. Treatment of <u>E</u>. <u>coli</u> with
MNNG and chloramphenicol results in a ten to fifty fold increase in
the number of mutants recovered [30]. This chloramphenicol effect
is most probably due to itsinhibition of enzyme induction, since
the level of O^6-methylguanine in cultures incubated in the presence
of chloramphenicol is approximately 20 times that of cultures incubated in its absence, and the level of mutation measured at three
loci is also correspondingly higher (Table 1.). One problem with
such experiments is that the system is induced so rapidly that it
is difficult to obtain a zero time control value for reactivity;
even after 10 min incubation in the absence of chloramphenicol, the
ratio of 7-methylguanine to O^6-methylguanine compared to that observed at 40 min indicates that enzyme has already been produced

TABLE 1

ALKYLATION PRODUCTS IN THE PRESENCE AND ABSENCE OF CHLORAMPHENICOL

MNNG treatment	7-N-Methylguanine			O6-Methylguanine			3-N-Methylguanine			DNA recovered (mg)c	Mutationd		
	DNA (dpm/mg)	Prod (%)	No. adducts genome	DNA (dpm/mg)a	Prod (%)b	No. adducts genome	DNA (dpm/mg)	Proc (%)	No. adducts genome		No. mutants/ no. scored	Proportion of mutants	No. mutationse genome
10 min, 2.5 µg/ml	6911	76.1	392	164	2.72	14	86	0.96	5.0	7.77			
40 min, 1.25 µg/ml	4731	81.1	268	43	1.50	5	12	0.21	0.7	7.05	2/2516	0.0008	0.08
40 min, 1.25 µg/ml, + chloramphenicol	6606	61.6	373	705	12.9	79	52	0.49	3.0	7.40	23/1550	0.015	1.5
40 min, 2.5 µg/ml	15425	83.9	876	133	1.16	12.1	21	0.11	1.1	6.27	10/983	0.010	1.3
40 min, 2.5 µg/ml, + chloramphenicol	20654	69.6	1173	2549	13.8	233	130	0.44	7.4	5.07	79/648	0.122	15

aRadioactivity is not corrected for column recovery.

bAmount of O6-methylguanine is corrected for column recovery (95% of 3-meA and 7-meG are recovered and were not corrected).

cDetermined from the absorbancy of guanine in column eluates.

dMutation to ara, aceAB, arg, and met determined by replica plating.

eCalculated by multiplying the average number of mutations per locus by 4000 (possible number of genes which could mutate).

and is removing O[6]-methylguanine residues. This rapid induction can
be observed by treating cultures with MNNG and then, at intervals,
adding chloramphenicol (Fig. 6). Mutation frequency remains high
when chloramphenicol is added during the first 10 min of MNNG treatment but drops precipitously as chloramphenicol addition is
delayed, presumably because sufficient enzyme has already been induced to remove O[6]-methylguanine adducts.

This rapid induction of enzyme may be the reason why MNNG mutagenesis is observed to be greatest at or near DNA growing points [6].
Mutation presumably occurs as the result of mispairing as the DNA
replication fork passes over an O[6]-methylguanine residue. If induction occurs rapidly, and if there is any delay in replication as a
result of the MNNG treatment, then it will be only near the growing
point at the time of treatment that any appreciable number of O[6]-
methylguanine residues will be present at the time of replication.
Given a 10-min induction time and a 40-min period for replication
of DNA [6], some concentration of mutations at the growing point is
inevitable.

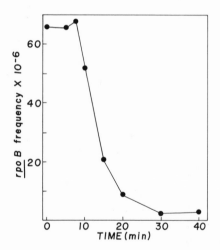

Fig. 6.   Effect of time of chloramphenicol addition on the yield of
MNNG-induced mutation.   Exponential E. coli ABAA cells were treated
with 2.5 µg/ml MNNG, and chloramphenicol (50 µg/ml) was added at the
time indicated after the addition of MNNG.   After 40 min from the
initial addition of MNNG, treated cultures were washed, grown in
M9 medium with aeration until stationary phase was reached, and then
plated on tryptone plus yeast extract medium containing rifampin
(100 µg/ml).

Rec A mutants of E. coli are mutagen-stable [36] and do not
produce increased numbers of mutations after UV irradiation. Nonetheless, their response to MNNG is almost quantitatively equivalent
to the wild type at low doses, and they do give a typical chloramphenicol enhancement of mutation. An effect of rec A on MNNG-induced
mutation can be demonstrated in E. coli. One characteristic feature
of MNNG-induced mutagenesis is the production of numerous, closely
linked multiple mutations. Such closely linked multiple mutations
might be thought of as a necessary result of growing point mutagenesis resulting from multiple alkylations at or near the growing
point. However, it appears that a separate mechanism is involved.

We measure multiple mutation by selecting for rifampin-resistant
E. coli and then scoring for the closely linked acetate AB mutations
leading to inability to use acetate as a carbon source. An excess
of aceAB mutations is observed in the selected population of rifampin
resistant MNNG-treated cells over that in unselected cells and the
increase in the proportion of aceAB mutants as a function of MNNG
dose is linear in both selected and unselected populations, suggesting that a single event is responsible for the multiple mutational
events. There is a constant excess of about three times the unselected value in selected populations of bacteria.

Although chloramphenicol increases the frequency of single site
mutations, it does not produce a comparable increase in multisite
mutations [30]. Neither the rec A nor the uvr E strain responds to
MNNG with the production of a high frequency of closely linked mutations (Table 2) although both do respond to chloramphenicol with an
increased frequency of single site mutations. The lexA mutant gives
normal levels of closely linked mutation after MNNG treatment, and
we have therefore concluded that the process requires only constitutive levels of the rec A gene product [36]. We suspect that a process requiring recombination (and the rec A gene product) includes
a repair step in which synthesis catalyzed by the uvr E gene product
results in errors. This is certainly a minor mutational pathway in
E. coli since some rec A mutants give normal single site mutation
frequencies after MNNG treatment. However, it may be that the relative importance of mutation pathways differs among organisms. Some
years ago mutagen stable strains of B. subtilis unable to respond to
methylating agents were isolated in this laboratory [11], and similar
radiation-sensitive, chemical mutagen-stable mutants have been isolated in yeast [20]. It is possible that the closely linked mutation
pathway which is minor in E. coli may turn out to be a major mode for
MNNG-induced mutagenesis in other organisms, including eukaryotes.

DEVELOPMENT OF AN IN VITRO SYSTEM

Dissection of the molecular events in mutation depends on the
availability of mutants blocked at various stages of the process.

TABLE 2

CLOSELY LINKED MUTATION PRODUCTION IN REPAIR-DEFICIENT STRAINS

Strain	Frequency rpoB	AceAB mutants/ no. scored	Proportion of mutants	χ^2 (p value)[a]
AB1157	2.4×10^{-5}	24/965	0.025	0.005
	Unselected	7/996	0.007	
ABAA	2.7×10^{-5}	12/753	0.016	0.018
	Unselected	1/595	0.002	
rec F	1.6×10^{-5}	18/1116	0.016	0.005
	Unselected	2/1131	0.002	
rec B, C	3.6×10^{-5}	14/435	0.032	0.009
	Unselected	8/808	0.010	
lexA3	2.2×10^{-5}	29/900	0.032	0.005
	Unselected	9/920	0.010	
uvrA	5.9×10^{-6}	15/500	0.030	0.01
	Unselected	6/700	0.009	
uvrD (RS11)	2.6×10^{-6}	17/1609	0.011	0.01
	Unselected	4/1566	0.003	
mutH (RS55)	2.0×10^{-5}	27/1450	0.019	0.005
	Unselected	4/1345	0.003	
recL	1.4×10^{-5}	15/926	0.016	0.02
	Unselected	4/934	0.004	
recA13	5.9×10^{-5}	8/615	0.013	0.50
	Unselected	8/978	0.008	
recA13 (repeat)	1.2×10^{-5}	9/834	0.011	0.63
	Unselected	7/578	0.012	
recA12	8.1×10^{-6}	5/1361	0.004	0.55
	Unselected	9/1494	0.006	
recA12 (repeat)	1.7×10^{-5}	7/1485	0.005	0.96
	Unselected	8/1454	0.006	
uvrE502 (RS14)	1.7×10^{-5}	20/1546	0.013	0.77
	Unselected	23/1612	0.014	
uvrE502 (repeat)	1.5×10^{-5}	14/1396	0.010	0.67
	Unselected	17/1356	0.013	

[a]Calculated as $\chi^2 = (|f - F| - 0.5)^2 \sum_{i=1}^{4} \frac{1}{F_i}$, where f is the number of mutants observed and F is the number expected. Values of p less than 0.05 are considered significant.

The analysis would also be greatly aided by the development of biochemical models which permitted the in vitro reconstruction of systems able to mutate. The availability of methods for mapping DNA
molecules by restriction analysis and for sequencing the restriction
fragments has already led to a number of in vitro mutation systems
[13, 29]. We have adopted a system using the bacteriophage ØX174
DNA for our work. This small viral DNA has been completely sequenced
by Sanger and his group [22] and has been used for the analysis of
the effect of treatment with polynuclear aromatic hydrocarbons [12],
UV [33], and for the analysis of the fidelity of different DNA polymerases [8]. The principle of our method is shown in Fig. 7.
Replicative form ØX174 DNA is prepared and cut with the restriction
enzyme Hae II. The restriction fragments are separated by gel electrophoresis, and a single isolated fragment is then annealed with
single-stranded ØX174 DNA which has been previously reacted with
acetoxyacetylaminofluorene (AAAF), anti-benzpyrene diolepoxide
(anti-BPDE), or with UV. The restriction fragment serves as a primer
at a known nucleotide position for in vitro DNA synthesis using a
DNA polymerase and a mixture of deoxynucleoside triphosphates, one
of which is labeled with ^{32}P. Synthesis proceeds unless and until
blocked by an AAF, UV, or anti-BPDE adduct. The reaction mixture is
then treated with Hae II to separate primer from newly synthesized
DNA, the product is denatured and analyzed on a polyacrylamide gel.
Separate reaction mixtures with dideoxy chain terminators [23], or
with cytosine arabinoside triphosphate, are run alongside to provide
a sequence standard. The net result after autoradiography of the
gel is a film showing a series of bands indicating the nucleotide
sites at which DNA synthesis has been blocked.

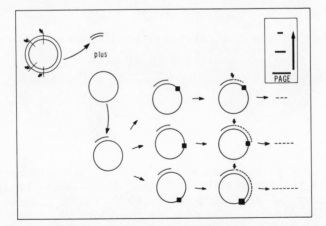

Fig. 7.   Principle of the method using ØX174 DNA to locate the site
of lesions. Single circles, ØX174 DNA; double circles, replicative
form: solid squares, site of a lesion; dashed line, newly synthesized DNA; PAGE, polyacrylamide gel electrophoresis.

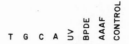

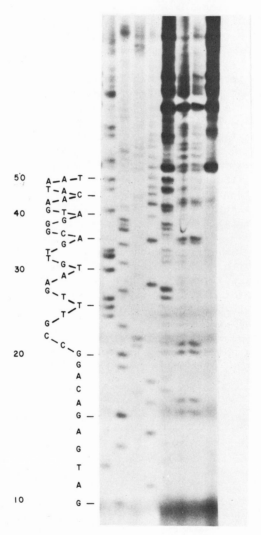

Fig. 8.   Polyacrylamide gel analysis of the products synthesized by
polI on DNA templates reacted with AAAF or anti-BPDE or irradiated
with UV.   About 265 AAAF adducts or 140 anti-BPDE adducts were present per ØXDNA molecule.   The DNA for the UV template was irradiated
with 1000 J/m^2 of UV at a DNA concentration of 100 µg/ml.   The primer
used was Hae II fragment 5.   Lanes A, C, G, T are sequence standards.
Numbering is from the center of the Hae II recognition site.   The
reaction conditions are as previously published [18].

Using DNA polymerase I (Klenow fragment lacking 5'-3' nuclease
activity), DNA synthesis is blocked at a level one and two nucleotides before the reacted site on the DNA template [18] (Fig. 8).
It is most likely that the major reaction site for AAAF [16] and
anti-BPDE is guanine [35]. The formation of pyrimidine dimers is the
most likely product of UV irradiation [27], and the position of the
bands (Fig. 8) indicates this difference in specificity.

At least two hypotheses account for the failure of E. coli pol I
to insert a stable base in newly synthesized DNA at the level of the
reacted G in the AAAF-treated template. Either the conformational
change induced by reaction with AAAF [34] (or with UV or anti-BPDE)
alters the template sufficiently so that an entering nucleotide
cannot base pair, or a "wrong" nucleotide is first inserted and then
removed by the 3'-5'-nuclease of polymerase I as would be expected
if this nuclease had a major editing or "proof-reading" function.
Weinstein and Grunberger [34] have studied the effect of AAF modification of guanine in synthetic oligonucleotides on translation of
neighboring bases and have shown that the inhibitory effect on translation was "limited mainly to the base immediately adjacent to the
modified G residue" in GAAAA oligomers, although there was no effect
in a GUUU template. Therefore it is possible that purely steric
effects can account for the site of inhibition.

We have studied this question using two additional enzymes, a
DNA polymerase α prepared from Daudi human lymphoma cells and AMV
reverse transcriptase obtained from Dr. Joseph Beard by courtesy of
the National Cancer Institute, NIH. With UV- and with anti-BPDE-
treated templates, the AMV reverse transcriptase-catalyzed pattern
and the DNA polymerase α pattern is identical to that obtained by
using E. coli polymerase I (Fig. 9). Since careful determination
failed to demonstrate any 3'-5' or 5'-3' nuclease activity in our
DNA polymerase α preparation and since AMV reverse transcriptase is
reported only to have RNase H activity [32], the results indicate
that DNA polymerases can be blocked at sites adjacent to UV- or
anti-BPDE reacted nucleotides without the aid of an editing nuclease.
The results obtained with AAAF-treated templates are more complex.
When AAF-DNA is used as a template with reverse transcriptase as a
polymerase, a nucleotide is inserted in the newly synthesized strand
at the level of the reacted nucleotide in the template (Fig. 9).
DNA polymerase α appears to behave like AMV reverse transcriptase
at some sites and like DNA polymerase I at others. We therefore
conclude that the polymerase itself, the nature of the alteration
and its site play important roles in determining the exact site of
inhibition. We are now attempting to find out what base (or bases)
is inserted by AMV reverse transcriptase opposite the site of a
lesion in the template strand.

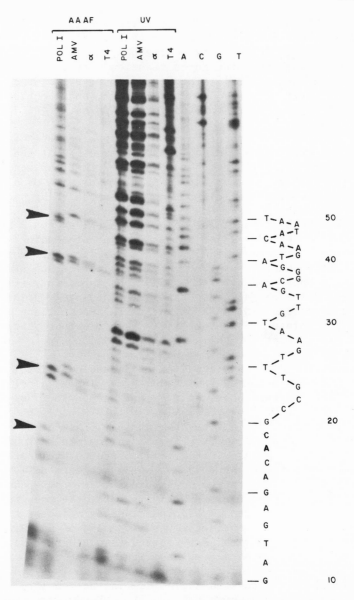

Fig. 9.   Sites of inhibition of in vitro DNA synthesis on UV-
irradiated and AAAF-treated ∅X174 DNA templates. Treated ∅X DNA templates were prepared as described in the legend to Fig. 8.   In vitro
DNA synthesis was catalyzed by either E. coli polymerase I (pol I),
AMV reverse transcriptase (AMV), DNA polymerase α from the Daudi lymphoma line (α) or T4 DNA polymerase (T4).   The reaction products were
analyzed by polyacrylamide gel electrophoresis as previously described [18]. Arrows indicate the site of obvious differences in
the site of inhibition.

Our methodology is not as yet able to detect "readthrough" by
these enzymes by analysis of the gel patterns. Furthermore, there
are considerable data in the literature indicating that reverse
transcriptase is more likely to make errors during replication [8],
but we do not know whether our observation is related to these
experiments. The problem of readthrough is of the greatest importance because of its relationship to the problem the cell has in
"bypassing" lesions. A temporary halting of synthesis at the site
of a lesion would, we suppose, result in a band on the gels and so
seeing such bands does not necessarily demonstrate an absolute block
to synthesis. We would like to be able to unequivocally reproduce
a "readthrough" or "bypass" phenomenon with our ØX174 system. The
purity of the system used is critical for such work, since oligonucleotides, present in the reaction mixture, can lead to illegitimate reinitiation. We think this particular problem has been solved
and we are now attempting to construct model systems.

One suggestion as to how synthesis can proceed on a damaged
template is for polynucleotidyl transferase to add nucleotides in a
non-template specified manner to circumvent the block. Random base
pairing might then provide a suitable double stranded structure to
extend the chain normally. We have accomplished a part of this plan
(Fig. 10). A reaction mixture of AAF-treated DNA with polymerase I
was inactivated by heating. Addition of polynucleotidyl transferase
resulted in the disappearance of a number of the bands as would be
expected if synthesis had proceeded on the previously terminated
chains (Fig. 10). Readdition of polymerase I to the polynucleotidyl
transferase reaction mixture then restored the original pattern of
bands. The most conservative explanation of this last finding is
that the 3'-5' exonuclease activity of the polymerase resulted in
digestion of the unpaired nucleotides back to the original blocked
position. Since addition of terminal deoxynucleotidyl transferase
had no effect on the end position of the bands, we are only part
way towards a system which will bypass lesions in vitro.

Our results imply that numerous factors may affect the behavior
of a DNA synthesizing system as it meets a base with an adduct. Not
only does the nature of the lesion affect the response but the properties of the polymerase as well. Additional factors of importance
are the site of the lesion in a sequence, just what bases are nearby
and probably also the relative amount of enzyme and substrate. We
do not know the role of single strandedness of the overall template;
for example, the effect of a pyrimidine dimer may be greater in such
a template than in double-stranded DNA. We do not understand why
we often see two bands at some lesions, although often we see only
one. Nonetheless we think that this system will eventually permit
us to understand some of the factors involved in the in vivo bypass
of adducts and how errors can be generated in such reactions.

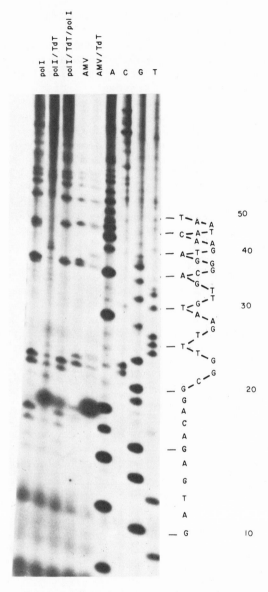

Fig. 10.   Effect of terminal deoxynucleotidyl transferase (TdT) on
the length of DNA synthesized on an AAAF reacted template.   AAAF-
reacted DNA was prepared as in the legend to Fig. 8.   The reaction
mix was incubated 30 min with pol I or AMV reverse transcriptase as
indicated and the pol I reaction mixtures were inactivated by heating
8 min at 65°C.   TdT was then added where indicated followed in one
mix by additional pol I.   The reaction products were analyzed by
gel electrophoresis.

ACKNOWLEDGEMENT

This work was supported by grants from the National Institutes of Health (GM07816, CA 14599, CP85669) and the Department of Energy (EY765-02-2040). We are particularly appreciative of the help of the NCI Carcinogenesis Research Program in providing radioactive anti-BPDE.

K. Tatsumi is a Fellow of the Leukemia Research Society of America, R. Sklar is a trainee of a program supported by the National Institutes of Health (GM 0090; CA09273), and K. Ayres is a trainee in a Pathobiology Program of the National Institute of General Medical Sciences (T32-GM7190).

REFERENCES

1. Altamirano-Dimas, M., R. Sklar, and B. Strauss, Selectivity of the excision of alkylation products in a xeroderma-pigmentosum-derived lymphoblastoid line, Mutat. Res., 60 (1979) 197-206.
2. Ames, B., Identifying environmental chemicals causing mutations and cancer, Science, 204 (1979) 587-593.
3. Andrews, A., J. Robbins, K. Kraemer, and D. Buell, Xeroderma pigmentosum long term lymphoid lines with increased ultra-violet sensitivity, J. Natl. Cancer Inst., 53 (1974) 691-693.
4. Beerman, T., and I. Goldberg, DNA strand scission by the anti-tumor protein Neocarzinostatin, Biochem. Biophys. Res. Comm., 59 (1974) 1254-1261.
5. Bose, K., P. Karran, and B. Strauss, Repair of depurinated DNA in vitro by enzymes purified from human lymphoblasts, Proc. Natl. Acad. Sci. (U.S.), 75 (1978) 794-798.
6. Cerdá-Olmedo, E., P. Hanawalt, and N. Guerola, Mutagenesis of the replication point by nitrosoguanidine: map and pattern of replication of the Escherichia coli chromosome, J. Mol. Biol., 33 (1968) 705-519.
7. D'Andrea, A., and W. Haseltine, Sequence specific cleavage of DNA by the antitumor antibiotics neocarzinostatin and bleomycin, Proc. Natl. Acad. Sci. (U.S.), 75 (1978) 3608-3612.
8. Gopinathan, K., L. Weymouth, T. Kunkel, and L. Loeb, Mutagenesis in vitro by DNA polymerase from an RNA tumour virus, Nature, 278 (1979) 857-859.
9. Hatayama, T., I. Goldberg, M. Takeshita, and A. Grollman, Nucleotide specificity in DNA scission by neocarzinostatin, Proc. Natl. Acad. Sci. (U.S.), 75 (1978) 3603-3607.

10. Higgins, N. P., and B. Strauss, Differences in the ability of
    human lymphoblastoid lines to exclude bromodeoxyuridine and
    in their sensitivity to methyl methanesulfonate and to in-
    corporated (^{3}H) thymidine, Cancer Res., 39 (1979) 312-320.
11. Hill, T., L. Prakash, and B. Strauss, Mutagen stability of
    alkylation-sensitive mutants of <u>Bacillus</u> <u>subtilis</u>, J.
    Bacteriol., 110 (1972) 47-55.
12. Hsu, W., E. Lin, R. Harvey, and S. Weiss, Mechanism of phage
    ΦX174 DNA inactivation by benzo(a)pyrene-7,8-dihydrodiol-
    9,10 epoxide, Proc. Natl. Acad. Sci. (U.S.), 74 (1977)
    3335-3339.
13. Hutchinson, C., S. Phillips, M. Edgell, S. Gillam, P. Jahnke,
    and M. Smith, Mutagenesis at a specific position in a DNA
    sequence, J. Biol. Chem., 253 (1978) 6551-6560.
14. Jeggo, P., M. Defais, L. Samson, and P. Schendel, An adaptive
    response of <u>E</u>. <u>coli</u> to low levels of alkylating agent:
    comparison with previously characterized DNA repair path
    ways, Mol. Gen. Genet., 157 (1977) 1-9.
15. Karran, P., N. P. Higgins, and B. Strauss, Intermediates in
    excision repair by human cells: Use of Sl nuclease and
    benzoylated naphthoylated cellulose to reveal single-strand
    breaks, Biochemistry, 16 (1977) 4483-4490.
16. Kriek, E., J. Miller, V. Juhl, and E. Miller, 8-(N-2-Fluorenyl-
    acetamido)-guanosine, and arylamidation reaction product of
    guanosine and the carcinogen N-acetoxy-N-2-fluorenylaceta-
    mide in neutral solution, Biochemistry, 6 (1967) 177-182.
17. Maaloe, O., and N. Kjeldgaard, Control of Macromolecular
    Synthesis, W. A. Benjamin, New York, 1966.
18. Moore, P., and B. Strauss, Sets of inhibition of in vitro DNA
    synthesis in carcinogen and UV-treated ΦX174 DNA, Nature,
    278 (1979) 664-666.
19. Poon, R., T. Beerman, and I. Goldberg, Characterization of DNA
    strand breakage in vitro by the antitumor protein Neocar-
    zinostatin, Biochemistry, 16 (1977) 486-493.
20. Prakash, L., The relation between repair of DNA and radiation
    and chemical mutagenesis in Saccharomyces cerevisiae,
    Mutat. Res., 41 (1976) 244-248.
21. Samson, L., and J. Cairns, A new pathway for DNA repair in
    <u>Escherichia</u> <u>coli</u>, Nature, 267 (1977) 281-283.
22. Sanger, F., G. Air, B. Barrell, N. Brown, A. Coulson, J. Fiddes,
    C. Hutchinson, P. Slocombe, and M. Smith, Nucleotide se-
    quence of bacteriophage ΦX174 DNA, Nature 265 (1977)
    687-697.
23. Sanger, F., S. Nicklen, and A. Coulson, DNA sequencing with
    chain terminating inhibitors, Proc. Natl. Acad. Sci. (U.S.),
    74 (1977) 5463-5467.
24. Sato, K., R. Slesinski, and J. Littlefield, Chemical mutagenesis
    at the phosphoribosyltransferase locus in cultured human
    lymphoblasts, Proc. Natl. Acad. Sci. (U.S.), 69 (1972
    1244-1248.

25. Schendel, P., and P. Robins, Repair of 06-methylguanine in
    adapted Escherichia coli, Proc. Natl. Acad. Sci. (U.S.),
    75 (1978) 6017-6020.

26. Scudiero, D., E. Henderson, A. Norin, and B. Strauss, The
    measurement of chemically-induced DNA repair synthesis in
    human cells by BND-cellulose chromatography, Mutat. Res.,
    29 (1975)

27. Setlow, R., Cyclolbutane-type pyrimidine dimers in polynucleo-
    tides, Science, 153 (1966) 379-386.

28. Sharp, P., B. Sugden, and J. Sambrook, Detection of two
    restriction endonuclease activities in Haemophilus parain-
    fluenzae using analytical agarose-ethidium bromide electro-
    phoresis, Biochemistry, 12 (1973) 3055-3063.

29. Shortle, D., and D. Nathans, Local mutagenesis: A method for
    generating viral mutants with base substitutions in pre-
    selected regions of the viral genome, Proc. Natl. Acad.
    Sci. (U.S.), 75 (1978) 2170-2174.

30. Sklar, R., Enhancement of nitrosoguanidine mutagenesis by
    chloramphenicol in Escherichia coli K-12, J. Bacteriol.,
    136 (1978) 460-462.

31. Tatsumi, K., Unpublished data.

32. Verma, I., The reverse transcriptase, Biochim. Biophys. Acta,
    473 (1977) 1-38.

33. Villani, G., S. Boiteux, and M. Radman, Mechanism of ultra-
    violet-induced mutagenesis: Extent and fidelity of in
    vitro DNA synthesis on irradiated templates, Proc. Natl.
    Acad. Sci. (U.S.), 75 (1978) 3037-3041.

34. Weinstein, I. G., and D. Grunberger, Structural and functional
    changes in nucleic acids modified by chemical carcinogens,
    In: Chemical Carcinogenesis, Part A, P. Ts'o and J.
    DiPaolo, Eds., Marcel Dekker, New York, 1974, pp. 217-235.

35. Weinstein, I., A. Jeffrey, K. Jennette, S. Blobstein, R. Harvey,
    C. Harris, H. Autrup, H. Kasai, and K. Nakanishi, Benzo (a)-
    pyrenediol-epxoides as intermediates in nucleic acid
    binding in vitro and in vivo, Science, 193 (1976) 592-595.

36. Witkin, E., Ultraviolet mutagenesis and inducible DNA repair
    in Escherichia coli, Bacteriol. Rev., 40 (1976) 869-907.

K. Tatsumi's present address is Department of Internal
Medicine, Division of Hematology and Immunology, Kanzawa Medical
University, Uchinada-machi Kahoku-gun, Ishikawa 920-02, Japan.

CHAPTER 3

DNA REPAIR PATHWAYS

R. B. SETLOW

Biology Department, Brookhaven National Laboratory
Upton, New York   11973 (U.S.A.)

SUMMARY

Our knowledge about DNA repair mechanisms in mammalian cells is
reviewed. Ways of measuring excision repair are summarized, and
various modes of excision repair are described in terms of mechanisms
that yield patch sizes of 0, 1, a few (short patch), and many (long
patch) bases. The biological and molecular ways of measuring the
effects of replication on a damaged template are presented, as are
various models of postreplication repair.

INTRODUCTION

There have been a large number of recent reviews on the topics
of DNA repair [5, 11, 12, 16, 26, 31, 33]. The interested reader
should consult these, in particular the works of Hanawalt et al.
[11, 12] and subsequent articles in this volume for details not
documented here.

There are a number of reasons why it is useful to study DNA
repair: (1) DNA repair is an aspect of nucleotide metabolism and is
of intrinsic interest in its own right.   (2) Cells and people [3, 29]
deficient in repair respond in completely different ways than wild-
type cells or normal individuals to physical or chemical environmental
mutagens. For example, one can show from the dose-response relations
for skin cancer in normal humans and in xeroderma pigmentosum individuals that repair in normal individuals removes greater than 85%
of the UV-induced carcinogenic lesions [30],   (3) A knowledge of DNA
repair kinetics is probably crucial in estimating dose response relations at low doses.   (4) Studies of DNA repair may identify potentially sensitive subsets of the human population [1].

EXCISION REPAIR

Excision repair is described as either nucleotide or base excision repair, depending upon whether the initial step is an attack on the polynucleotide's backbone or on an altered base itself [12, 33].

Nucleotide Excision Repair

Figure 1 shows the sequence of steps in nucleotide excision repair of the prototype damage, i.e., UV-induced pyrimidine dimers. Since such dimers can be reversed photochemically or by photoenzymatic means, it is one of the few damages that has been identified as having biological consequences. The steps exemplified in Fig. 1 need no elaboration except to indicate that the initial endonucleolytic step seems to be the rate-limiting one and that exonuclease and polymerase steps are not necessarily separated temporally. Repair complexes are thought to be involved in the process. A labile endonuclease specific for dimers has been isolated from calf thymus [34], but none have been reported from other mammalian systems.

Complications in the interpretations of the kinetics of nucleotide excision may arise because thymine dimers are not randomly distributed in tracts of thymine (but are if some cytosine is in the tracts) [36]. Moreover, some reports indicate large changes in dimer yields through the cell cycle or in DNA to be replicated shortly after irradiation [32, 35]; but another report finds no cell cycle effect [4]. A further complication arises because the initial rate of excision is high in the internucleosome region as compared to the DNA in the nucleosomes themselves and it is not clear how rapidly the nucleosomes rearrange.

The damages arising from treatment with a number of carcinogenic chemicals mimic UV, in that they are poorly repaired in cells defective in excision repair of UV damage as well as for other reasons [30]. Some ways in which some chemical damage mimics UV damage in human cells are:

(1) UV-sensitive cells (XP) are more sensitive to the chemical than normal cells
(2) Chemically treated viruses show a higher survival on normal cells than on XP cells
(3) XP cells deficient in repair of UV damage are also deficient in excision of chemical damage
(4) Excision repair of UV and of chemical damage involves long patches (approx. 100 nucleotides)

It was reasonable to suppose that a common endonuclease step was the basis for the coordinate deficiency in repairing many agents; however, this does not seem to be the case. A UV mimetic, such as

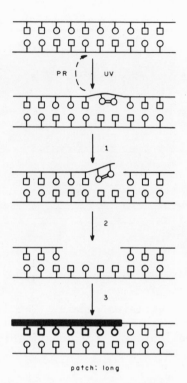

patch: long

Fig. 1.   Steps in nucleotide excision repair following UV irradiation that makes pyrimidine dimers (0=0). Enzymatic photoreactivation
(PR) can monomerize the dimers. The steps are (1) specific endonuclease; (2) exonuclease; (3) polymerase and ligase. The bases
and DNA backbone inserted by repair are shown by the darker symbols
and line.

N-acetoxy-AAF, does not inhibit UV excision repair in normal human
cells even at saturating doses [2]. On the other hand, the chemical
severely inhibits the residual excision repair of UV damage observed
in xeroderma pigmentosum cells [2]. This is an additional reason
for supposing that the repair scheme illustrated in Fig. 1 is more
complex than just the independent action of a number of enzymatic
activities.

Base Excision Repair

The several documented pathways are shown in Fig. 2. Pathway a
involves the demethylation of a methylated base [24] and hence
involves the excision of only part of a base. Note that it would be
difficult to detect this pathway by many of the conventional ways of

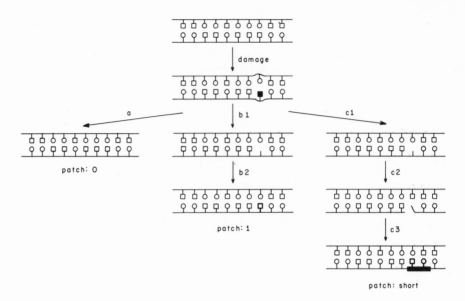

Fig. 2.   Steps in base excision repair. The damage (■) may be an
alkylated base: (a) dealkylation; (b) depurination followed by
insertion of the proper purine; (c) depurination followed by endonuclease, polymerase, and ligase.

detecting repair (see below). Pathway b involves a glycosylase [16]
followed by an insertase [8, 17]. Pathway c also involves a glycosylase, but its action is followed by an apurinic/apyrimidinic endonuclease, which in turn is followed by polymerase and ligase to result
in a short patch [25].

    The kinetics of base excision repair have not been extensively
studied in human cells. It is an intriguing observation that E. coli
is able to adapt to treatment with low levels of alkylating agents
(MNNG) so that a subsequent treatment with radioactive MNNG results
in the removal of O^6-methylguanine at high speed [28]. A mammalian
analog of this system might be the observation that chronic long-term
treatment of animals with low doses of nitrosamines speeds up the
removal of O^6-methylguanine following a subsequent small radioactive
dose [18]. In E. coli the mediator of this response appears to be
consumed in the reaction [27]. Such an observation could explain why
in animals large doses of nitrosamines, given shortly before a small
radioactive dose, inhibit removal of the radioactive O^6-methylguanine
[23]. An alternative explanation is that the large dose saturates
the rate limiting step in one of the enzymatic reactions in base
excision repair [23].

Methods of Measuring Excision Repair

Some of the techniques employed in measuring excision repair of
parental DNA are:

1. Host cell reactivation of treated viruses (need a repair
   deficient host or a heavily treated host).
2. Specific loss of products (products must be identified).
3. Loss of sites sensitive to specific endonucleases (endonucleases must be available and characterized).
4. Incorporation of bases into parental DNA.
   a. Unscheduled DNA synthesis.
   b. Repair replication.
   c. Photolysis of incorporated BrdUrd.
5. Appearance and/or disappearance of single strand breaks.
   a. Sedimentation in alkali.
   b. Alkaline elution.
   c. Sedimentation of nucloids.
   d. BND-cellulose chromatography.
   e. Sensitivity to S1 nuclease.
   f. Inhibition of initiation of clusters of replicons.

Host cell reactivation is the most general technique, but even
though it sidesteps the problem of whether a resistant cell is
resistant because a chemical does not enter it, it still needs a
repair deficient host to compare with a repair proficient one. The
proper biochemical way to measure repair is by the specific loss of
products, but unfortunately most of the crucial products have not
been identified uniquely. Recently, sensitive immunological techniques have been devised for measuring the presence of products in
DNA, for example a radioimmunoassay can measure concentrations of
O^6-ethylguanine in DNA at levels of 1 μM [19]. The loss of sites
sensitive to specific endonucleases (method 3) is supersensitive
[22], but relatively few specific endonucleases are available.
Method 4 represents different ways of measuring effectively the same
thing, and where tested they have been found to give consistent
results [2]. The appearance and/or disappearance of single-strand
breaks (method 5) has very high sensitivity using the alkaline elution technique - a technique that is also capable of measuring
crosslinks and DNA protein links in treated cells [10]. The sedimentation of nucloids can be made supersensitive. If cells after UV
irradiation are incubated in the presence of inhibitors such as
ara-C, changes in sedimentation resulting from approximately 0.01
J/m^2 can be detected [37]. The latter dose makes one pyrimidine
dimer in 2-5 $\times$ 10^9 daltons.

REPLICATION ON A DAMAGED TEMPLATE

When replication takes place before excision has been accomplished, the replication occurs on a damaged template and the consequences for cells may be bad. Some of these consequences are (1) mutations in treated cells or viruses; (2) reactivation of UV-irradiated viruses by treatment of cells; (3) enhanced viral mutagenesis by treatment of cells; (4) inhibition of DNA synthesis; (5) nascent DNA smaller than normal and chased into normal sizes (post replication repair); (6) (enhancement of postreplication repair by small doses before a challenge dose?) The article by Kimball [13] concentrates on the first three items. The last three items concern the macromolecular correlates of this replication. Many damages inhibit DNA synthesis by inhibiting the initiation of clusters of replicons as a result of direct strand breaks or breaks introduced in repair [20]. Damage such as the presence of pyrimidine dimers acts as an inhibitor of the motion of replication forks [9]. It is not clear how this latter inhibition is overcome, or the molecular nature of the DNA synthesized on a damaged template [15]. Figure 3 presents two possible pictures. In one--modified after the bacterial case--gaps remain opposite lesions, and the gaps are filled in by de novo synthesis, or by cross-overs and subsequent branch migration [14]. In the other, only one strand stalls; the other continues for a way, migrates, and acts as a template for the stalled strand [33]. There is experimental evidence for both models. Even more controversial is the interpretation of the enhancement of post-replication repair. Small doses of UV or chemical, given several hours before a higher challenge dose, result in a daughter DNA that becomes parental size sooner than from cells given only the challenge dose [7]. Painter [21] presented sedimentation data indicating that the observed increase in postreplication repair, might be explained by a change in the distribution of replicon sizes, brought about by the first small dose; hence, he argued that it was not necessary to invoke an enhancement phenomenon to explain such results. However, the rate of DNA fork motion determined autoradiographically is greater after the split dose than after the single dose [9]. Moreover, if the first dose is given in the G2 phase of the cell cycle there is an appreciable observed enhancement in early S phase, even though there has been little opportunity for elongation of replicons [6]. Biological experiments have not been done that indicate whether enhanced postreplication is real or not, and if real what, if any, is its biological importance.

CONCLUSION

One or more DNA repair mechanisms have been found in all species investigated. There is little doubt that DNA repair has played an important role in evolution, and that organisms defective in repair are killed more readily by environmental agents. We understand poorly

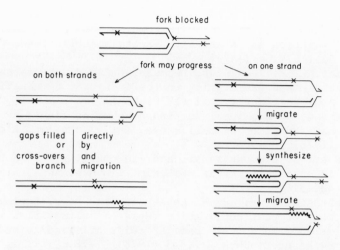

Fig. 3.   Replication on a damaged template: Daughter strand repair.
Two models for postreplication or replication repair [5, 9, 15, 33].

the details of the steps in repair and the kinetics of repair in both
prokaryotes and eukaryotes. Even though the organization of DNA in
eukaryotes is very different from that in prokaryotes, nevertheless,
it is important to analyze prokaryotic systems well so as to get hints
and leads as to how to attack the more difficult eukaryotic systems.

The kinetics of repair after low doses – doses we receive in the
real world – must be known for any quantitative risk assessment. We
could extrapolate from high doses to low doses, but the extrapolation
assumes we have molecular models that we believe in. Such is not yet
the case.

The role of DNA repair in mutagenesis is the subject of the
remainder of this volume.

ACKNOWLEDGEMENT

This research was carried out at Brookhaven National Laboratory
under the auspices of the U.S. Department of Energy.

REFERENCES

1. Abo-Darub, J. M., R. Mackie, and J. D. Pitts, DNA repair
      deficiency in lymphocytes from patients with actinic
      keratoses, Bull. Cancer (Paris), 65 (1978) 357-362.

2. Ahmed, F. E., and R. B. Setlow, DNA repair in xeroderma pigmentosum cells treated with combinations of ultraviolet
   radiation and N-acetoxy-2-acetylaminofluorene, Cancer Res.,
   39 (1979) 471-479.
3. Arlett, C. F., and A. R. Lehmann, Human disorders showing
   increased sensitivity to the induction of genetic damage,
   Ann. Rev. Genet., 12 (1978) 95-115.
4. Clarkson, J. M., The induction of thymine dimers by U.V. light
   as a function of cell stage, Int. J. Radiat. Biol., 34
   (1978) 583-586.
5. Cleaver, J. E., DNA repair and its coupling to DNA replication
   in eukaryotic cells, Biochim. Biophys. Acta, 516 (1978)
   489-516.
6. D'Ambrosio, S. M., P. M. Aebersold, and R. B. Setlow, Enhancement of post replication repair in ultraviolet light
   irradiated Chinese hamster cells by irradiation in G_2 or
   S-phase, Biophys. J., 23 (1978) 71-78.
7. D'Ambrosio, S. M., and R. B. Setlow, Defective and enhanced
   post replication repair in classical and variant xeroderma
   pigmentosum cells treated with N-acetoxy-acetyl amino-
   fluorene, Cancer Res., 38 (1978) 1147-1153.
8. Deutsch, W. A., and S. Linn, DNA binding activity from cultured
   human fibroblasts that is specific for partially depurinated
   DNA and that inserts purines into apurinic sites, Proc. Natl.
   Acad. Sci. (U.S.), 76 (1979) 141-144.
9. Doniger, J., DNA replication in ultraviolet light irradiated
   Chinese hamster cells: The nature of replicon inhibition
   and post-replication repair, J. Mol. Biol., 120 (1978)
   433-446.
10. Fornace, A. J., Jr., and J. B. Little, DNA-protein cross-linking
    by chemical carcinogens in mammalian cells, Cancer Res., 39
    (1979) 704-710.
11. Hanawalt, P. C., P. K. Cooper, A. K. Ganesan, and C. A. Smith,
    DNA repair in bacteria and mammalian cells, Ann. Rev.
    Biochem., 48 (1979) 783-836.
12. Hanawalt, P. C., E. C. Friedberg, and C. F. Fox, DNA Repair
    Mechanisms, Academic Press, New York, 1978
13. Kimball, R. F., Relationship between repair processes and
    mutation induction in bacteria, This volume, p. 1.
14. Lavin, M. F., A model for postreplication repair of UV damage
    in mammalian cells, In: DNA Repair Mechanisms, P. C.
    Hanawalt, E. C. Friedberg, and C. F. Fox, Eds., Academic
    Press, New York, 1978, pp. 509-512.
15. Lehmann, A.R., Post replication repair of DNA in UV-irradiated
    mammalian cells, In: DNA Repair Mechanisms, P. C. Hanawalt,
    E. C. Friedberg, and C. F. Fox, Eds., Academic Press,
    New York, 1978, pp. 617-623.
16. Lindahl, T., DNA glycosylases, endonucleases for apurinic/
    apyrimidinic sites, and base excision-repair, Progr. Nucl.
    Acid Res. Mol. Biol., 22 (1979) 135-192.

17. Livneh, Z., D. Elad, and J. Sperling, Enzymatic insertion of
    purine bases into depurinated DNA in vitro, Proc. Natl.
    Acad. Sci. (U.S.), 76 (1979) 1089-1093.
18. Montesano, R., H. Bresil, and G. P. Margison, Increased
    excision of O^6-methylguanine from rat liver DNA after
    chronic administration of dimethyl nitrosamine, Cancer Res.,
    39 (1979) 1798-1802.
19. Mueller, R., and M. F. Rajewsky, Sensitive radioimmunoassay for
    detection of O^6-ethyldeoxyguanosine in DNA exposed to the
    carcinogen ethylnitrosourea in vivo or in vitro, Z.
    Naturforsch., 33C (1978) 897-901.
20. Painter, R. B., DNA synthesis inhibition in HeLa cells as a
    simple test for agents that damage DNA, J. Environ. Pathol.
    Toxicol., 2 (1978) 65-78.
21. Painter, R.B., Does ultraviolet light enhance post replication
    repair in mammalian cells?, Nature, 275 (1978) 243-245.
22. Paterson, M. C., Use of purified lesion-recognizing enzymes to
    monitor DNA repair in vivo, Advan. Rad. Biol., 7 (1978)
    1-53.
23. Pegg, A. E., Effect of pretreatment with other dialkylnitro-
    samines on excision from hepatic DNA of O^6-methylguanine
    produced by dimethylnitrosamine, Chem.-Biol. Interact., 22
    (1978) 109-116.
24. Pegg, A. E., Enzymatic removal of O^6-methylguanine from DNA by
    mammalian cell extracts, Biochem. Biophys. Res. Commun.,
    84 (1978) 166-173.
25. Regan, J. D., and R. B. Setlow, Two forms of repair in the DNA
    of human cells damaged by chemical carcinogens and mutagens,
    Cancer Res., 34 (1974) 3318-3325.
26. Roberts, J. J., The repair of DNA modified by cytotoxic,
    mutagenic, and carcinogenic chemicals, Advan. Rad. Biol.,
    7 (1978) 211-436.
27. Robins, P., and J. Cairns, The numerology of the adaptive
    response to alkylating agents, Nature, 280 (1979)
    74-76.
28. Schendel, P. F., and P. E. Robins, Repair of O^6-methylguanine
    in adapted Escherichia coli, Proc. Natl. Acad. Sci. (U.S.),
    75 (1978) 6017-6020.
29. Setlow, R. B., Repair deficient human disorders and cancer,
    Nature, 271 (1978) 713-717.
30. Setlow, R. B., Different basic mechanisms in DNA repair, Arch.
    Toxicol., in press.
31. Setlow, R. B., and J. K. Setlow, Effects of radiation on poly-
    nucleotides, Ann. Rev. Biophys. Bioeng., 1 (1972) 293-349.
32. Slor, H., and J. E. Cleaver, Repair replication in replicating
    and nonreplicating DNA after irradiation with UV light,
    Nucl. Acid Res., 5 (1978) 2095-2098.
33. Strauss, B., K. Tatsumi, P. Karran, N. P. Higgins, E. Ben-Asher,
    M. Altamirano-Dimas, L. Rosenblatt, and K. Bose, Mechanisms
    of DNA excision repair in human cells, Polycyclic Hydro-
    carbons Cancer, 2 (1978) 177-201.

34. Waldstein, E. A., S. Peller, and R. B. Setlow, UV-endonuclease
         from calf thymus with specificity toward pyrimidine dimers
         in DNA, Proc. Natl. Acad. Sci. (U.S.), 76 (1979) 3746-3750.
35. Watanabe, M., and M. Horikawa, Analysis of differential sensi-
         tivities of synchronized HeLa S3 cells to radiations and
         chemical carcinogen during the cell cycle: (II) Ultraviolet
         light, Biochem. Biophys. Res. Commun., 58 (1974) 185-191.
36. Wilkins, R. J., The non-random distribution of pyrimidine
         dimers in ultra-violet-irradiated DNA, Int. J. Rad. Biol.,
         35 (1979) 381-385.
37. Yew, F. F.-H., and R. T. Johnson, Ultraviolet-induced DNA
         excision repair in human B and T lymphocytes. II. Effects
         of inhibitors and DNA precursors, Biochim. Biophys. Acta,
         562 (1979) 240-251.

CHAPTER 4

MUTAGEN-SENSITIVE MUTANTS IN NEUROSPORA

ALICE L. SCHROEDER and LOREE D. OLSON

Program in Genetics, Washington State University
Pullman, Wash. 99164 (U.S.A.)

SUMMARY

Initial work on the fungus Neurospora crassa has shown that at
least two DNA-repair systems exist in this eukaryote: excision
repair and a mutation-prone repair. The evidence suggests that there
is also a third repair system. Recently, new mutagen-sensitive
strains have been isolated in several laboratories, but they are not
yet fully characterized. A hunt for cytoplasmically inherited UV
sensitivity has failed to turn up any such mutants among 25 new UV-
sensitive isolates.

INTRODUCTION

With the first experiments demonstrating excision repair of DNA
in Escherichia coli [1, 23] and with the isolation of mutants showing
an association between recombination and DNA repair [4], a number of
laboratories began to seek similar mutants in eukaryotes. They hoped
both to establish the existence of DNA repair systems in eukaryotes
and to obtain mutants defective in recombination.

In Neurospora, UV or ionizing radiation-sensitive mutants representing at least eight different loci were soon isolated. Most were
obtained by forward selection procedures in which conidia (vegetative
spores) from colonial strains were mutagenized, grown, and replica-
plated with velveteen with one of the replicas being exposed to ultraviolet light (UV) or γ-rays. Colonies which failed to grow on replica
plates after UV or γ-ray treatment were isolated from the original
plates and the sensitivity of their conidia tested further [2, 14,
19, 20, 26]. One mutant, uvs-2, arose spontaneously in a wild-type
strain [25], and another, nuc-2, was isolated on the basis of its
nuclease deficiency [10].

The properties of these radiation-sensitive mutants have already been reviewed in detail [21] and so will be discussed only briefly here. Two of the mutants, uvs-2 and upr-1, are clearly defective in pyrimidine dimer excision [28]. A third mutant, uvs-3, has a large number of properties in common with the recA mutants of E. coli. A fourth mutant, uvs-6, has a number of properties in common with polA (DNA polymerase I) mutants of E. coli. However, crude extracts of uvs-6 mutants do have wild-type levels of DNA polymerases as do crude extracts of uvs-1, uvs-2, uvs-3, and uvs-4. Lack of a reliable method for separation of Neurospora DNA polymerases has so far prevented examination of the levels of the individual polymerases [11, 22].

The remaining mutants do not fit any of the patterns seen in E. coli. Two unmapped isolates, gs3 and gs20 are sensitive to γ-rays but not to UV [14], a similar class of mutants is found in yeast [17].

Three important conclusions can be drawn from these studies. There are at least two DNA repair pathways in Neurospora: excision repair and a mutation-prone pathway [21]. There may be a third major repair pathway. This possibility is supported both by the appearance of new classes of mutants and by the relatively low UV sensitivity of the Neurospora mutants. The most sensitive mutant, uvs-2, is 20 times as sensitive to UV as the wild type. None of the other mutants are more than 4 times as sensitive to UV than wild type, while the uvrA mutants of E. coli are about 60 times as sensitive, and the recA mutants as much as 160 times as sensitive to UV than wild-type E. coli [9]. Finally, there appears to be a major difference in excision-repair. The Uvr mutants of E. coli are not sensitive to ionizing radiation while the Neurospora excision-repair defective mutants, uvs-2 and upr-1, both show significant sensitivity. This difference suggests that the enzymes controlled by these two genes have different capabilities than those controlled by the Uvr genes of E. coli or that ionizing radiation is producing excision repairable damage in Neurospora but not in E. coli. The much greater protein content of eukaryote chromosomes makes the latter quite possible.

The hope of obtaining recombination defective mutants was not fulfilled. The most promising mutants, uvs-3 and uvs-6, are homozygous sterile [16, 19]. However, the sterility cannot be assigned to a failure of recombination since meiosis never begins in these strains [18, 19].

NEWLY ISOLATED MUTAGEN-SENSITIVE MUTANTS

Recently, workers in several laboratories have isolated a number of new radiation sensitive mutants. Several techniques have been used.

Mei-3

The most thoroughly characterized new mutant is the mei-3 mutant. It was discovered because of its ability to increase the instability of duplications [15]. The mei-3 mutant represents a new locus. It is UV-sensitive at high temperatures. In addition, mei-3 resembles uvs-3 and uvs-6, in that growth is inhibited by histidine and it is homozygous sterile [16]. It may be a true recombination-defective mutant, as meiosis is blocked in homozygous crosses by a disruption of pairing in Zygotene [18].

Nuclease-Deficient Mutants

A method for isolating mutants with low levels of nuclease release has been developed by Käfer and Fraser [13]. Colonies from mutagenized conidia are tested on DNA containing agar and/or minimal agar with a DNA overlay. After an appropriate incubation period, 1 N HCl is added to precipitate the DNA. Areas where nuclease action has hydrolyzed the DNA appear clear. The mutants isolated can be assigned to eight genes. Because studies of an endo-exo nuclease in Neurospora indicated that this nuclease could be involved in DNA repair [6], these mutants were tested for UV sensitivity and known mutagen-sensitive mutants were tested for nuclease release. One of the newly isolated mutants is UV-sensitive and appears to be an allele of uvs-3 [8, 13]. Two of the previously discovered mutants, uvs-3 and uvs-6, show a marked reduction in nuclease release both on DNA agar and in liquid culture [7].

MMS-Sensitive Mutants

Käfer [12] has developed a procedure for testing methyl methane-sulfonate (MMS) sensitivity in Neurospora. The uvs-2, uvs-3, uvs-4, and uvs-6 mutants are sensitive to MMS, while the upr-1 mutant is not. Thus, the two excision-defective mutants uvs-2 and upr-1 clearly differ in this property.

Recently, Käfer has isolated a number of MMS-sensitive mutants by replica plating [12]. These fall into several classes: some are sensitive only to MMS; others also show sensitivity either to UV light or to ionizing radiation but not both; finally, some are sensitive to all three agents. The multiple patterns of cross-sensitivity and the relatively low UV and ionizing radiation sensitivities of all these mutants provide further evidence that there must be more than two DNA repair pathways in Neurospora. These mutants are discussed in greater detail by Fraser and Käfer [8].

Sterility Mutants

In our laboratory, we have tested the male sterile mutants iso-
labed by Weijer and Vigfusson [27] for UV sensitivity. One mutant
(10528A) is 1.6 times as sensitive to UV as wild type. Unfortunately,
it is sterile as either parent.

SCREENING FOR CYTOPLASMIC FACTORS CONTROLLING UV SENSITIVITY

Recently, we have isolated 25 new UV-sensitive mutants by a
method based on a technique developed by D. E. A. Catcheside (personal
communication). In this method, conidia from the colonial temperature-sensitive strain, cot-1, are mutagenized and plated on agar
containing the UV-absorbing agent p-aminobenzoic acid (PABA). They
are incubated at 25°C (growth permissive temperature) until a small
colony forms, then overlaid with 2.5 ml soft agar containing PABA.
The plates are incubated again at 25°C until the hyphae grow up
through the overlay and spread into a small colony. The colonies are
then exposed to a dose of UV (210 J/m^2) and incubated at 34°C, a
temperature which causes a short, distinctive branching in cot-1
which makes each hypha look like a tiny bottle brush. The plates are
scanned under a microscope. Non-UV-sensitive colonies survive the UV
dose and are recognized by the presence of bottle brush hyphae in
both the upper and lower layers of the colony. UV-sensitive colonies
can be easily recognized because the upper layer of hyphae die and
remain unbranched while the lower layers are protected by the PABA
containing agar and become branched. They can be rescued and tested
further for mutagen sensitivity, allelism, etc.

In the earlier mutant isolations of Chang et al. [3] and
Schroeder [22], four isolates did not transmit UV-sensitivity to
their progeny when used as the conidial (male) parent. However, the
possibility that UV-sensitivity was controlled by a cytoplasmic factor
in these could not be tested since the strains used for the mutant
isolation were female sterile.

A major reason for undertaking the current study was to search
for mutants with cytoplasmically determined UV-sensitivity. As can
be seen in Table 1, a number of the 25 UV-sensitive mutants isolated
did show low or no transmission of the UV-sensitive trait to their
progeny when used as the male (conidial) parent. However, in no case
when the mutant was used as the female (protoperithecial) parent was
the trait transmitted to all or even most of the progeny as expected
for a cytoplasmic trait [5]. If UV-sensitive progeny recovered from
this first generation cross were then used in a cross to a non-UV-
sensitive strain, segregation of UV-sensitive to nonsensitive progeny
approached that expected for a single Mendelian gene in most cases.
By the second backcross, all isolates had the segregation values
expected if the UV-sensitivity trait were slightly disadvantageous

TABLE 1

SEGREGATION OF ULTRAVIOLET SENSITIVITY AND NONSENSITIVITY IN
PROGENY OF RECIPROCAL HETEROZYGOUS CROSSES OF UV-SENSITIVE MUTANTS
TO NONSENSITIVE STRAINS[a]

Mutant	Cross[c]	UV-sensitive strain used as protoperithecial parent (♀)[b]		UV-sensitive strain used as conidial parent (♂)	
		uvs$^+$	uvs$^-$	uvs$^+$	uvs$^-$
Slow germinating class					
1-68	1	17	3	23	2
	2			15	5
2-6	1	29	6	26	0
2-8	1	21	5	28	0
3-54	1	3	5	12	0
	2			13	7
UV-sensitive class					
3-8	1	58	37	9	2
	2	35	30		
3-14	1	60	10	9	2
	2	45	27		
3-79	1	60	9	26	0
	2	40	15		
3-83	1	51	35	25	0
	2	39	26		
4-7	1	53	34	13	4
	2	65	41		
4-23	1	27	3	20	0
	2	40	17		
4-33	1	65	29	14	2
	2	26	33		

[a]Methods were as described in Schroeder [19].

[b]All uvs mutants were induced in the strain 74-OR31-16A, provided by Dr. F. J. de Serres. This strain contains the markers al-2 (Y112M38), cot-1 ([C102(t)], and pan-2 (Y387-15.7a).

[c]In the first generation the non-UV-sensitive parent was cot-1 [C102(t)]. In subsequent generations either the standard wild types 74-OR23-1A or 74-OR81a or the nic-3 (Y31881) strain backcrossed to these wild types was used. These strains were provided by Dr. E. Käfer.

and controlled by one or at the most two Mendelian genes. Thus,
cytoplasmic mutations leading to UV sensitivity are relatively rare
or nonexistent in Neurospora, or this method of isolation selects
against their recovery. The reason for the low transmission of the
trait in the first generation is not known. The most plausible
hypothesis is that the original isolates were heterokaryons, since
multinucleate conidia were mutagenized, and that there was strong
selection for the non-UV-sensitive component in crosses. Partial
dominance of UV-sensitivity would enhance this possibility. Partial
dominance has been seen in the uvs-6 mutant [24].

Of the mutants isolated, several appear to have UV-delayed
conidial germination rather than reduction of survival. Eleven of
the 25 isolates were sufficiently UV-sensitive to warrant further
study. The number of previously unobserved loci they represent is
not yet known. Our results so far indicate that this method of isolation may select for a certain class of UV-sensitive mutants. All
the mutants show a relatively low UV sensitivity (maximum sensitivity
3-fold). Also, most of the other mutants that have been isolated by
non-selective techniques are sensitive to MNNG, and many are sensitive
to MMS and/or ionizing radiation. Most of our new mutants show only
a slight sensitivity to MNNG, two are sensitive to ionizing radiation,
and none are sensitive to MMS.

CONCLUSION

Studies of mutagen sensitive mutants in Neurospora have shown
that a large number of genes control mutagen sensitivity. So far all
are nuclear. Some definitely control steps in DNA-repair processes
similar, but probably not identical, to the excision-repair and post-
replication repair systems of E. coli. Some of the others may be
involved in one or more DNA-repair processes unique to eukaryotes.

ACKNOWLEDGEMENTS

We thank Mr. Douglas Ferro for testing the UV sensitivity of the
10528A mutant of Weijer and Vigfusson, and Drs. E. Käfer and
D. Stadler for their helpful discussions. This work was supported
by NCI grant 5-R01CA22587 to Alice L. Schroeder.

REFERENCES

1. Boyce, R. P., and P. Howard-Flanders, Release of ultraviolet
       light-induced thymine dimers from DNA in E. coli, Proc.
       Natl. Acad. Sci. (U.S.), 51 (1964) 293-300.

2. Chang, L. T., and R. W. Tuveson, Ultraviolet-sensitive mutants
    in Neurospora crassa, Genetics, 56 (1967) 801-810.
3. Chang, L. T., R. W. Tuveson, and M. H. Munroe, Non-nuclear
    inhertiance of UV sensitivity in Neurospora crassa, Can. J.
    Genet. Cytol., 10 (1968) 920-927.
4. Clark, A. J., and A. D. Margulies, Isolation and characterization
    of recombination-deficient mutants of Escherichia coli K-12,
    Proc. Natl. Acad. Sci. (U.S.), 53 (1965) 451-459.
5. Fincham, J. R. S., and P. R. Day, in: Fungal Genetics, 3rd ed.,
    Botanical Monographs, Vol. 4, Blackwell Scientific, Oxford-
    Edinburgh, 1971, pp. 314, 320.
6. Fraser, M. J., S. Kwong, D. M. Galer, and T. Y.-K. Chow, Regu-
    lation by proteinases of a putative Rec$^-$ nuclease of Neuro-
    spora, in: DNA Repair Mechanisms, P. C. Hanawalt, E. C.
    Friedberg, and C. F. Fox, Eds., Academic Press, New York,
    1978, pp. 441-444.
7. Fraser, M. G., Alkaline deoxyribonucleases released from
    Neurospora crassa mycelia: two activities not released by
    mutants with multiple sensitivities to mutagens, Nucl. Acids
    Res., 6 (1979) 231-246.
8. Fraser, M. J., T. Y.-K. Chow, and E. Käfer, Nucleases and their
    control in wild-type and nuh mutants of Neurospora, This
    volume, p. 63.
9. Howard-Flanders, P., and R. P. Boyce, DNA repair and genetic
    recombination: studies on mutants of Escherichia coli
    defective in these processes, Radiat. Res. (Suppl.), 6
    (1966) 156-181.
10. Ishikawa, T., A. Toh-e, I. Unc, and K. Hasunuma, Isolation and
    characterization of nuclease mutants of Neurospora crassa,
    Genetics, 63 (1969) 75-95.
11. Joester, W., K.-E. Joester, B. van Dorp, and P. H. Hofschneider,
    Purification and properties of DNA-dependent DNA-polymerases
    from Neurospora crassa, Nucl. Acids Res., 5 (1978) 3043-
    3055.
12. Käfer, E., Sensitivity to methyl-methane-sulfonate in Neurospora,
    Neurospora Newsl., 25 (1978) 19.
13. Käfer, E., and M. Fraser, Isolation and genetic analysis of
    nuclease halo (nuh) mutants of Neurospora crassa, Mol. Gen.
    Genet., 169 (1979) 117-127.
14. Mehta, R. D., and J. Weijer, U.V. mutability in gamma-ray-
    sensitive mutants of Neurospora crassa, in: Symposium on
    Use of Radiation and Radioisotopes for Genetic Improvement
    of Industrial Microorganisms, International Atomic Energy
    Agency, Vienna, 1971, pp. 63-71.
15. Newmeyer, D., and D. R. Galeazzi, The instability of Neurospora
    duplication Dp(I1→IR) H4250 and its genetic control,
    Genetics, 85 (1977) 461-487.
16. Newmeyer, D., A. L. Schroeder, and D. R. Galeazzi, An apparent
    connection between histidine recombination and repair in
    Neurospora, Genetics, 89 (1978) 271-279.

17. Prakash, L., The relation between repair of DNA and radiation
        and chemical mutagenesis in Saccharomyces cerevisiae,
        Mutat. Res., 41 (1976) 241–248.
18. Raju, N. B., and D. D. Perkins, Barren perithecia in Neurospora
        crassa, Can. J. Genet. Cytol. 20 (1978) 54–59.
19. Schroeder, A. L., Ultraviolet-sensitive mutants of Neurospora,
        I. Genetic basis and effect on recombination, Mol. Gen.
        Genet., 107 (1970) 291–304.
20. Schroeder, A. L., Ultraviolet-sensitive mutants of Neurospora,
        II. Radiation studies, Mol. Gen. Genet., 107 (1970) 305–320.
21. Schroeder, A. L., Genetic control of radiation sensitivity and
        DNA repair in Neurospora, in: Molecular Mechanisms for
        Repair of DNA, P. C. Hanawalt and R. B. Setlow, Eds.,
        Part B, Plenum Press, New York, 1975, pp. 567–576.
22. Schroeder, A. L., and S. L. Norton, unpublished data.
23. Setlow, R. B., and W. L. Carrier, The disappearance of thymine
        dimers from DNA: an error correcting mechanism, Proc. Natl.
        Acad. Sci. (U.S.), 51 (1964) 226–231.
24. Shelby, M. D., F. J. de Serres, and Gerald J. Stine, Ultra-
        violet-inactivation of conidia from heterokaryons of
        Neurospora crassa containing UV-sensitive mutations, Mutat.
        Res., 27 (1975) 45–58.
25. Stadler, D. R., and D. A. Smith, A new mutation in Neurospora
        for sensitivity to ultraviolet, Can. J. Genet. Cytol., 10
        (1968) 916–919.
26. Tuveson, R. W., Genetic and enzymatic analysis of a gene
        controlling UV sensitivity in Neurospora crassa, Mutat. Res.,
        15 (1972) 411–424.
27. Weijer, J., and N. V. Vigfussion, Sexuality in Neurospora crassa,
        I. Mutations to male sterility, Genet. Res., 19 (1972)
        191–204.
28. Worthy, T. E., and J. L. Epler, Biochemical basis of radiation
        sensitivity in mutants of Neurospora crassa, Mutat. Res.,
        19 (1973) 167–173.

CHAPTER 5

NUCLEASES AND THEIR CONTROL IN WILD-TYPE AND <u>nuh</u> MUTANTS

OF NEUROSPORA

M. J. FRASER, T. Y.-K. CHOW, and E. KÄFER

Departments of Biochemistry and Biology, McGill
University, Montreal, Quebec, Canada, H3G 1Y6

SUMMARY

A review of all of the work on Neurospora nucleases strongly
suggests that five nucleases, originally isolated on the basis of
markedly different properties, may actually be derived from a single
inactive precursor polypeptide via different routes of proteolysis.
One of these nucleases may be involved in DNA repair and/or
recombination. Two repair-deficient mutants of Neurospora, <u>uvs-3</u>
and <u>nuh-4</u>, may have a lesion in protease(s) which control the
level of this nuclease or in some function which regulates the
protease(s). Both of these mutants map in the same gene region
and they may be defective in recombination, since they are sensitive
to various mutagens and to mitomycin C and they show high frequency
of spontaneous, but not radiation-induced, recessive lethal
mutations and/or deletions.

INTRODUCTION

Nuclease halo (<u>nuh</u>) mutants of Neurospora fail to secrete
normal amounts of alkaline deoxyribonuclease (DNase) activity when
grown on solid agar in the presence of sorbose [9]. Among the
various <u>nuh</u> mutants, some have been found also to affect the levels
of secreted and/or intracellular nucleases when grown in liquid
culture [2, 3]. The most interesting mutants in this group are
sensitive to a broad spectrum of mutagens, including ultraviolet
light (UV), x-rays, methyl-methane sulfonate (MMS), and nitrosoguanidine (NG), and are also usually sensitive to mitomycin C [1,
9]. Only one repair-deficient mutant was isolated originally as
a <u>nuh</u> mutant (<u>nuh-4</u>), but several other mutants with the Nuh

63

phenotype were detected among a number of mutants sensitive to MMS [8] and to UV [9]. Two UV-sensitive mutants that were later found to have the Nuh phenotype, uvs-3 and uvs-6, were originally isolated by Schroeder [20, 21] and shown to be homozygous sterile and to increase the frequency of somatic loss of heterozygosis for mating type. In addition, they both affect spontaneous and radiation-induced mutagenesis [22]. Other repair-deficient mutants with the Nuh phenotype, especially nuh-4, have been shown to produce extremely high frequencies of recessive lethals [8]. Nuh-4 may be allelic to uvs-3, but it is less sensitive to x-rays and to mitomycin C and has a considerably higher viability than uvs-3.

Other types of repair-deficient mutants of Neurospora, e.g., uvs-2 and upr-1, which are deficient in the excision of pyrimidine dimers in vivo [26], and several MMS-sensitive mutants which have normal fertility and mutation rates do not have the Nuh phenotype and are usually not sensitive to mitomycin C [except uvs-2 (recent unpublished result)].

NATURE OF NUCLEASES

Several nuh mutants which were found to contain reduced levels of intracellular single-strand DNase (ss-DNase) activity [2] have been examined in detail for both the secretion of alkaline DNases from mycelia grown in sorbose-containing liquid culture medium [3] and their contents of major intracellular alkaline DNases [2]. These are the repair-deficient mutants uvs-3, uvs-6, and nuh-4 and a mutagen-insensitive mutant (nuh-3). The results are summarized in Table 1.

Three major alkaline DNases (see summary of properties in Table 2) were secreted in sucrose- and in sorbose-containing media. Sorbose enhanced the Nuh phenotype by increasing the secretion of total ss-DNase activity (14-fold for the wild-type [3]) without altering the proportions of the three DNases that were secreted. Two of these activities were shown to be identical to nucleases that had been previously isolated from Neurospora [3]. The first was a single-strand specific exonuclease (ss-exonuclease) identical to that purified from conidia [17, 23] but not found in mycelia [15] (see Table 2). The second was endo-exonuclease [4] which was purified from mycelia where it has been found in both active and inactive precursor forms [5, 10]. The precursor is converted to the active enzyme by both endogenous and exogenous proteases. Evidence was obtained [3] that "ageing" of crude preparations of extracellular ss-exonuclease resulted in a conversion of ss-exonuclease to endo-exonuclease. This was seen as an appearance of ds-DNase activity and a change in the mode of degradation of ss-DNA from an exonucleolytic to an endo-nucleolytic mode. The third enzyme released from wild-type mycelia, DNase A, has not been previously described in Neurospora (Table 2).

TABLE 1

SUMMARY OF SECRETIONS AND INTRACELLULAR LEVELS OF ALKALINE DNases OF MYCELIA OF REPAIR MUTANTS AND THE MUTAGEN-INSENSITIVE nuh-3 MUTANT OF NEUROSPORA

Strain	Secretion of DNase A, ss-exonuclease, and endo-exonuclease	Levels of intracellular nucleases relative to wild type[a]			Ratios of precursor to total active DNase (ss-DNase)[b]
		D1	D2	D3	
Wild type	normal	100%	100%	100%	2.7
uvs-3	very low DNase A and endo-exonuclease	29%	67%	18%	7.8
uvs-6	low DNase A	78%	72%	74%	3.4
nuh-4	low ss-exonuclease very low endo-exonuclease	59%	83%	46%	4.6
nuh-3	very low ss-exonuclease low endo-exonuclease	78%	22%	39%	7.5

[a]Calculated from the data of Chow and Fraser [2]. Only the values underlined are considered to be significantly different from wild type.
[b]Calculated from the data of Chow and Fraser [2]. The specific ss-DNase activities were determined in crude extracts before and after activation of the precursor with trypsin. The level of precursor is taken as the difference between these values.

TABLE 2

PROPERTIES OF NEUROSPORA NUCLEASES ACTIVE IN THE pH RANGE 7-9

Enzyme		Substrate	Mode of degradation [b]	Divalent metal ion	Inhibitors [c]	Comments
Type	M_{app} [a]					
ss-Endonuclease [11-13]	—	ss-DNA ds-DNA ss-RNA	Endo No activity Endo	Co^{2+} bound? Mg^{2+}, Ca^{2+} stimulation	ATP [16] EDTA Thiols	Intracellular enzyme an end-product of proteolysis of endo-exonuclease [4] Heat stable at 50°C
Mitochondrial nuclease [14]	75K [2]	ss-DNA ds-DNA RNA	Endo Endo Endo	Mg^{2+}	Ca^{2+}, EDTA [c] PHMB	Intracellular enzyme Heat-sensitive at 50°C
ss-Exonuclease [17, 23]	—	ss-DNA ds-DNA RNA	{ Low endo, high exo No activity Endo	Mg^{2+} (no Mg^{2+})	Ca^{2+}, EDTA	Secreted enzyme found in mycelia [15] Heat-sensitive at 50°C
Endo-exonuclease [4, 10]	60-75K	ss-DNA ds-DNA RNA	Endo, exo Exo Endo	Mg^{2+}, (Ca^{2+})	ATP [4] EDTA	Intracellular and secreted enzyme Heat-stable at 50°C Also found in inactive precursor form, M_{app} 90K [5, 10]
D1 [2]	75K	ss-DNA ds-DNA RNA	Endo, exo Exo Endo	Mg^{2+}	EDTA	Intracellular enzyme Heat-stable at 50°C Binds to ss-DNA cellulose
DNase A [3]	65K	ss-DNA ds-DNA RNA	Endo Endo No activity	Ca^{2+}	EDTA	Secreted enzyme

[a] Apparent molecular weight (M_{app}) in kilodaltons as determined by sedimentation in linear sucrose density gradients.

[b] "Endo" and "Exo" refer to endonucleolytic and exonucleolytic modes of degradation.

[c] EDTA is ethylenediaminetetraacetic acid and PHMB is p-hydroxymercuribenzoate.

DNase A is a Ca^{2+}-dependent endonuclease of apparent molecular weight (M_{app}) of 65K with no specificity for ss- or ds-DNA and no RNase activity [3]. DNase A has not been found intracellularly as yet.

The secretions of both DNase A and endo-exonuclease from uvs-3 were greatly reduced relative to the wild type (see summary in Table 1 and Fraser [3]). For nuh-4, the secretions of both ss-exonuclease and endo-exonuclease were greatly reduced relative to the wild type. On the other hand, for uvs-6 the secretion of only DNase A was appreciably reduced relative to the wild-type. The mutagen-insensitive nuh-3 mutant failed to secrete mainly ss-exonuclease, but the secretion of endo-exonuclease was also somewhat reduced relative to the wild type [3]. Thus, in three out of four cases, for uvs-3, nuh-4, and nuh-3, the mutations affected the release of at least two different DNases.

The major intracellular alkaline DNase activities of the wild-type and mutants, referred to below as D1, D2, and D3, were resolved by chromatography [2] of extracts in turn on DEAE-Sepharose (which resolved D3 from D1 and D2) and on phosphocellulose (which resolved D1 from D2). D1, D2, and D3 made up respectively 16%, 34%, and 50% of the total ss-DNase activity in crude extracts of the wild type. A 2.7-fold increase in ss-DNase activity was observed on treating wild-type extracts with trypsin, due to the activation of endo-exonuclease precursor (Table 1). Based on their unique properties (Table 2), D2 and D3 were identified respectively as the mitochondrial nuclease, first described by Linn and Lehman [14], and endo-exonuclease, first isolated and characterized in our own laboratory [4]. Although even partially purified preparations of D2 and D3 have ds-DNase activity, neither enzyme expressed this activity appreciably in crude extracts. A protein inhibitor has been isolated from the D1 plus D2 fraction (from DEAE-Sepharose) by chromatography of aged preparations on DEAE-cellulose [2]. A low molecular weight (M_{app} of 22K) DNase inhibitor has also been isolated from Aspergillus [24], but it is not known whether it differentially inhibits the ds-DNase versus the ss-DNase activity of analogous nucleases.

D1 has not been identified previously in Neurospora. Fresh preparations of D1 from DEAE-Sepharose initially expressed only single-strand specific endo-nuclease (ss-endonuclease) activity. However, ds-DNase activity was unmasked in three ways: (1) by chromatography on DEAE-cellulose or (2) by chromatography on ss-DNA cellulose, where in both cases the ds-DNase activity expressed was exonucleolytic in character and the enzyme behaved like D3 (endo-exonuclease); or (3) by "ageing" at 0-4°C for a few days, in which case the ds-DNA activity expressed was endonucleolytic in character and the preparation behaved like D2 (the mitochondrial nuclease). In fact, D2 was separated from "aged" D1 preparations by re-chromatography on phosphocellulose. When the D1 plus D2 fraction from DEAE-Sepharose was chromatographed on ss-DNA cellulose, over 80% of the ss-DNase activity bound strongly and was separated from most of the protein. The activity recovered from ss-DNA cellulose was stable over a period of at least three weeks. Rather than a mixture of D1 and D2, it resembled endo-exonuclease (D3) in several properties, e.g., the expression of ss-endonuclease and ds-exonuclease activities, low ratio (2.0) of activity with ss-DNA versus ds-DNA, sedimentation rate (see below), sensitivity to EDTA and dependence on Mg^{2+} for activity. On the other hand, unlike endo-exonuclease, the purified D1 was not inhibited by ATP and did not show any activity in the presence of Ca^{2+}. These properties, however, appeared when D1 was treated with trypsin. If D1 is a precursor form of endo-exonuclease, it would be predicted that trypsin treatment would also abolish the binding to ss-DNA. This prediction has now been tested and confirmed. It is interesting to note that a trypsin-sensitive ss-DNA-binding activity was previously co-purified with endo-exonuclease (D1-like) activity [4]. The above properties suggest that D1 is closely related to endo-exonuclease (D3), perhaps a form of the enzyme intermediate between the inactive precursor and endo-exonuclease. In contrast, purified D1 from ss-DNA cellulose behaved quite differently when chromatographed on phospho-cellulose and, when eluted, behaved in every respect (cf. Table 2) like the micochondrial nuclease (D2). It is not understood what causes this striking conversion, but the observation suggests that a "converting factor" has also bound to ss-DNA cellulose and is somehow triggered to act when the fraction is passed through phospho-cellulose. These results suggest that when the D1 plus D2 fraction is passed through phosphocellulose to separate D1 and D2, the amount of D2 recovered may reflect the level of "converting factor" present, i.e., D2 may arise, at least partially, as an artifact of chromato-graphy on phosphocellulose. On the other hand, characterization of the unresolved D1 plus D2 fraction indicated that at least some of the D2 component was present before resolution on phosphocellulose [2] and is likely a true intracellular nuclease. The above results indicate that D1 is not only a "precursor" of D3, but of D2 as well, a nuclease with markedly different properties than endo-exonuclease (D3).

The sedimentation behavior of the partially purified intra-cellular nucleases has been studied in linear sucrose gradients (see Fig. 1). Freshly isolated D2 (from phosphocellulose) and D3 (from DEAE-Sepharose or phosphocellulose) both sedimented with apparent molecular weights (M_{app}) each of 75K. The M_{app} of D3 is higher than those found for the trypsin-activated precursor (M_{app} of 61K [5]) or for the least degraded form of endo-exonuclease isolated previously (peptide molecular weight of 53K [10]) and for the Neurospora ss-endonuclease (M_{app} of 55K [11]) which is likely an end-product of proteolysis of endo-exonuclease [4]. Thus, the intracellular form described here is either a less modified form of the nuclease or is associated with other protein(s) such as the

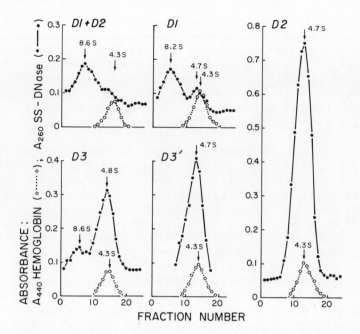

Fig. 1.   Sedimentation of various intracellular alkaline DNase
fractions derived from log phase Neurospora mycelia in linear 5-20%
sucrose gradients with bovine hemoglobin (4.3S) as a marker for
(clockwise from the top left):   (D1 + D2) the D1 plus D2 fraction
freshly isolated from DEAE-Sepharose;   (D1) the D1 fraction from
phosphocellulose "aged" 1 week at 0-4°C;   (D2) freshly prepared D2
from phosphocellulose;   (D3) D3 which had been chromatographed on
DEAE-cellulose and then on phosphocellulose;   (D3') D3 freshly
derived from DEAE-Sepharose.   The ss-DNase activity (●) was
determined in each gradient fraction by measuring the release of
acid-soluble material (A_{260}) from ss-DNA at pH 8.0 in a fixed
period of time [2, 3];   hemoglobin (○) was determined by
measuring the absorbance of each fraction at 440 nm (A_{440}).

ds-DNase inhibitor.   The sedimentation behavior of D1 varied,
depending on which fraction was examined.   In crude extracts, all
of the ss-DNase activity sedimented with an M_{app} of 75K, as did the
purified D1 from ss-DNA cellulose (data not shown).   However, in
the D1 plus D2 fraction from DEAE-Sepharose, most of the ss-DNase
activity sedimented with an M_{app} of approximately 180K, while D1
from phosphocellulose showed both 180K and 75K components in
variable amounts (see Fig. 1).   This behavior indicated that D1 was
associating with other protein(s) or with itself (dimer formation)
in addition to relatively low molecular weight protein(s) such as
ds-DNase inhibitor [24] to yield the 180K species.

D1 was found to be very heat-stable at (50-60°C, 10 min), like
the endo-exonuclease (D3) and its precursor. On the other hand, D2
was rapidly inactivated at 50°C. In this respect, the ss-DNase
activity of D1 plus D2 (from DEAE-Sepharose) behaved like a mixture
of D1 and D2 as well as in response to inhibitions by EDTA and PHMB
and activations with divalent metal ions [2]. Again, it seems
likely then that D2 exists intracellularly per se and is not simply
an artifact of chromatography on phosphocellulose (see above).

The recoveries of freshly isolated intracellular nucleases, D1,
D2, and D3, from the repair-deficient mutants and nuh-3 relative
to the wild-type are reported in Table 1. The uvs-3 and nuh-4
mutants which are possibly allelic [9] were found to be deficient
in both D1 and D3. Both of these mutants also secreted only low
amounts of endo-exonuclease (D3). However, although the differences
in x-ray and mitomycin C sensitivities and in levels of intracellular
nucleases were only quantitative, there was a striking qualitative
difference in the secretion of DNases from the two mutants: uvs-3
failed to secrete appreciable amounts of DNase A, while nuh-4
secreted normal amounts of this enzyme [3]. The third repair-
deficient mutant (uvs-6) was not appreciably deficient in any of
the major alkaline nucleases, but secreted only low amounts of
DNase A [3], an enzyme which has not been detected intracellularly
and is apparently not related to the other nucleases. DNase A
could be a minor intracellular activity, or possibly it is not
solubilized by our extraction procedures. The intracellular levels
of both D2 and D3 were low in the mutagen-insensitive nuh-3 mutant,
but the level of D1 is near normal, unlike in uvs-3 and nuh-4.
The observations suggest that low levels of D1 may result in
mutagen sensitivity and could implicate this enzyme in DNA repair
and/or recombination. The near normal level of D1 in the mutagen-
sensitive uvs-6 mutant can be interpreted to mean that other
factor(s) affecting mutagen-sensitivity are altered in this mutant.

An enzyme with many properties in common with the Neurospora
ss-endonuclease and endo-exonuclease has been implicated in
recombination in Ustilago maydis [6, 7]. It is interesting that
second form of this activity with some properties in common with D1
(including strong binding to ss-DNA-cellulose) is associated through
several steps of purification with an ATPase which is inhibited by
both ss- and ds-DNA [18]. The similarities in enzymological
properties between the Neurospora endo-exonuclease and the ATP-
dependent bacterial rec-nucleases have been pointed out [4]. It
seems possible that D1 may be a fungal rec-nuclease with
ATP-dependent nuclease and DNA-dependent ATPase activities which
have become "uncoupled" as a result of exposure to protease(s)
during isolation procedures.

The results summarized above strongly suggest to us that all
of the nucleases (those enzymes acting on both DNA and RNA) which

have been isolated from Neurospora to date [ss-endonuclease,
mitochondrial nuclease (D2), ss-exonuclease, endo-exonuclease (D3)
and D1], despite wide differences in properties, are nevertheless
related and likely derived from the same inactive precursor. This
novel "working hypothesis" is presented in schematic form in Fig. 2.
All five active forms of enzyme involved have been shown to have
endonuclease activity with ss-DNA and RNA (Table 2), and at least
three of them have been shown to produce oligonucleotides with 5'-p
and 3'-OH termini [13, 14, 17]. In this scheme, the precursor is
depicted as having two blocked active sites, an endonuclease site
for DNA and RNA and an exonuclease site for DNA only. The precursor
is a hydrophobic protein as determined from its affinity for octyl-
and phenyl-Sepharose [5, 10], a property which is lost when it is
activated in vitro with trypsin. This behavior is consistent with
its being a preproenzyme, at least some of which is destined for
secretion. Perhaps the primary secretion product is ss-exonuclease
which could be produced from the precursor by the action of plasma
membrane protease(s) and extracellular proteases. The extracellular
ss-exonuclease has a M_{app} of 75K which is close to that of the
single polypeptide isolated from conidia [17]. The enzyme would
have only a partially accessible endonuclease site (low ss-endonuclease activity) and a partially accessible exonuclease site
allowing attack only on ss-DNA. Further extracellular proteolysis
could convert ss-exonuclease to endo-exonuclease (M_{app} 65K) [3] or
the conversion could be direct from the precursor by the action of
plasma membrane protease(s).

     Intracellularly, the first product of processing is likely D1
which is depicted as having only a partially accessible endonuclease
site, the exonuclease site being blocked by the ds-DNase inhibitor
shown as part of the D1 structure. D1 in this form can dimerize or
associate with other proteins to form a fast-sedimenting species
(M_{app} 180K). It can also lose the ds-DNase inhibitor portion of its
structure, perhaps, through further proteolysis. In this case
endo-exonuclease would be the product of processing. Another type
of proteolysis might be involved in the conversion of D1 to D2
(mitochondrial nuclease). This would require the destruction of the
exonuclease site and a loosening of the endonuclease site to make
it accessible to ds-DNA. In the cell these modifications could
occur at different intracellular sites, e.g., conversion of D1 to
endo-exonuclease (D3) by protease(s) associated with microsomal
membranes or the nucleus and conversion of D1 to D2 by protease(s)
associated with the mitochondria. Further processing of D3 to
ss-endonuclease would presumably occur through the action of
lysosome-like protease(s) during massive protein breakdown as occurs
under starvation conditions. This would destroy the exonuclease
site leaving a single-strand specific endonuclease "core" enzyme.
Such "processing" by endogenous Neurospora protease(s) has been
seen in vitro [4] and constitutes part of the evidence for the two

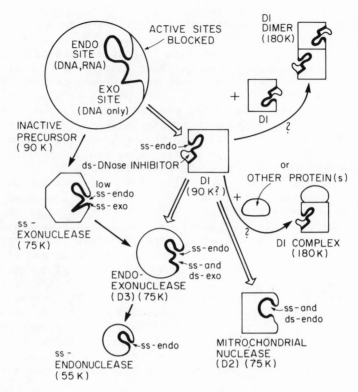

Fig. 2.   Schematic representation of the possible relationships
between five Neurospora nucleases [ss-endonuclease, mitochondrial
nuclease (D2), ss-exonuclease, endo-exonuclease (D3) and D1] and
how they may derive from a single inactive precursor (see text for
explanation).   The scheme also shows how D1 may either dimerize or
combine with other protein(s) to form the observed 180K species.

active sites model for endo-exonuclease [4].   Our hypothesis
predicts that there would be immunological cross-reactivity between
the various purified nucleases and common tryptic peptides.   It
also suggests that proteases associated with different membrane
fractions may convert the precursor into different end products.
These aspects of the model are under test.

A further implication of this model is that proteases are
involved in regulating the levels of precursor and various active
forms of nucleases in Neurospora.   This implication is particularly
relevant for the uvs-3 mutant which exhibits not only mutagen
sensitivities and abnormal mitotic recombination, but is also
deficient in UV-induced mutagenesis [22].   At least two types of

proteases, the rec A and lon or deg gene products, have been associated with control of mutagenesis in Escherichia coli [19, 25].

REFERENCES

1. Chow, T. Y.-K., and M. J. Fraser, Sensitivity of DNA-repair deficient mutants of Neurospora to histidine and to mitomycin C, Microbiol. Genet. Bull., 45 (1978) 4-5.
2. Chow, T. Y.-K., and M. J. Fraser, The major intracellular alkaline deoxyribonuclease activities expressed in wild-type and rec-like mutants of Neurospora crassa, Can. J. Biochem., 57 (1979), 889-901.
3. Fraser, M. J., Alkaline deoxyribonucleases released from Neurospora crassa mycelia: two activities not released by mutants with multiple mutagen sensitivities, Nucl. Acids Res., 6 (1979) 231-246.
4. Fraser, M. J., R. Tjeerde, and K. Matsumoto, A second form of the single-strand specific endonuclease of Neurospora crassa which is associated with a double-strand exonuclease, Can. J. Biochem., 54 (1976) 971-980.
5. Gáler, D. M., Purification and properties of Neurospora endo-exonuclease precursor, M. Sc. thesis, McGill University, 1978, pp. 1-117.
6. Holloman, W. K., Studies on a nuclease from Ustilago maydis. II. Substrate specificity and mode of action of the enzyme, J. Biol. Chem., 248 (1973) 8114-8119.
7. Holloman, W. K., and R. Holliday, Studies on a nuclease from Ustilago maydis. II. Purification, properties and implication in recombination of the enzyme, J. Biol. Chem., 248 (1973) 8107-8113.
8. Käfer, E., unpublished results.
9. Käfer, E., and M. Fraser, Isolation and genetic analysis of nuclease halo (nuh) mutants of Neurospora crassa, Mol. Gen. Genet., 169 (1979) 117-127.
10. Kwong, S., and M. J. Fraser, Neurospora endo-exonuclease and its inactive (precursor?) form, Can. J. Biochem., 56 (1978) 370-377.
11. Linn, S., An endonuclease from Neurospora crassa specific for polynucleotides lacking an ordered structure, In: Methods in Enzymology, Vol. 12A, L. Grossman and K. Moldave (Eds.), Academic Press, New York, 1967, pp. 247-255.
12. Linn, S., and I. R. Lehman, An endonuclease from Neurospora crassa specific for polynucleotides lacking an ordered structure. I. Purification and properties of the enzyme, J. Biol. Chem., 240 (1965) 1287-1293.
13. Linn, S., and I. R. Lehman, An endonuclease from Neurospora crassa specific for polynucleotides lacking an ordered structure. II. Studies of enzyme specificity, J. Biol. Chem., 240 (1965) 1294-1304.

14. Linn, S., and I. R. Lehman, An endonuclease from mitochondria
    of Neurospora crassa, J. Biol. Chem., 241 (1966) 2694-2699.
15. Mills, C., and M. J. Fraser, Different chromatographic forms
    of Neurospora crassa nucleases specific for single-stranded
    nucleic acids, Can. J. Biochem., 51 (1973) 888-895.
16. Rabin, E. Z., M. Mustard, and M. J. Fraser, Specific inhibition
    by ATP and other properties of an endonuclease of
    Neurospora crassa, Can. J. Biochem., 46 (1968) 1285-1291.
17. Rabin, E. Z., H. Tenenhouse, and M. J. Fraser, An exonuclease
    of Neurospora crassa specific for single-stranded nucleic
    acids, Biochim. Biophys. Acta, 259 (1972) 50-68.
18. Rusche, J. R., T. C. Rowe, and W. K. Holloman, DNA-polymerase
    and topoisomerase from Ustilago have associated ATPase
    activities, Fed. Proc., 38 (1979) 485.
19. Sedgwick, S. G., A. Levine and A. Bailone, Induction of rec A+
    -protein synthesis in Escherichia coli, Mol. Gen. Genet.,
    160 (1978) 267-276.
20. Schroeder, A. L., Ultraviolet sensitive mutants of Neurospora.
    I. Genetic basis and effect on recombination, Mol. Gen.
    Genet., 107 (1970) 291-304.
21. Schroeder, A. L., Ultraviolet sensitive mutants of Neurospora.
    II. Radiation studies, Mol. Gen. Genet., 107 (1970) 305-
    320.
22. Schroeder, A. L., Genetic control of radiation sensitivity in
    Neurospora, In: Molecular Mechanisms for Repair of DNA,
    Part B, P. C. Hanawalt and R. B. Setlow (Eds.), Plenum
    Press, New York, 1975, pp. 567-576.
23. Tenenhouse, H., and M. J. Fraser, The ribonuclease activities
    of single-strand specific nucleases of Neurospora crassa,
    Can. J. Biochem., 51 (1973) 569-580.
24. Uozumi, T., K. Ishino, T. Beppu, and K. Arima, Purification
    and properties of the nuclease inhibitor of Aspergillus
    oryzae and kinetics of its interaction with crystalline
    nuclease 0, J. Biol. Chem., 251 (1976) 2808-2813.
25. Witkin, E. M., Ultraviolet light mutagenesis and inducible
    DNA repair in Escherichia coli, Bact. Rev., 40 (1976)
    869-907.
26. Worthy, T. E., and J. L. Epler, Biochemical basis of radiation-
    sensitivity in mutants of Neurospora crassa, Mutat. Res.,
    19 (1973) 167-173.

CHAPTER 6

MUTATION-INDUCTION IN REPAIR-DEFICIENT STRAINS OF NEUROSPORA

FREDERICK J. DE SERRES

Office of the Director, National Institute of
Environmental Health Sciences, Research Triangle Park,
North Carolina   27709 (U.S.A.)

SUMMARY

Various mutants sensitive to UV-induced inactivation have been
used to study the process of spontaneous and induced mutation in
the ad-3 region of Neurospora crassa. Studies on haploid strains
have shown that the process of mutation-induction in the ad-3 region
is under genetic control. Studies on two-component heterokaryons
have shown that this control effects both point mutations and multilocus deletions. Comparisons made between an excision-repair
deficient two-component heterokaryon (59) have shown that the level
of effect is markedly mutagen-specific. All possible effects on
the process of mutation-induction in the ad-3 region have been found
in the strains tested.

INTRODUCTION

Studies with various repair-deficient strains of Neurospora
[24] have shown that the process of mutation-induction at specific
loci is under genetic control. In this paper I will review the
studies which show that these repair-deficient mutations not only
influence the recovery of specific locus mutants quantitatively,
but qualitatively as well. We have used the induction of ad-3
mutants as our assay system in both haploid strains and two-component heterokaryons of Neurospora.   In the former case we can recover
and analyze point mutations at two closely linked loci, ad-3A and
ad-3B.   In the latter case, in two-component heterokaryons, multilocus (chromosomal or interstitial) deletions can also be recovered
which cover the ad-3A locus, the ad-3B locus, or both loci simultaneously (as well as another closely linked locus nic-2) [10]. Point
mutations at the ad-3B locus show allelic complementation [1, 4, 9],
and there is a high correlation between complementation pattern and

genetic alteration at the molecular level [15, 18-21]. Thus, tests
for allelic complementation can provide evidence for qualitative
differences in the spectra of genetic alterations among samples of
ad-3B mutants induced in wild-type or repair-deficient mutant
strains. Genetic analysis of ad-3 mutants by heterokaryon tests
makes it possible to characterize these mutants and to resolve the
initial induction-curve for ad-3 mutants into its various components
as indicated in Fig. 1 for either haploid strains or two-component
heterokaryons.

Haploid Strains

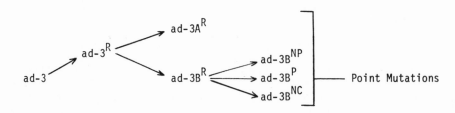

Two-Component Heterokaryons

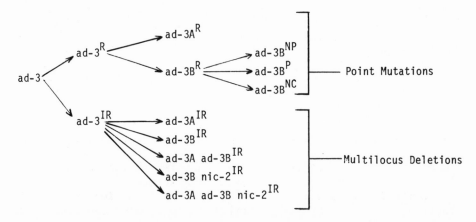

Fig. 1.   Comparison of the classes of ad-3 mutants identified by
various genetic tests in experiments with either haploid strains or
by two-component heterokaryons of Neurospora: IR = irreparable;
R = reparable (will grow as haploid in the presence of appropriate
nutrients);   NP = nonpolar;   NC = noncomplementing;   C = complementing;   P = polarized.

MUTATION–INDUCTION IN HAPLOID STRAINS

All of the repair-deficient strains described by Schroeder [24]
were obtained by us and crossed into a common genetic background
(wild-type OR74A). This procedure made it possible, then, to test
the effect of each repair-deficient mutation on the process of
mutation-induction at the ad-3A and ad-3B loci both quantitatively
and qualitatively. All strains (uvs-1, uvs-2, uvs-4, uvs-5, uvs-6
and upr-1) have the same spontaneous mutability as wild-type,
whereas uvs-3 is at least 5-10 times higher [2, 7, 8].

Comparisons of mutation-induction between wild-type and repair-
deficient strains after UV [2], γ rays [11], MNNG, ICR-170 and
4NQO [13, 14] have shown striking quantitative differences as summarized in Table 1.

All possible effects on mutation-induction were found in these
strains ranging from no significant increase over spontaneous background (uvs-3 after UV or 4NQO), reduced frequencies (uvs-4 after
UV or γ rays, uvs-5 after all treatments), no difference from wild-
type (uvs-6 after all treatments) and enhanced frequencies (upr-1
after UV, γ rays, MNNG and 4NQO). Of particular interest is the
fact that both upr-1 and uvs-2 are excision-repair deficient [25]
and respond similarly to all mutagenic treatments except ICR-170
[12]. In these cases, rather than the enhanced recoveries found
with both strains after UV, γ-rays, MNNG, or 4NQO, upr-1 showed the
same mutant frequencies found with the wild-type strain, whereas
mutant recovery with uvs-2 was markedly reduced.

GENETIC ANALYSIS OF ad-3 MUTANTS IN HAPLOID STRAINS

The genetic analysis of ad-3 mutants recovered after UV treatment has shown marked qualitative differences in the spectra of
ad-3B mutants induced in both upr-1 and uvs-2 from that found in
the wild-type strain [3]. In these experiments lower percentages
of ad-3B mutants with non-polarized complementation patterns were
found, and higher frequencies of non-complementing mutants, with no
change in the frequencies of mutants with polarized patterns. These
data have been interpreted as indicating [5] that lesions that would
normally be processed to produce base-pair substitutions (with non-
polarized patterns) are being converted in the excision-repair
deficient strains to frameshift mutations, giving rise instead to
noncomplementing mutants.

TABLE 1

COMPARATIVE SENSITIVITY OF RADIATION-SENSITIVE MUTANTS
TO INACTIVATION AND MUTATION-INDUCTION AT THE ad-3A
AND ad-3B LOCI IN NEUROSPORA CRASSA[a]

	UV	γ-Rays	MNNG	ICR-170	4NQO
Inactivation					
uvs-1	+	n.t.	n.t.	n.t.	n.t.
uvs-2	++++	++	++	+	+++
uvs-3	+++	+++	++	+	++
uvs-4	+++	0	n.t.	n.t.	n.t.
uvs-5	++	0	+++	+	0
uvs-6	+++	++++	+++	+	++
upr-1	+++	+	+	+	++
Mutation Induction					
uvs-1	0	n.t.	n.t.	n.t.	n.t.
uvs-2	++	++	++	R	+++
uvs-3	–	R	R	R	–
uvs-4	R	R	n.t.	n.t.	n.t.
uvs-5	R	R	R	R	R
uvs-6	0	0	0	0	0
upr-1	++	++	+	0	++

[a]Legend: 0 = same sensitivity as wild-type; + to
+++ = increasing degrees of sensitivity; R = reduced sensitivity; – = not mutable; n.t. = not tested.

MUTATION-INDUCTION IN TWO-COMPONENT HETEROKARYONS

By inducing ad-3 mutants in two-component heterokaryons it is
possible to determine whether the excision-repair deficiency in
uvs-2, for example, would influence the relative frequencies of
point mutations in the ad-3 region versus multilocus deletions
(Fig. 2). A comparison has been made between heterokaryon 12 [9]
which is heterozygous in the ad-2 region (ad-3A⁺ ad-3B⁺ / ad-3A
ad-3B) and is repair-sufficient, with heterokaryon 59 [6] which has
the same genetic composition as heterokaryon 12 except that it is
repair-deficient (uvs-2/uvs-2). Comparisons of the genetic effects
of methyl methanesulfonate (MMS), N-methyl-N'-nitro-N-nitrosoguani-
dine (MNNG), and aflatoxin (AFL-B) have shown that all chemicals
induce higher frequencies of multilocus deletions in heterokaryon
59 than in heterokaryon 12 [7, 8]. Similar results were found with
2-aminopurine (2-AP), but no difference was found between the

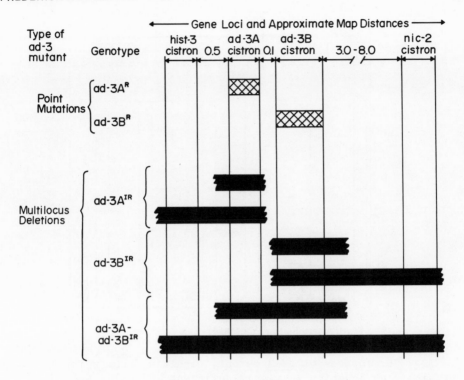

Fig. 2.   Comparison of the extent of genetic damage in various
point mutations and multilocus deletion mutations in the ad-3 region
in two-component heterokaryons of Neurospora.

relative frequencies of these two classes of ad-3 mutations after
treatment with actinomycin D (ACT-D) [7, 8].

The apparent conversion of genetic damage which would normally
produce point mutations in heterokaryon 12 to multilocus deletions
in heterokaryon 59 is illustrated in Figs. 3 and 4. The level of
effect is mutagen-dependent and must depend upon the production of
a particular type of genetic lesion which is processed differently
in heterokaryon 59 to produce multilocus deletion mutants rather than
point mutants. With 2-AP, for example, where a comparison is made
between ad-3 mutants induced at comparable forward-mutation frequencies, only about 12% of the mutants are multilocus deletions in
heterokaryon 12 whereas 68% are of this type in heterokaryon 59.

Data similar to that found with the haploid strains resulted
from UV, 4NQO, β-propiolactone, MMS, MNNG, or AFL-B1 treatment of
two-component heterokaryons [7. 8]. In all cases lower percentages
of ad-3B mutants with nonpolarized complementation patterns were
found in the samples induced in heterokaryon 59 than in those

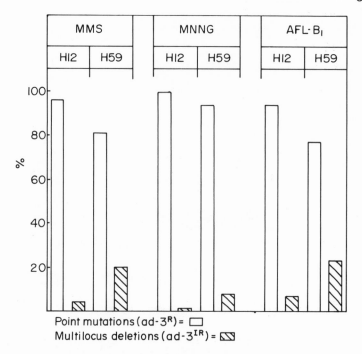

Fig. 3.   Percentages of ad-3 mutants resulting from point mutation
and multilocus deletion in repair-deficient and wild-type two-
component heterokaryons of Neurospora crassa induced by 2-amino-
purine (2-AP) or Actinomycin D (ACT-D).

induced in heterokaryon 12 (and higher percentages of noncomplementing mutants in heterokaryon 59 than in heterokaryon 12).

GENERAL IMPLICATIONS FOR HIGHER EUKARYOTES INCLUDING MAN

      The data obtained from comparisons of mutation-induction in
wild-type and excision-repair deficient heterokaryons may be particularly relevant to risk-estimation if the excision-repair deficiency in lower eukaryotes is comparable to that found in the human
population, for example, in xeroderma pigmentosum (XP) patients.
Such individuals are not only at a higher risk from cancer and such
genetic damage as the production of chromosome aberrations [23], but
our data support the idea that they might also be at a higher risk
for the production of gene mutations. The latter point has already
been shown with experiments comparing mutation-induction at specific
loci between normal and xeroderma pigmentosum cells in culture [16,
17] but the Neurospora data provide information beyond the quantitative effects found with the experiments on mammalian cells in
culture.

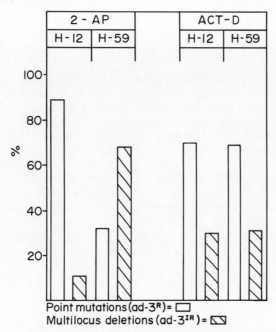

Fig. 4. Percentage of ad-3 mutants resulting from point mutations and multilocus deletions after mutagenic treatment of wild-type and excision-repair deficient two-component heterokaryons of Neurospora crassa induced by methyl methanesulfonate (MMS), N–methyl–N'–nitro-nitrosoguanidine (MNNG) and aflatoxin B₁ (AFL–B₁).

The marked qualtiative effects in Neurospora which show that genetic damage resulting in point mutations in wild-type strains can be converted to multilocus deletions in excision-repair deficent strains has serious implications, if direct extrapolation to man is possible. If exposure to a mutagenic agent which results in pre-dominantly point mutations in normal individuals is converted to multilocus deletions in xeroderma pigmentosum patients, then XP patients are at a much higher risk genetically.

Our concern is that genetic damage at loci which would produce recessive point mutations (which might not be expressed for many generations) could show immediate expression in the F$_1$ generation if this damage is converted to multilocus deletions. In mice, for example, the experiments of Russell [22] have shown that multilocus deletions in the dilute, short-ear region can show immediate expression in the F$_1$ progeny in terms of lethality, reduced birth weight, etc.

FUTURE COURSE

In Neurospora it will be possible to construct two-component heterokaryons heterozygous for uvs-2 (+/uvs-2) and to determine whether such heterokaryons are more like homozygous sufficient (+/+) or deficient (uvs-2/uvs-2) strains. Since heterozygotes for xeroderma pigmentosum occur at even higher frequencies in the human population than the homozygous recessives, this new line of work will provide some assessment of the relative sensitivities of normal, heterozygous and homozygous recessive individuals. Similar studies should, of course, be done with human cells in culture, but the data from experiments with two-component heterokaryons of Neurospora have shown that important qualitative differences in the spectra of genetic alterations are not revealed until genetic analysis of induced mutants has been performed. Unfortunately, it is still difficult, if not impossible, to subject specific locus mutation in mammalian cells in culture to this more rigorous type of genetic analysis.

REFERENCES

1. de Serres, F. J., Carbon dioxide stimulation of the ad-3 mutants Neurospora crassa, Mutat. Res., 3 (1966) 420-425.
2. de Serres, F. J., Mutability of the UV-sensitive strains of Neurospora crassa, Genetics, 68 (1971) 14-15.
3. de Serres, F. J., Mutagenic specificity of chemical carcinogens in microorganisms. In: Proceedings of Workshop on Approaches to Assess the Significance of Experimental Chemical Carcinogenesis Data for Man, December 10-12, 1973, Brussels, Belgium (IARC Scientific Publication 10), IARC, Lyon, 1974, pp. 201-211.
4. de Serres, F. J., The utilization of leaky ad-3 mutants of Neurospora crassa in heterokaryon tests for allelic complementation, Mutat. Res., 3 (1966) 3-12.
5. de Serres, F. J., Qualitative effects of UV-sensitive strains of Neurospora crassa on mutation induction at the ad-3B locus, Mutat. Res., 21 (1973) 216-217.
6. de Serres, F. J., Unpublished data.
7. de Serres, F. J., H. E. Brockman, C. Y. Hung, and T. M. Ong, Comparison of the mutagenic effects of chemical mutagens in excision-repair deficient and wild-type two-component heterokaryons of Neurospora crassa. Presented at the 9th Annual Meeting, Environmental Mutagen Society, San Francisco, California, March 9-13, 1978, Program and Abstracts Book, pp. 51-52.
8. de Serres, F. J., H. E. Brockman, C. Y. Hung, and T. M. Ong, Comparison of the mutagenic effects of 2-aminopurine and actinomycin D in excision-repair deficient and wild-type two-component heterokaryons of Neurospora crassa, Environ. Mut., 1 (1979) 132.

9. de Serres, F. J., H. E. Brockman, W. E. Barnett, and H. G.
    Kolmark, Allelic complementation among nitrous acid-induced
    ad-3B mutants of Neurospora crassa, Mutat. Res., 4 (1967)
    415-424.
10. de Serres, F. J., and H. V. Malling, Measurement of recessive
    lethal damage over the entire genome and at two specific
    loci in the ad-3 region of a two-component heterokaryon of
    Neurospora crassa, In: Chemical Mutagens: Principles and
    Methods for their Detection, Vol. II, A. Hollaender, Ed.,
    Plenum Press, New York, 1971, pp. 311-342.
11. de Serres, F. J., and M. E. Schüpbach, Mutagenesis at the ad-3A
    and ad-3B loci in haploid UV-sensitive strains of Neurospora
    crassa. II. Comparison of γ-ray induced inactivation and
    mutation-induction dose-response curves, Mutat. Res., in
    press.
12. Inoue, H., T. M. Ong, and F. J. de Serres, Inactivation and
    mutation induction by ICR-170 in UV-sensitive strains of
    Neurospora crassa, Mutat. Res., 38 (1976) 379.
13. Inoue, H., T. M. Ong, and F. J. de Serres, Lethal and mutagenic
    effects of 4-nitroquinoline-1-oxide in UV-sensitive strains
    of Neurospora crassa, Mutat. Res., 53 (1978) 82-83.
14. Inoue, H., T. M. Ong, and F. J. de Serres, Lethal and mutagenic
    effects of N-methyl-N'-nitro-N-nitrosoguanidine in UV-
    sensitive strain of Neurospora crassa, Mutat. Res., 31
    (1975) 307-308.
15. Kilbey, B. J., F. J. de Serres, and H. V. Malling, Identifica-
    tion of the genetic alteration at the molecular level of
    ultraviolet light-induced ad-3B mutants in Neurospora
    crassa, Mutat. Res., 12 (1971) 47-56.
16. Maher, V. M., J. J. McCormick, P. L. Grover, and P. Sims, Effect
    of DNA repair on the cytotoxicity and mutagenicity of poly-
    cyclic hydrocarbons derivatives in normal and xeroderma
    pigmentosum human fibroblasts, Mutat. Res., 43 (1977)
    117-138.
17. Maher, V. M., L. M. Ouellette, R. D. Curren, and J. J.
    McCormick, Frequency of ultraviolet light-induced mutations
    is higher in xeroderma pigmentosum variant cells than in
    normal cells, Nature 261 (1976) 593-595.
18. Malling, H. V., and F. J. de Serres, Correlation between base-
    pair transition and complementation pattern in nitrous acid-
    induced ad-3B mutants of Neurospora crassa, Mutat. Res., 5
    (1968) 359-371.
19. Malling, H. V., and F. J. de Serres, Identification of genetic
    alterations induced by ethylmethanesulfonate in Neurospora
    crassa, Mutat. Res., 6 (1968) 181-193.
20. Malling, H. V., and F. J. de Serres, Identification of the
    spectrum of x-ray-induced intragenic alterations at the
    molecular level in Neurospora crassa, Rad. Res., 31 (1967)
    637-638.

21. Malling, H. V., and F. J. de Serres, Relation between comple-
         mentation patterns and genetic alterations in nitrous acid-
         induced ad-3B mutants of Neurospora crassa, Mutat. Res., 4
         (1967) 425-440.
22. Russell, L. B., Definition of functional units in a small chro-
         mosomal segment of the mouse and its use in interpreting
         the nature of radiation-induced mutation, Mutat. Res., 11
         (1971) 107-123.
23. Sasaki, M. S., DNA repair capacity and susceptibility to
         chromosome breakage in xeroderma pigmentosum cells, Mutat.
         Res., 20 (1973) 291-293.
24. Schroeder, A. L., Genetic control of radiation sensitivity and
         DNA repair in Neurospora, In: Molecular Mechanisms for
         Repair of DNA, Part B, P. C. Hanawalt and R. B. Setlow,
         Eds., Plenum Press, New York, 1975, pp. 567-576.
25. Worthy, T. E., and J. L. Epler, Biochemical basis of radiation-
         sensitivity in mutants of Neurospora crassa, Mutat. Res.,
         19 (1973) 167-173.

CHAPTER 7

GENETIC AND PHYSIOLOGICAL FACTORS AFFECTING REPAIR AND

MUTAGENESIS IN YEAST

JEFFREY F. LEMONTT

Biology Division, Oak Ridge National Laboratory
Oak Ridge, TN   37830 (U.S.A.)

SUMMARY

Current views of DNA repair and mutagenesis in the yeast
Saccharomyces cerevisiae are discussed in the light of recent data
and with emphasis on the isolation and characterization of
genetically well-defined mutations that affect DNA metabolism in
general (including replication and recombination). Various
"pathways" of repair are described, particularly in relation to
their involvement in mutagenic mechanisms. In addition to genetic
control, certain physiological factors such as "cell age," DNA
replication, and the regulatory state of the mating-type locus are
shown to also play a role in repair and mutagenesis.

INTRODUCTION

Since the realization that DNA repair and mutagenesis in
E. coli are closely related, enzymatically controlled cellular
processes [8, 59, 174, 177], there has been a great deal of interest
in determining whether repair mechanisms proposed for prokaryotes
might also apply to eukaryotic cells. The axiomatic belief held by
many that these more highly evolved cells would prove to be more
complex in every way no doubt influenced many investigators to focus
attention upon the unicellular uninucleate budding yeast
Saccharomyces cerevisiae. This organism is among the simplest of
all eukaryotes and offers several advantages over not only simpler
prokaryotic systems but also more complex eukaryotic systems. These
include: (1) ease of handling and low cost; (2) sophisticated
genetic manipulation; (3) well-defined mitotic cell cycle in stable
haploid, diploid, and polyploid strains; (4) relatively high

tolerance of certain aneuploidies; (5) conjugation and meiotic
development; (6) a nucleosome-dependent chromosomal organization;
(7) a wealth of genetic and biochemical information concerning both
nuclear-specific and mitochondrial-specific cellular processes [3,
5, 20, 51, 54, 118, 125, 151, 152, 156].

Attempts to explain the phenotypic traits of uvr, lex, rec, and
other mutants of Escherichia coli, most notable of which is enhanced
mutagen cytotoxicity, led inescapably to the hypothesis that this
increased lethality is caused by the failure to repair DNA damage,
provided that the genomes suffer the same number of initial lesions
[68, 174]. Moreover, the proposal by Witkin in 1967 [175] that
different pathways of repair could represent either an accurate
(error-proof or error-free) or an inaccurate (error-prone or
mutagenic) molecular restoration of genetic information proved to be
an important turning point in the way geneticists interpreted
experiments concerning repair effects on induced mutagenesis. Today,
error-prone repair of UV damage in bacteria is believed to have an
inducible component involving alteration or inhibition of the editing
(nucleolytic) function of a DNA polymerase [78, 178].

In spite of efforts to extend the concept of error-prone repair
to eukaryotic organisms, we still know very little about the nature
of this repair, much less how the errors are made. Thus, it should
be emphasized that without direct error frequency assays involving
defined damaged-DNA substrates and purified repair enzymes, the
error-prone repair concept represents only a descriptive albeit
useful construct, just as it did in 1967. The evidence for error-
prone repair depends upon the identification of one or more mutant
genes conferring both increased mutagen sensitivity and defective
induced mutability, compared with a wild type. Similarly, error-free
repair in wild-type strains is inferred by virtue of its apparent
absence in well-defined hypersensitive mutants that are also hypermutable (presumably because more lesions are repaired by error-prone
repair). Obviously, these concepts cannot apply when chemical
mutagens are subject to cellular metabolism unless numbers of DNA
lesions are quantitated in both mutant and wild-type cells. This is
one reason physical agents, particularly UV light and to a lesser
extent ionizing radiations, have been so useful for quantitative
studies of repair and mutagenesis.

There now exists a considerable body of information on repair
and mutagenesis in Saccharomyces cerevisiae. Although certain
aspects of this subject have been reviewed in the past [19, 56, 121,
166], the present summary attempts to broaden our current understanding not only by including more recent genetic data, but also
by emphasizing the interrelation between cellular processes that
involve DNA metabolism, namely repair, mutagenesis, recombination,
and replication; also included are developmental systems regulating
the sexual cycle which affect chromatin indirectly.

ISOLATION OF MUTANTS WITH ENHANCED MUTAGEN SENSITIVITY

In 1967 Nakai and Matsumoto [122] were the first to describe
radiosensitive mutants in yeast. They identified two separate mutant
loci, now called rad1 and rad2 [38], that caused a significant loss
of UV resistance; another, now called rad51 [37, 42], led primarily
to x-ray sensitivity with only a slight effect on UV sensitivity.
Snow [159] then reported six UV-sensitive mutants, each carrying
different mutant loci, four of which were also hypersensitive to
nitrous acid (NA), but with a different rank order. Snow hypothesized
that although repair of lesions inflicted by UV and NA would likely
occur by nonidentical enzymatic reactions, the different repair enzymes might represent components of one general repair system. Cox
and Parry [22] then deliberately attempted to "saturate" the yeast
genome with mutations conferring UV sensitivity in an effort to estimate the total number of independent genes responsible. Genetic
analysis of 96 isolates revealed 22 separate mutant loci, five of
which were also responsible for increased x-ray sensitivity. Subsequent isolations (Table 1) have revealed a large number of genetic
loci controlling mutagen sensitivity, including 22 new genes detected
in mutants selected for methyl methanesulfonate (MMS) sensitivity by
Prakash and Prakash [137]. Of these, only five conferred MMS sensitivity alone, while others caused either UV (6) or x-ray (5) sensitivity as well, and six others led to cross-sensitivity to both
radiations.

Ananthaswamy et al. [1] recently attempted to "saturate" the
yeast genome with N-methyl-N'-nitro-N-nitrosoguanidine (MNNG)-induced
mutations controlling x-ray sensitivity and found 15 new complementation groups, each complementing the existing rad set. Among such
x-ray-sensitive mutants all but four were cross-sensitive to MMS,
while none was cross-sensitive to UV. Although allelism tests to mms
strains have not been performed, it is likely that several new unique
genes are represented because the combined x-ray- and MMS-sensitivity
phenotype of these 11 is expressed by only five of 22 mms loci.

To summarize thus far, UV-sensitive mutants comprise at least
19 genetic loci (rad1,2,3,4,7,10,13,14,16,19,20,21,22 and mms3,6,
10,13,18,19); x-ray-sensitive mutants comprise 26-31 loci (rad50,
51,52,53,54,55,56,57, xs3, xrs2,4, mms8,9,14,16,20, and an estimated
10-15 others); UV- and x-ray-sensitive mutants comprise 15 loci
rad5,6,8,9,11,12,15,17,18 and mms7,11,12,15,17,21); and, finally,
mutants sensitive to MMS but not to radiations comprise five loci
(mms1,2,4,5,22). Since many but not all of the above 65-70 mutations
have been shown to recombine with one another in meiosis, it is
important to bear in mind the distinction between allelism and genetic
complementation in estimating numbers of genetic loci. On the other
hand, complementing repair-deficient mutants at the same chromosomal
locus have not been reported.

TABLE 1

YEAST MUTANTS SELECTED FOR HYPERSENSITIVITY TO MUTAGENS

Enrichment (pre-screen)	Isolation (screen)	Genetic loci[a]	Cumulative total (new loci)	Reference
UV	—	rad1	1	Nakai and Matsumoto, 1967 [122]
UV	UV	rad2, rad51	3	Snow, 1967 [159 and unpublished]
EMS	UV	rad1,...,5, 10,14	8	
EMS, UV	UV	rad1,...,17,19,...,22,50	23	Cox and Parry, 1968 [22]
NA	UV,X	rad1,2,18,52,53,xs3	27	Resnick, 1969 [142]
UV	UV	rad1	27	Moustacchi, 1969 [120]
UV	UV	rad2,rad4,uvs2	28	Zakharov et al., 1970 [179]
—	X	rad50,51,54,xrs2,xrs4	31	Suslova and Zakharov, 1970 [162]
MNNG	UV	rad2,rad9,r$_1^s$	32	Averbeck et al., 1970 [2]
—	X	rad5,9,18,50,52,...,57	35	Snow [unpublished]; Mortimer [unpublished]; Game and Mortimer, 1974 [42]
UV	MMS	rad1,4,6,52,55,57, mms1,...,22	57	Prakash and Prakash, 1977 [137]
MNNG	X	rad5,17,50,53,54, + 15 new isolates	61-72	Ananthaswamy et al., 1978 [1]

[a] Standardized rad locus assignments are based upon interlaboratory allelism tests [37, 38, 39]; rad50 and higher confer only ionizing radiation sensitivity; rad1,...,rad49 have been reserved for those that confer only UV sensitivity or sensitivity to both UV and ionizing radiation; others have not been tested for complementation or assigned to rad loci; ellipses (...) refer to consecutive locus numbers implied by the series.

Does this very large number of genes represent a reasonably
accurate estimate for all possible mutants of this type? Although
the answer to this question is not known, it does not seem likely
to be a resounding "yes" for several reasons. On statistical grounds
(based on the distribution of allelic repeats observed at 22 loci),
Cox and Parry [22] estimated an additional 8-15 undetected mutable
rad loci. With respect to the 22 new mms loci, Prakash and Prakash
[137] have calculated a maximum likelihood estimate of 48 ± 15 (S.D.)
loci responsible for MMS sensitivity. Table 1 shows that mutants at
some loci (e.g., rad1 or rad2) have been more readily detectable
than others. Doubtless, this results from many factors, including
the original strain employed (genetic background), the dose and type
of mutagen used to enrich the mutant population prior to screening,
the dose and type of mutagen used for screening hypersensitive
strains, the conditions of treatment, and the level of effect
arbitrarily chosen as a criterion for isolation. For example, the
extreme UV sensitivity or rad1 and rad2 strains, a result of defective pyrimidine dimer excision repair [131, 164, 168], is probably
a major reason such mutants have been repeatedly reisolated. Moreover, Prakash and Prakash [137] screened for the inability to grow
in the continual presence of 0.5% MMS and found three loci (mms2,10,
22) that did not confer MMS hypersensitivity when cells were exposed
to brief MMS treatments in buffer. Thus, the permeability of MMS in
such strains may be different under different conditions and in
different genetic backgrounds. Since mms10 also enhances UV sensitivity, repair processes may be involved. Since mms2 and mms22
confer only enhanced MMS sensitivity (under certain conditions),
MMS-specific repair processes may exist, or, alternatively, genetically altered MMS transport into the cell nucleus may be involved,
again underscoring the need to compare strains having the same
initial DNA damage.

ISOLATION OF MUTANTS AFFECTED IN MUTAGENESIS AND RECOMBINATION

Early recognition of the interrelation between DNA repair,
mutagenesis, recombination, and replication in bacteria [68, 176]
stimulated a number of yeast geneticists to ask whether these
processes have anything in common in eukaryotic organisms. In
particular: (1) Are mutagenesis and recombination in yeast genetically controlled? (2) If so, how many genes are involved? (3) Do
any of these genes function in repair-associated mechanisms? Table 2
shows that a number of genes have been identified in mutants
selected for various genetic end points other than enhanced mutagen
sensitivity. These include spontaneous and induced mutation as well
as spontaneous and induced mitotic recombination.

TABLE 2

YEAST MUTANTS SELECTED FOR ALTERED MUTAGENESIS OR MITOTIC RECOMBINATION

Selection phenotype	Genetic loci	Reference
Decreased UV reversion of arg4-17 (i.e. UV hypo-mutable)	rev1,rev2,rev3	Lemontt, 1971 [93]
Decreased UV forward mutation of CAN1 (UV hypo-mutable)	umr1,...,umr7	Lemontt, 1973 [96]; 1977 [100]
Decreased X-ray-induced gene conversion at arg4 (X-ray hypo-rec)	rec1,...,rec5,2D11, 2C16	Rodarte-Ramon and Mortimer, 1972 [149]
Increased spontaneous reversion of lys1-1 (mutator)	mut1,...,mut5,MUT6, mut9,mut10	von Borstel et al., 1973 [167]; Hastings et al., 1976 [55]
Increased spontaneous gene conversion at arg4 (hyper-rec)	—	Maloney and Fogel, 1976 [108]
Increased spontaneous mutation of CAN1 (mutator)	rem1	Golin and Esposito, 1977 [46]
Decreased spontaneous reversion of lys1-1 (antimutator)	—	Quah et al., 1977 [140]

UV Reversion-Defective Mutants

Using the vigorous UV-induced revertibility of the arg4-17 ochre allele to monitor induced mutability, Lemontt [93] screened clones, derived from cells surviving ethyl methanesulfonate (EMS) treatment, for defective UV reversion. Upon genetic analysis 20 such isolates were found to comprise single recessive alleles of only three genes, called rev1, rev2, and rev3; rev2 was subsequently found to be allelic with UV-sensitive mutants isolated by Snow [159] and by Cox and Parry [22] and has since been renamed rad5 [38]. Mutations at any one of these three loci cause varying degrees of enhanced sensitivity to UV, x-rays, and EMS, implicating their involvement in some form of DNA repair. This suggests that UV mutagenesis in yeast is genetically controlled by an error-prone repair process, as had already been proposed for E. coli by Witkin [177].

The rev1 and rev3 genes were shown to cause large reductions in UV mutation frequencies compared with the wild type, not only for reversion of arg4-17 (ochre), lys1-1 (ochre), and arg4-6 (putative missense) [93], but also for forward mutation at biosynthetic loci across the genome leading to auxotrophic requirements and for forward mutation at two specific ADE loci (ade1 or ade2) [150] causing red-pigmented clones [95]. Conversely rev2 had much smaller effects at arg4-17 and lys1-1 and at biosynthetic loci yet had no significant effect at all on UV reversion of arg4-6 or on forward mutation at the ADE loci [93, 95]. Moreover, the average effect of rev1 across the genome (4% of the wild-type response) was much greater than at the two selected ade genes (19% of wild type), whereas the effect of rev3 was large in both cases (4 and 2% of wild type, respectively) [95]. This was one of the first indications that UV mutagenesis might not be acting uniformly at all genetic sites, i.e., a hot-spotting effect or a specificity of interaction between certain mutagenic (error-prone repair) enzymes and particular genomic regions or particular types of DNA damage. It was also suggested that the rev2 block is highly specific, perhaps affecting only UV reversion of ochre alleles.

More recently, extensive data of Lawrence and Christensen concerning the effect of rev genes on UV reversions of well-defined cyc1 (iso-1-cytochrome c) alleles have for the most part confirmed these earlier suggestions of specificity and nonrandomness of UV mutagenesis [88, 89, 91]. In addition, they have identified several other mutant rad loci that reduce UV mutagenesis [87]: rad6, rad8, rad9, and rad18. These all cause enhanced sensitivity to both UV and x-rays, like the rev genes and like recA and lex genes of E. coli. [177]. Unlike lexA, however, which is dominant over the wild-type allele [119], rad and rev genes involved in UV mutagenesis are all recessive in their effects on survival and induced mutation, suggesting the loss of required enzymatic steps in the mutagenic mechanism.

Forward Mutation at the CAN1 Locus

Unlike reversion, recessive forward mutation usually results in
the loss of an essential cellular function and, in principle, can
derive from various mutational alterations. Many systems used to
quantitate forward mutation (e.g., auxotrophy, pigmented clones,
lethals) have limited utility mainly because they are nonselective
and therefore relatively inconvenient. Many systems measure mutation
at any one of a large number of genetic loci. Forward mutation at
CAN1, however, represents a convenient, selective drug-resistance
system that is sensitive to many physical and chemical mutagens [11,
45, 49, 83, 84, 99, 100, 141, 170].

Recessive can1 mutants become resistant to the highly toxic
arginine analogue, canavanine, by mutational alteration of CAN1 on
chromosome V, believed to be the structural gene for the arginine-
specific permease enzyme [49, 170]. Since this permease transports
virtually all exogenous arginine (and canavanine) into the cell under
normal conditions of ammonia repression when general amino-acid
permeases are inactive, all such canavanine-resistant mutants map at
this one genetic locus [47-49]. Intragenic (interallelic) complementation has not been observed even among a large number of unique
dihybrids, suggesting that arginine permease is functional as a
single polypeptide [170]. Fine-structure mapping of alleles yielding
the greatest recombination is suggestive of enough DNA to code for a
protein as large as 260,000 daltons [170]. The molecular weight of
arginine permease is not known, but it could be considerably less if
(1) the correspondence between gene and protein for this mapping
method [81, 110, 124] is unreliable for CAN1 (the largest gene presumed to exist in yeast), as appears to be the case for very small
genome intervals [115, 116], or if (2) certain portions of the gene
are non-structural and are subject to post-transcriptional or post-
translational processing critical for functional integration of the
permease into the cell membrane. Thus, mutations in noncoding but
critical sequences could also result in inactive permease; and
unlike most mutable genes used in mutation studies, which usually
affect soluble enzyme activities, CAN1 is responsible for the
activity of an important membrane protein that must be synthesized
(presumably on cytoplasmic ribosomes) and subsequently transported
and integrated into the cell envelope in some specific way.

In wild-type yeast grown to stationary phase in a yeast-extract-
peptone-dextrose (YEPD) complex broth, it is observed that many mutagens, including UV, cause vigorous induction of can1 mutants and that
these are readily expressed on selective agar containing the drug,
presumably before canavanine toxicity becomes too great [45, 99-101].
These findings are believed to be due in part to a relatively high
turnover rate of the permease such that mutational expression is
strongly influenced by the cellular level of endogenous free arginine
(dependent upon type of growth medium) rather than by the ability to

undergo residual divisions on the plate [45]. This is consistent
with the general observation that canavanine cytotoxicity is dependent upon the exogenous ratio of canavanine to arginine such that
defective canavanyl proteins are eventually synthesized. Thus, for
pregrowth in YEPD broth media the free arginine pool is presumably
high enough to prevent significant toxicity during a period when the
permease activity is decaying rapidly.

UV Forward Mutation-Defective Mutants

In an effort to identify new genes controlling UV mutagenesis
or its expression at CAN1, Lemontt screened for clones (YEPD pregrowth) with less than wild-type levels of UV mutation to canavanine
resistance [96]. Such ultraviolet mutation-resistant isolates were
subsequently characterized and found to carry one of seven nonlinked
recessive umr alleles [100]. The umr loci did not cause canavanine
resistance and were not linked to can1, nor could they be explained
by an extra (disomic) copy of chromosome V. Unlike rev or rad
mutants, four of these genes (umr4, umr5, umr6, umr7) had no significant effect on either the UV sensitivity or the UV revertibility of
three ochre mutations, his5-2, lys1-1, and ura4-1. Diploids homozygous for umr5, umr6, or umr7 all failed to sporulate, suggesting
a meiotic defect [100]. The umr7 locus, known to be allelic with
and mapping in the same region as tup1 and cyc9 on chromosome III,
has an exceedingly rich pleiotropic phenotype with effects on conjugation (α-specific poor mating ability), the cell surface (extreme
flocculence or cell clumping and "self-shmooing"), and membrane-
associated functions (dTMP uptake and unusually high levels of
iso-2-cytochrome c) [100, 104, 105, 153, 171]. The UMR4, UMR5, UMR6
and UMR7 genes may be more concerned with expression of can1
mutations rather than with mechanisms of mutagenesis directly [101].
On the other hand, umr1, umr2 and umr3 mutants were slightly more
UV-sensitive than the wild type and were affected to varying degrees
in UV revertibility of one or another of the three ochre alleles
[100]. This is consistent with the idea that one or more of these
latter three UMR genes are concerned with highly specific branches of
mutagenic pathways, those contributing very little to the overall
repair potential of the cell. Homozygotes of umr2 and umr3 failed
to sporulate. However, since all umr loci except umr1 also led to
increased canavanine toxicity, and since UV-induced can1 mutation
frequencies may be boosted if selected is delayed and preceded by a
period of cell division in growth medium [101], it is possible that
there has been a genetic alteration either in the arginine pool size
or in the rate or quality of arginine permease turnover processes.
Thus, UMR1 seems most likely to be involved in mutagenic repair
pathways; this is further supported by the finding that umr1 rad2
and umr1 rad6 double-mutant haploids are much more UV-sensitive
(synergistic) than the respective single rad strains [103]. On the

other hand, the involvement of UMR2 and UMR3 in mutagenic pathways
remains more tentative.

Hypo-rec, Hyper-rec, and Mutator Strains

In 1964 Holliday [62] proposed a molecular model for gene
conversion in fungi implicating a role for repair enzymes such as
nucleases, polymerases, and ligases. The model involves breakage
and reannealing of complementary DNA strands of homologous chromatids
to generate a "hybrid" region. If the region includes a heterozygous
mutation, this hybrid DNA will contain one or more mispaired bases
(mismatched or heteroduplex DNA), a substrate for repair. Recombination-deficient mutants of E. coli were found to be radiation
sensitive [18]. Radiation-sensitive mutants of Ustilago maydis [63]
were recombination-deficient [64]. Further, post-replication repair
of daughter-strand gaps in DNA [154] appeared to require recA+-
dependent recombination ability [158]. All these findings had the
effect of intensifying the search for genes affecting recombination
in yeast. It should be emphasized that recessive rec mutants are
not easily selected by conventional genetic means since single
mutational events in one chromosome are not expressed in heterozygous
diploids. Instead, radiation-sensitive mutants were routinely
examined (in homozygous condition) for effects on either meiotic or
mitotic recombination. Early indications were that many rad genes
had no effect in meiosis, whereas rad/rad mitotic cells generally
expressed higher levels of radiation-induced recombination than
comparable RAD/RAD or RAD/rad diploids at equal exposures, suggesting
that unrepaired radiation damage to DNA is recombinogenic [94, 160].

In a more direct approach Rodarte-Ramon and Mortimer [148, 149]
selected rec mutants directly on the basis of defective x-ray-
induced mitotic gene conversion at arg4. They constructed a strain
disomic (n + 1) and heteroallelic for arg4 on chromosome VIII,
thereby permitting expression of rec genes on any of the other haploid
chromosomes. Seven genes were identified, two of which conferred
x-ray sensitivity, one of which caused UV and x-ray sensitivity, and
four of which had no effect on radiation survival; rec2 (x-ray
sensitive) was later found to be allelic with rad52 [43]. It was
suggested that enzymatic steps required for induced recombination in
yeast might also be shared by certain repair pathways.

With a similar system Maloney and Fogel [108] screened heteroallelic arg4 disomics for enhanced spontaneous mitotic gene
conversion. Several genes have been identified and are believed to
be affected in a regulatory mechanism that normally keeps mitotic
recombination at a low level. (There exists genetic evidence for
such repression of mitotic intragenic recombination [33]). Some of
these mutants exhibit enhanced sensitivity to MMS, UV, or x-rays,
implicating a role of DNA repair in the regululation of spontaneous

mitotic recombination. This is supported by the results of Prakash and Prakash [138], who found that homozygotes of mms8, mms9, mms13, or mms21 exhibit a hyper-rec phenotype (increased spontaneous mitotic segregation from CAN1/can1 to can1/can1); rad18 also shows the hyper-rec phenotype [7].

As summarized in a review by Resnick [144], it should be emphasized that mitotic recombination of alleles within a gene is observed to be predominantly a nonreciprocal process (i.e., gene conversion) rather than a result of reciprocal crossing-over events, whereas the reverse is generally true of intergenic recombination, particularly after the frequency has been raised by exposure to external agents [123]; and, most mutagens are good recombinogens. In either case, mutational alteration of one homolog occurs much too infrequently to account for mitotic recombination in yeast and other fungi. The implications for mammalian somatic cell mutagenesis should be clear: The induction of autosomal recessive "mutants" in cell lines believed to be already heterozygous [16] may in fact be induction of mitotic crossing-over anywhere between the genetic locus and its centromere, or, to a lesser extent, gene conversion (assuming that chromosome loss, deletion, and nondisjunction can be excluded).

Probing the potential relation between DNA repair and spontaneous mutability, von Borstel and his co-workers found that the spontaneous mutation rate is increased by several rad genes - rad18, rad52, xs3 [165], and, more recently, rad3, rad6, rad51 [55]. In direct screening for such mutators [167], at least eight genetic loci have been identified [55]; one, MUT6, is dominant and without effect on UV, x-ray, or MMS sensitivity; among the other seven recessive mut loci, all but one (mut1) sensitize cells to one or more of these mutagens; mut5 has been reported to be allelic with rad51. These authors believe that spontaneous DNA lesions (including replication errors) are susceptible to repair by systems having several steps in common with systems that repair mutagen-induced DNA damage. The isolation of antimutator strains has also been reported [140]. In addition, rev3 has antimutator activity [139].

Previous work with bacteriophage T4 mutator [161] and anti-mutator [28] strains has suggested that the exonucleolytic activity associated with the polymerase has a proofreading or editing function that normally corrects (repairs) spontaneous replicative errors, presumably mismatched bases [58, 155]. The inducible component of UV-induced mutagenesis in E. coli also appears to be associated with some process that permits the replicase (DNA polymerase III) to make errors at higher than normal frequency [9]. Whether yeast and higher eukaryotic cells have the same or a similar mechanism is not known. It does seem clear, however, that spontaneous mutability is genetically controlled in a complex way that is not entirely inde-pendent of repair mechanisms.

There is evidence that spontaneous mutagenesis and mitotic recombination are under joint genetic control in yeast. Using a procedure to select dominant or recessive mutations affecting spontaneous forward mutability at CAN1, Golin and Esposito [46] have described a semidominant mutation, reml-1, that elevates the spontaneous rates of both mutagenesis and mitotic recombination. Meiotic recombination is not affected by this mutation even when homozygous, but ascopore viability is reduced, suggesting a meiotic defect in chromosomal integrity or disjunction. These authors feel that spontaneous mutation and recombination are enhanced as a result of an increase in specific DNA structures such as mismatched base pairs or single-stranded regions. A previously selected meiotic mutation, spo7-1, isolated as sporulation deficient has been shown to be responsible for both antimutator activity (mitotic) and defective pre-meiotic DNA synthesis [31]. There is now a good correlation between meiotic deficiencies and certain x-ray-sensitive rad mutants [42, 44]; sporulative ability is reduced in homozygotes of rad51 and rad55; rad50, rad52, and rad57 homozygotes do sporulate, but nearly all meiotic products are inviable, analogous to mei mutants of Drosophila [4] and rec mutants of Ustilago [66, 67]. Sporulation is completely abolished by rad6-1. Recent results by Game et al. [44] show that RAD50, RAD52, and RAD57 are not required for early and late meiotic events (namely premeiotic DNA synthesis and sporulation, respectively) but are required for successful meiotic recombination.

To summarize, there are now a large number of genes in yeast believed to control various aspects of DNA repair, mutagenesis, and recombination. Mutants selected on the basis of one altered property often turn out to be pleiotropic with respect to another phenotypic trait. To this extent certain yeast mutants appear analogous to bacterial mutants affected in some aspect of DNA metabolism. Clearly, not all of these genes may be concerned with DNA repair directly, as discussed by previous authors [22, 56, 137]. The challenge to define in molecular terms cellular functions gone awry in nearly 100 (and potentially more) mutants underscores and provides evidence for the enormous complexity of eukaryotic DNA-related metabolism. The existence of dominant and semidominant mutations that jointly affect repair, mutagenesis, and recombination in yeast raises the possibility that induction of such mutations in somatic tissues of mammals, for example, might also serve to increase (by recombination) the overall rate of homozygosis of deleterious heterozygous recessive loci. In this way, induction of hyper-rec mutants might increase the cancer risk.

"PATHWAYS" OF REPAIR

It has been possible to characterize presumed repair-deficient mutations by their interactions in multiply-mutant haploid strains,

as developed by Game and Cox [39, 40] and by Haynes [56]. Howard-
Flanders et al. [69] were among the first to demonstrate the utility
of this approach for understanding DNA repair mechanisms by con-
structing a double mutant of E. coli carrying both uvrA and recA
and showing that the two mutations interacted synergistically with
regard to UV sensitivity. That is, UV survival of this double
mutant was very much less than what would have been expected on the
basis of an additive effect of the two single mutants; further,
the UV dose yielding an average of one lethal event (37% survival)
corresponded to approximately one pyrimidine dimer per cell. This
result suggested two important hypotheses: (1) that uvrA and recA
each block very different repair pathways acting on UV-damaged DNA;
(2) that these two major pathways could account for virtually all
of the UV resistance exhibited by the wild type. This agreed with
the finding that uvrA mutants lacked excision repair but recA
mutants did not [68]. Two or more mutations blocking DNA repair
along the same linear pathway are expected to interact epistatically
such that the multiple mutant is no more sensitive to the mutagen
than the most sensitive single mutant.

    Despite some inherent limitations of multiple mutant analysis,
as discussed in detail elsewhere [39, 40, 87], it has been possible
to gain a certain amount of information concerning mechanism of
repair in yeast from this kind of approach in conjunction with other
phenotypic traits expressed by repair-deficient mutants. On this
basis, there exist three so-called "epistasis groups" of rad loci
such that a strain carrying multiple mutations within a group
exhibits epistasis whereas a strain with mutations in different
groups exhibits either an additive or synergistic interaction. The
epistasis groups are suggestive of metabolic pathways [21].

                        Excision Repair of UV Damage

    The epistasis group defined by rad1, rad2, rad3, rad4, rad10,
and rad16 consists of mutants with a biochemical defect in excision
repair of UV-induced pyrimidine dimers [39, 131, 134, 135, 146, 147,
164, 168]; furthermore, rad22 is epistatic to rad1 with respect to
UV survival [87]. Thus, at least seven genes appear to be required
for excision repair in yeast. Excision repair acts only on nuclear
DNA and is not able to remove pyrimidine dimers from mitochondrial
DNA [131, 169]. In general, mutations in this pathway do not lead
to x-ray sensitivity, nor do they have any effect on recombination,
meiosis, or sporulation. Additionally, like uvr mutants of E. coli
[177], most if not all of these mutants exhibit enhanced frequencies
of UV mutagenesis compared with the wild type at equal UV doses, and
a significant fraction of the induced mutability is photoreversible
in both mutant and wild-type strains [2, 87, 92, 143, 179]. At
equal survival levels induced mutabilities are approximately the

same in RAD and rad2 strains [30]. Moreover, with respect to the
observed spectrum of base-pair changes inferred from amino-acid
replacements in iso-1-cytochrome c among UV revertants of ochre cyc1
alleles [9], and rad1 response is the same as that produced by the
wild type. All these findings have suggested that UV mutations are
produced predominantly from unexcised pyrimidine dimers in DNA by
a mutagenic process different from the excision repair pathway which
is considered to be essentially error-free.

Error-Prone Repair of UV Damage

The epistasis group defined by rad6, rad8, rad9, rad18, rev1,
rev2 (i.e. rad5), and rev3 consists of mutants with varying degrees
of both UV and x-ray sensitivity [21, 22, 40, 87, 93]. None except
rad9 significantly reduces mitotic recombination [82];   rad6
prevents sporulation [22];   and the others do not apparently affect
meiosis. The rad18 gene is synergistic with rad1, rad2, or rad3
but epistatic with rad6 [40]. All seven mutants of this group are
epistatic with rad6, suggesting that all are involved in one major
pathway concerned with repair of UV damage [87]. Mutants carrying
rad6 or rad9 are proficient in carrying out pyrimidine dimer
excision [135];   the others are also excision-proficient [19].

The most interesting property of mutants in this group is
defective UV mutagenesis, suggesting, by analogy to recA and lexA
mutants of E. coli [87, 96], that this single repair pathway is
error-prone for UV damage. From this point on, the analogy to
prokaryotic mechanisms of mutagenesis begins to break down.
Lawrence and Christensen [88, 90] have pointed out how many of the
observations in yeast are at best difficult to explain with the
one-step unitary model proposed for E. coli [12, 178], according to
which suppression of the editing function of DNA polymerase permits
replication past a pyrimidine dimer while two random, often
incorrect bases are inserted opposite the lesion. Thus, recA and
lexA mutations should prevent induction of mutations of all types
and at all genetic sites, and mutations induced in the wild type
should involve double base-pair changes [88, 90].

Lawrence et al. [92] have demonstrated that rad6 and rad18
affect UV mutagenesis not only quantitatively but also qualitatively
by altering the spectrum of base changes observed among induced
revertants of cyc1 nonsense alleles. Not all mutants defining
error-prone repair in yeast block UV-induced mutational changes of
all types and at all genetic sites;   and, double base-pair changes
are rare in yeast [90]. While rev3 and rad6 are non-specific and
prevent normal levels of UV mutagenesis at every genetic site tested,
the remaining mutants of this pathway have strong allele-specific
effects with respect to UV reversion (for examples see Table 3).

TABLE 3

ALLELE-SPECIFIC CONTROL OF UV MUTAGENESIS BY REV GENES[a]

Type	Allele	Codon		Position	UV Revertibility			
		Mutant	Normal		REV	rev1	rev2	rev3
Ochre	cyc1-9	UAA	GAA	2	+	−	−	−
	−2	UAA	CAA	21	+	−	+	
	−72	UAA	GAA	66	+	−	+	
Amber	cyc1-179	UAG	AAG	9	+	−	+	−
	−84	UAG	UGG	64	+	−	+	
	−76	UAG	GAG	71	+	−	+	
Initiation	cyc1-131	GUG	AUG	−1	+	+	+	(−)
	−133	AGG	AUG	−1	+	−	+	−
	−13	AUPy	AUG	−1	+	−		−
	−51	CUG	AUG	−1	+	−		−
Frameshift	cyc1-183	+A	AAA	10	+	+		−
	−239	−G	AAG	4	+	+	+	−
	−331	−A	GAA	2	+	+	+	−
Proline missense	cyc1-115	CCPy	CUPy	14	+	+	+	(−)
	−6	CCU	GCU	12	+	−		−

[a]Data from Lawrence and Christensen [87-89, 91].

The REV2 gene product appears to be concerned only with UV reversion of ochre alleles, yet, this clearly is not the case for all such alleles. Although the REV1 product may not be required for frameshift mutagenesis by UV, it is required for many but not all base-pair transitions and transversions. By inspection of the nearly complete base sequence information in the region of many cyc1 alleles and of their revertants, it has been possible to test the idea that the allele specificity of UV reversion (as typified by rev1) may be based upon one or more of the following factors;   (1) position within the gene, (2) kind of DNA triplet altered, (3) type of base-pair change (e.g. transition vs transversion, or AT to GC vs GC to AT), (4) variable recovery of reversions (5) non-random formation of dimers in regions rich in adjacent pyrimidines, (6) unusual kinds of premutational lesions, or (7) different ratios of mutagenic to non-mutagenic repair at different genetic sites. Lawrence and Christensen have concluded that none of these factors alone can satisfactorily account for the nonrandomness of UV reversion [88, 90]. Even in a wild-type strain the same ochre triplet occurring at different sites reverts with entirely different patterns of base-pair change, suggestive of some form of site (or sequence) specificity [157]. Moreover, UV reversion of the cyc1-131 allele by GC to AT transition, which does not require REV1 but which is nonetheless photoreversible, occurs within an alternating purine-pyrimidine nucleotide sequence, obviously a region where intrastrand pyrimidine dimers cannot be induced [88, 90]. Thus, we also need to understand how DNA damage at one site results in mutation at another.

Thus far, the best explanation for site-specific mutagenesis is a presumed nonrandom interaction between certain gene products (of error-prone repair) and DNA damage in particular genomic regions [90]. It is not known whether this surprising level of complexity is unique to yeast or to eukaryotes in general. Bacterial studies in the past have for the most part not been concerned with this question of specificity. Not until very recently have mutation-resistant ("rev-like") mutants of E. coli been selected directly [74]. If such apparent site-specific regulation of mutagenesis is found to be unique to eukaryotes, the molecular environment of the chromatin is likely to play a role.

Minor Repair Pathway for UV Damage

A third "minor pathway" for repair of UV damage appears to involve enzymatic steps whose major ostensible function is to repair ionizing radiation-damaged DNA. The rad50 and rad51 genes each confer slight UV sensitivity and are epistatic to one another, yet rad51 interacts synergistically with both rad3 and rad18 with respect to UV survival. One lethal event (37% survival) in rad3 rad18 double mutants corresponds to approximately six pyrimidine dimers per cell, whereas in rad3 rad18 rad51 triple mutants only one or two are needed to produce the same effect. This suggests that unrepaired dimers are lethal and that virtually all of the UV resistance expressed by the wild type can be accounted for by the action of these three pathways [21, 40]. The rad52 locus also acts in this minor pathway, but has little or no effect on UV reversion. In excision-defective strains, however, a rad52 rad1 strain is nearly 10-fold more UV hypermutable than a rad1 strain, suggesting that this minor pathway is essentially error-free for repair of UV damage [87].

Repair of Ionizing Radiation Damage

The major pathway for repair of ionizing radiation damage is controlled by RAD50, RAD51,..., RAD57; rad52 contributes the greatest gamma-ray hypersensitivity, which is also exhibited by all double mutants with rad52 [113]. Frequencies of gamma-ray reversion in mutants of this group are similar to that expressed by the wild type, suggesting an error-free mode of repair [112]. Since rad52 strains are defective in gamma-ray-induced mitotic gene conversion [148, 149] and are also unable to repair double-strand DNA breaks [60, 145], this RAD52 pathway may involve recombinational repair; rad52 strains also have increased x-ray-induced dominant lethality, suggestive of a defect in the repair of chromosome breaks [61].

With respect to ionizing radiation survival and mutagenesis, McKee and Lawrence [112, 113] have found that the single mutagenic repair system for UV is also responsible for mutagenic repair of ionizing radiation damage and requires the functions of the RAD6, RAD8, REV1, REV2, and REV3 genes. Although both radiations produce very different kinds of pre-mutational DNA damage, gamma-ray mutagenesis is efficiently blocked by mutations of these loci, all of which comprise a "rad6 epistasis group" for gamma-ray survival; rad9 and rad18 also belongs to this group but do not block gamma-ray mutagenesis significantly, suggesting that this RAD6 pathway consists of both error-free and error-prone repair processes. In addition, McKee and Lawrence [114] have observed in rev strains allele-specific gamma-ray reversion patterns that are very similar to those expressed after UV exposure. These authors have argued that the simple idea of an enzymatic pathway for mutagenic repair consisting of sequential gene-controlled steps, with separate branch points leading to mutational specificity, does not adequately explain the distinctive yet partially overlapping mutational phenotypes expressed by mutants of this "pathway."

Mutagenesis by several chemical agents also requires a functional repair system, specifically the RAD6 and RAD9 gene products [130, 132, 133]. McKee and Lawrence [114] argue that mutations of different kinds or at different sites that arise from potentially very different premutational lesions are produced by the coordinate action of a large number of partially independent sets of gene functions.

PHYSIOLOGICAL FACTORS AFFECTING REPAIR AND MUTAGENESIS

Early studies on the recovery of yeast from radiation and chemical damage showed that the degree of liquid-holding recovery, an indicator of repair activity, could be modified by different physiological conditions [128, 1]9]. More recent studies [127] not only have emphasized the importance of genetically controlled repair processes but also have expanded our view of the diversity of cellular factors that can affect repair. These include "cell age," DNA replication, and the mating-type-dependent regulatory system.

Cell Age

The term, cell age, as developed by Parry and co-workers [126], encompasses two different phenomena: either the position in the mitotic cell cycle of synchronous cultures or the transition of exponentially growing (log-phase) asynchronous cultures to a nutrient-limited stationary phase. The increased radiation resistance of the budding cell fraction of yeast cultures observed in early studies [6] is now understood to be a reflection of the hypersensitive G_1 and early S (DNA replication) stages, compared with the more resistant late S and G_2 periods [15, 26, 27]. In general, this pattern is similar to that first observed in mammalian cells [163]. The variations in UV resistance could be due to different amounts of initial DNA damage induced at different times in the cell cycle or to varying efficiencies of repair mechanisms throughout the cycle. Although S-phase cells suffer 30% fewer pyrimidine dimers per unit UV dose than do cells having minimal resistance [14], this factor is not likely to be responsible for the bulk of the observed variations in UV sensitivity [25]. An excision repair-deficient (radl) strain exhibits cyclic variations in UV sensitivity very similar to those found in wild type, suggesting that excision repair acts efficiently and uniformly throughout the cell cycle [13]. In contrast a rec5 strain, defective in UV-induced mitotic recombination, exhibits the same UV sensitivity in G_1 and G_2, a level comparable to the wild-type G_1 level. This suggests that the increased G_2 (over G_1) UV resistance expressed by the wild type is due to a recombinational repair process that requires the REC5 gene product [13].

Davies et al. [25] used a zonal rotor centrifugation method to isolate large yeast populations on the basis of bud size (correlated with progress in the cell cycle), an obvious improvement over the

use of perturbing treatments that induce cell synchronony. Their
results confirm earlier observations that, in the wild type, UV
resistance is minimal in G_1 and maximum in S and G_2; yields of UV-
induced mitotic recombination (intergenic and intragenic) were
maximum in G_1 and minimum in S and G_2, again suggesting a relationship between cell survival and recombination. Fabre [32] has shown
that UV-induced intragenic mitotic recombination can occur in G_1
before chromosome replication, confirming earlier results [172] and
suggesting that homologous chromosomal pairing does not require
duplicated chromatids. In contrast to UV survival, nitrous acid
survival exhibited a minimum during only one period, that of DNA
replication, while induced mitotic recombination occurred at all
stages but was maximum during S [25].

    Radiation and chemical mutagen sensitivity have also been
compared in log-phase vs. stationary-phase cultures [126]. As
asynchronous log-phase cultures enter a transition period before
entering stationary phase, cells tend to complete their cycles and
begin arresting as unbudded cells (in G_1 or more properly G_0) [54].
Stationary-phase cells are observed to be more sensitive to UV and
x-rays than log-phase cells, whereas just the reverse is true of
sensitivity to several chemical mutagens. During the transition
period, UV resistance begins to decrease in cultures that have
already begun to show a significant reduction in the frequency of
budded cells. While excision repair-defective (rad1 or rad2) strains
also become more UV sensitive, a rad50 strain failed to exhibit this
effect, suggesting a requirement for the RAD50 gene product. In
contrast to UV survival, cell survival following treatment with NA,
mitomycin C, and EMS increases in cultures beginning to show loss
of budded cells. A significant fraction of this differential
chemical mutagen sensitivity appears to be due to different numbers
of initial DNA lesions inflicted, since cellular uptake of tritium-
labeled EMS is seven-fold less in stationary cells compared with
log-phase cells [126].

                         DNA Replication

    Until recently very little information has been available on
the role of DNA replication in repair and mutagenesis of yeast.
The main reason for this has been that only a few temperature-
sensitive mutants have been described [52, 53, 72] that have large
effects in turning off DNA synthesis specifically and rapidly after
temperature shift. Some mutants also affect RNA synthesis; the
gene products of many well-defined mutations are not known. It has
been suggested that a "replication complex" with one defective
protein component might undergo slight conformational changes and
still have some polymerizing activity [72]. Another reason concerns
the fact that most in vivo studies eventually depend upon the

conventional end point of colony (or mutant colony) formation, which in turn is dependent upon genome replication and cell division.

Yeast strains carrying cdc8 are defective in DNA replication (elongation, not initiation) at 36°C but not at 23°C [52]. Prakash et al. [136] have reported recently that cdc8 reduces frequencies of UV reversion (at 25°C), even in rad1 or rad51 strains; they argue that CDC8 plays a role in error-prone repair.

There now exists evidence that the temperature-sensitive cdc9-1 mutant [24] is defective in DNA ligase activity [73]. At the restrictive temperature this mutant (1) accumulates many single-strand breaks in DNA, (2) exhibits enhanced UV sensitivity, and (3) produces enhanced frequencies of spontaneous mitotic recombination (hyper-rec phenotype) [41]. These recent findings underscore the multiple role of this enzyme in DNA replication, repair, and recombination in yeast. It is suggested [41] that the excess single-strand gaps in DNA are themselves recombinogenic, either directly or by means of the induction of a recombination-repair system.

An important question concerns the kinetics of induced mutagenesis: Does it occur before, during, or after DNA replication? One approach might involve the use of a probe that can monitor the appearance of mutant (or recombinant) gene product as soon as it becomes expressed, rather than the phenotypic scoring of mutant (or recombinant) clones many generations removed from the initial mutagenic (or recombinogenic) event. Such a system has been previously used in Ustilago maydis to allow in vivo enzymatic measurement of radiation-induced mutation [97, 98] or mitotic recombination [65]. Another approach involves unambiguous detection of the "strandedness" of induced mutations. That is, fixation of premutational damage in one strand of unreplicated (G_1-phase) DNA is expected to give rise to a mosaic colony because after completion of the first cell cycle there will be one mutant and one nonmutant cell. Damage fixed as mutation in both strands prior to replication should lead to a pure mutant clone. Premutational damage not fixed as mutation until after the first round of replication will also produce mosaic clones.

James and Kilbey [70] observed UV induction of recessive lethal mutations in mitotic pedigrees of irradiated G_1 diploid yeast cells. With this technique they found that after low exposures to UV, induced mutations were produced in an excision repair-proficient strain prior to the first round of post-irradiation DNA replication, and most mutations were two-stranded. In an excision repair-defective (rad1) strain, induced mutations affecting both strands were not observed; moreover, mosaics arose as frequently in the second post-UV generation as in the first [71]. In rad1 strains unexcised pyrimidine dimers were shown to be responsible for UV mutagenesis even after passing through several DNA replication cycles [76], as Bridges and Munson had shown many years ago for

E. coli [10]. Hannan et al. [50] had previously shown that G_1 RAD
haploid cells produced exclusively pure mutant clones after a UV
exposure leading to high survival (63%, on the survival curve
"shoulder"). Mosaics, however, were produced with increasing
frequency for UV doses corresponding to exponentially decreasing
survival, and they could not be explained by first-division lethal
sectoring. These findings support the idea that pure mutant clones
are associated with efficient heteroduplex repair activity such that
loss of efficiency at higher UV doses leads to the induction of
mosaics.

    Kilbey et al. [75] have proposed a dimer/gap model to account
for the different kinetics of UV mutagenesis in RAD and rad1 strains.
According to the model, mutation fixation by error-prone repair is
presumed to be initiated in both strains by a structure consisting
of a single-stranded gap opposite a pyrimidine dimer, although this
structure is produced in different ways by the two strains. In RAD
strains after UV exposure sufficient to induce dimers close together
on opposite complementary strands, the excision of one may often
leave a gap that exposes the other. Since prereplicative mutagenesis (presumably an error-prone gap-filling process) eventually
affects both DNA strands [70], excision repair must remove the dimer
or heteroduplex repair must recognize and repair the mismatched site.
In rad1 strains excision cannot occur, and replication presumably
generates daughter-strand gaps opposite pyrimidine dimers, followed
by gap-filling and heteroduplex repair. This model is consistent
with the observation that UV mutagenesis in RAD strains exhibits
dose-squared dependence (two dimers required) [75, 89, 100]
compared with a linear dependence at low doses in rad1 [75] or rad2
[29] strains. Yet, there exists at least one case of linear
induction in RAD strains [30]. It is not altogether clear just how
gap filling generates single base-pair changes, which are responsible
for the majority of UV mutations in yeast [90] rather than double
base substitutions, as presumed in the bacterial model [12, 178].
An error-prone gap-filling model must also accommodate in some way
the observations of nonrandom action (site specificity of repair)
and "mutation at a distance" [90].

    Recent studies by Lemontt [99] have suggested that exposure of
YEPD-grown stationary-phase yeast to hydrazine (HZ), a carcinogen and
mutagen in other organisms [77], results in premutational DNA damage
that becomes fixed as mutation at the time of DNA replication, as
appears to be the case in Haemophilus [79, 80]. Unlike several other
mutagens, HZ mutability at CAN1 is entirely dependent upon post-
treatment DNA replication and occurs over a dose range that leaves
cell viability unaffected. HZ exposure does not extend the 3- to
4-hr growth lag normally observed in post-treatment medium.
Prokaryotic studies have suggested that N^4-aminocytosine may
represent an important premutational DNA lesion to HZ-exposed cells
[77]. Thus, unlike nonpairable pyrimidine dimers, this cytosine

analog might be considered a pairable lesion (with perhaps less than complete fidelity) produced in situ. N^4-Aminocytosine is known to be mutagenic in lambda phage and in E. coli when used as a precursor for DNA replication [17]. Thus, HZ may induce mutations in yeast by a mechanism of base mispairing at replication in the absence of any ostensible inhibitory effect on the replicative process itself, as proposed for Haemophilus. Kimball has suggested that N^4-aminocytosine may be an intrinsically more efficient base-analog mutagen than 5-bromouracil because the hydrazino ($-NH_2NH_2$) substitution for the 4-amino group occurs at a base-pairing position on the pyrimidine ring, while the bromine substitution does not [78].

It has also been possible to obtain indirect evidence for prereplicative error-free repair of HZ-induced premutational damage [102]. As observed in Haemophilus [80], if post-treatment DNA replication or its initiation is delayed in growth medium (in yeast with hydroxyurea or cycloheximide, respectively), the maximum level of replication-dependent mutagenesis attainable after removal of inhibitors decreases (Table 4). Excision repair-defective rad2-1 strains also exhibit such loss of HZ mutability. These findings have suggested that premutational lesions are being removed by some error-free process different from excision repair of pyrimidine dimers. Since cycloheximide blocks protein synthesis (which is required for initiation of DNA replication in yeast [57, 173]), this repair process must be constitutive. It is possible to speculate that some form of mismatch repair may be operating. If it is assumed that N^4-aminocytosine is a major premutational lesion, the duplex distortion (presumed to occur by virtue of a hydrazino rather than an amino proton donor in hydrogen bonding to guanine) might also be correctable by specific cleavage of the terminal amino group, restoring normal base pairing without the need for strand breaks in the backbone. Examining HZ-treated Haemophilus, Kimball and Hirsch [80] failed to detect single-strand breaks (or alkali-labile sites) in unreplicated DNA, nor did they observe gaps in newly synthesized DNA.

Mating-Type Locus-Dependent Regulation

Normal conjugation in yeast occurs between cells of opposite mating type, either a or α. These two mating phenotypes segregate in meiosis as different alleles of the same locus, called the mating-type locus (MAT). There are now many lines of evidence supporting the idea that the genetic information at MAT has a regulatory function that plays a central role in controlling whether a cell may undergo sexual conjugation or pursue meiotic development. Diploids exhibit one of three possible functional states at MAT: a/a, α/α, or a/α. Like a or α haploids, homozygous a/a or α/α diploids (selected by mitotic crossing-over) are able to mate normally (and produce and respond to mating pheromones), exhibit

TABLE 4

PREREPLICATIVE REPAIR OF HZ-INDUCED PREMUTATIONAL DAMAGE[a]

Post-treatment medium[b] (time at 30°C)	Mutation frequency ($\underline{can1}/10^7$ viable cells)	
	Control[c]	HZ[c]
None	13.2	15.2
Y (3 hr)	24.0	32.0
YCH (3 hr)	9.5	14.5
Y (1 day)	9.6	159
YCH (1 day)	12.5	24.7
Y (3 hr) + Y (1 day)	12.1	160
YCH (3 hr) + Y (1 day)	15.5	88.0
Y (1 day) + Y (1 day)	12.8	174
YCH (1 day) + Y (1 day)	14.0	22.3

[a]Data from Lemontt [102].

[b]Y (YEPD) or YCH (YEPD + 1 μg/ml cycloheximide).

[c]Control or HZ treatment in neutral buffer; 0.2 M, 1 hr.

medial bud initiation in mitosis, but cannot initiate meiosis and
sporulation when challenged to do so in the appropriate medium.
Such homozygotes exhibit a-specific or α-specific functions expressed
by haploids. Diploids heterozygous (a/α) at MAT are repressed in
mating ability (and fail to produce or respond to mating pheromones),
exhibit polar bud initiation, and have gained meiotic and sporulative
capacity. The a/α state appears not only to turn off certain haploid
functions, but also to turn on certain new diploid functions.
Moreover, the expression of these a-specific, α-specific, and a/α-
specific functions may be altered by various mutations in several
genes unlinked to MAT (mating-type-specific functions have been
reviewed recently [23, 107, 109]). Thus, in mitotic cells the
existence of phenotypic differences expressed by MAT homozygotes
compared with the "normal" (after normal a × α mating) MAT heterozygotes constitutes evidence for MAT regulation.

DNA repair, mitotic recombination, and mutagenesis all appear to be modulated to some degree by MAT. Although diploids are much more x-ray-resistant than haploids (the ploidy effect [117]), MAT homozygotes are more sensitive than a/α cells [85, 117], suggesting that a fraction of the extra diploid resistance is due to MAT heterozygosity. Liquid-holding recovery in buffer after x-ray exposure (which does not occur in haploids) is believed to be controlled in part by a MAT-dependent process (Hunnable and Cox, cited by Crandall et al. [23]). Moreover, Game and Mortimer [43] have found that some mutants (rad50, rad57) in the RAD52 pathway for repair of ionizing radiation damage exhibit a MAT effect (a/α more resistant than a/a or α/α), while others (rad52, rad54) do not. Thus, RAD52 and RAD54 may act prior to MAT dependent repair steps, whereas RAD50 and RAD57 may control subsequent MAT-independent steps [43]. A MAT effect for MMS sensitivity has also been reported [106].

Although UV survival does not show the MAT effect [86], UV-induced mitotic recombination does [36]. Frequencies of induced mitotic gene conversion in a/a or α/α diploids were as much as 100-fold lower than in a/α strains, again suggesting that the a/α regulatory state is required for maximal expression of induced mitotic recombination.

There is evidence that MAT regulation can affect UV mutagenesis. Martin et al. [111] have found that although mms3 causes UV sensitivity in haploids and diploids, a/α mms3/mms3 diploids exhibit defective UV reversion of arg4-17 or lys2-1, compared with a/α mms3/MMS and a/α MMS/MMS diploids; mms3 haploids have wild-type UV revertibility. In addition, a/a or α/α derivatives of the a/α mms3/mms3 strain were resotred to normal UV mutability. This shows that the a/α genetic configuration is responsible for the diploid-specific defective UV mutability.

Finally, α umr7-1 haploids fail to express several α-specific haploid functions (such as mating ability, α-factor production, a-factor response), while at the same time they have apparently turned on some a-specific functions ("shmoo" morphology, a-factor proteolysis [34, 35]); on the other hand, a umr7 haploids express normal a-specific functions [104, 105]. Both types of umr7 strains are enormously flocculent (clumpy) but can be dispersed by distilled-water washing [100]. Although these strains are defective in UV mutagenesis at CAN1 [100], it seems likely that this is due to an aberrant cell envelope which interferes in some way with normal expression of mutant arginine permease. This is supported by the observation that non-clumpy revertant derivatives exhibit wild-type levels of UV mutability at CAN1 [104].

ACKNOWLEDGEMENT

This research was sponsored by the Office of Health and
Environmental Research, U. S. Department of Energy, under contract
W-7405-eng-26 with the Union Carbide Corporation.

REFERENCES

1. Ananthaswamy, H. N., T. J. McKey, and R. K. Mortimer, Isolation
    and characterization of additional x-ray sensitive mutants
    of Saccharomyces cerevisiae (abs.), Ninth International
    Conference on Yeast Genetics and Molecular Biology,
    Rochester, N.Y., 1978, p. 45.
2. Averbeck, D., W. Laskowski, E. Eckardt, and E. Lehmann-Brauns,
    Four radiation sensitive mutants of Saccharomyces.
    Survival after UV- and x-ray-irradiation as well as UV-
    induced reversion rates from isoleucine-valine dependence
    to independence, Mol. Gen. Genet., 107 (1970) 117-127.
3. Bacila, M., B. L. Horecker, and A. O. M. Stoppani (Eds.),
    Biochemistry and Genetics of Yeast, Academic Press, New
    York, 1978.
4. Baker, B., A. T. C. Carpenter, M. S. Esposito, R. E. Esposito
    and L. Sandler, The genetic control of meiosis, Ann. Rev.
    Genet., 10 (1976) 53-134.
5. Bandlow, W., R. J. Schweyen, K. Wolf, and F. Kaudewitz (Eds.),
    Mitochondria 1977. Genetics and Biogenesis of Mitochondria,
    Walter de Gruyter, New York, 1977.
6. Beam, C. A., R. K. Mortimer, R. G. Wolfe, and C. A. Tobias,
    The relation of radioresistance to budding in Saccharomyces
    cerevisiae, Arch. Biochem. Biophys., 49 (1954) 110-122.
7. Boram, W. R., and H. Roman, Recombination in Saccharomyces
    cerevisiae: A DNA repair mutation associated with elevated
    mitotic gene conversion, Proc. Natl. Acad. Sci. (U.S.), 73
    (1976) 2828-2832.
8. Bridges, B. A., Mechanisms of radiation mutagenesis in cellular
    and subcellular systems, Ann. Rev. Nucl. Sci., 19 (1969)
    139-178.
9. Bridges, B. A., R. P. Mottershead, and S. G. Sedgwick, Mutagenic
    DNA repair in Escherichia coli. III. Requirement for a
    function of DNA polymerase III in ultraviolet-light muta-
    genesis, Mol. Gen. Genet., 144 (1976) 53-58.
10. Bridges, B. A., and R. J. Munson, The persistence through
    several replication cycles of mutation-producing pyrimidine
    dimers in a strain of Escherichia coli deficient in
    excision-repair, Biochem. Biophys. Res. Commun., 30 (1968)
    620-624.
11. Brusick, D. J., Induction of cycloheximide-resistant mutants in
    Saccharomyces cerevisiae with N-methyl-N'-nitro-N-nitroso-
    guanidine and ICR-170, J. Bacteriol., 109 (1972) 1134-1138.

12. Caillet-Fauquet, P., M. Defais, and M. Radman, Molecular
     mechanisms of induced mutagenesis. Replication in vivo of
     bacteriophage φX174 single-stranded, ultraviolet light-
     irradiated DNA in intact and irradiated host cells, J.
     Mol. Biol., 117 (1977) 95-112.
13. Chanet, R., M. Heude, and E. Moustacchi, Variations in UV-
     induced lethality and "petite" mutagenesis in synchronous
     culture of Saccharomyces cerevisiae. II. Responses of
     radiosensitive mutants to lethal damage, Mol. Gen. Genet.,
     132 (1974) 23-30.
14. Chanet, R., R. Waters, and E. Moustacchi, The induction of
     pyrimidine dimers in nuclear DNA after UV-irradiation during
     the synchronous cycle of Saccharomyces cerevisiae, Int. J.
     Radiat. Biol., 27 (1975) 481-485.
15. Chanet, R., D. H. Williamson, and E. Moustacchi, Cyclic
     variations in killing and "petite" mutagenesis induced by
     ultraviolet light in synchronized yeast strains, Biochim.
     Biophys. Acta, 324 (1973) 290-299.
16. Chasin, L. A., Mutation affecting adenine phosphoribosyl
     transferase activity in Chinese hamster cells, Cell, 2
     (1974) 37-41.
17. Chu, B. C. F., D. M. Brown, and M. G. Burdon, Effect of
     nitrogen and of catalase on hydroxylamine and hydrazine
     mutagenesis, Mutat. Res., 20 (1973) 265-270.
18. Clark, A. J., and A. D. Margulies, Isolation and characteri-
     zation of recombination-deficient mutants of Escherichia
     coli K12, Proc. Natl. Acad. Sci. (U.S.), 53 (1965) 451-459.
19. Cox, B. S., Pathways of UV repair and mutagenesis in
     Saccharomyces cerevisiae, In: Research in Photobiology,
     A. Castellani (Ed.), Plenum Press, New York, 1976, pp.
     689-697.
20. Cox, B. S., and E. A. Bevan, Aneuploidy in yeast, New Phytol.,
     61 (1962) 342-355.
21. Cox, B. S., and J. Game, Repair systems in Saccharomyces,
     Mutat. Res., 26 (1974) 257-264.
22. Cox, B. S., and J. M. Parry, The isolation, genetics and
     survival characteristics of ultraviolet light-sensitive
     mutants in yeast, Mutat. Res., 6 (1968) 37-55.
23. Crandall, M., R. Egel, and V. L. MacKay, Physiology of mating
     in three yeasts, Adv. Microb. Physiol., 15 (1977)
     307-398.
24. Culotti, J., and L. H. Hartwell, Genetic control of the cell
     division cycle. III. Seven genes controlling nuclear
     division, Exp. Cell Res., 67 (1971) 389-401.
25. Davies, P. J., R. S. Tippins and J. M. Parry, Cell-cycle
     variations in the induction of lethality and mitotic
     recombination after treatment with UV and nitrous acid in
     the yeast, Saccharomyces cerevisiae, Mutat. Res., 51
     (1978) 327-346.

26. de Langguth, E. N., and C. A. Beam, Repair mechanisms and cell
        cycle dependent variations in x-ray sensitivity of diploid
        yeast, Radiat. Res., 53 (1973) 226–234.
27. de Langguth, E. N., and C. A. Beam, The effects of ploidy upon
        cell cycle dependent changes in x-ray sensitivity of
        Saccharomyces cerevisiae, Radiat. Res., 55 (1973) 501–506.
28. Drake, J. W., and E. F. Allen, Antimutagenic DNA polymerases
        of bacteriophage T4, Cold Spring Harbor Symp. Quant. Biol.,
        33 (1968) 339–341.
29. Eckardt, F., and R. H. Haynes, Kinetics of mutation induction
        by ultraviolet light in excision-deficient yeast, Genetics,
        85 (1977) 225–247.
30. Eckardt, F., and R. H. Haynes, Induction of pure and sectored
        mutant clones in excision-proficient and deficient strains
        of yeast, Mutat. Res., 43 (1977) 327–338.
31. Esposito, M. S., M. Bolotin-Fukuhara, and R. E. Esposito,
        Antimutator activity during mitosis by a meiotic mutant
        of yeast, Mol. Gen. Genet., 139 (1975) 9–18.
32. Fabre, F., Induced intragenic recombination in yeast can occur
        during the G_1 mitotic phase, Nature, 272 (1978) 795–798.
33. Fabre, F., and H. Roman, Genetic evidence for inducibility of
        recombination competence in yeast, Proc. Natl. Acad. Sci.
        (U.S.), 74 (1977) 1667–1671.
34. Finkelstein, D., personal communication.
35. Finkelstein, D. B., and S. Strausberg, Metabolism of α-factor
        by a mating type cells of Saccharomyces cerevisiae, J.
        Biol. Chem., 254 (1979) 796–803.
36. Friis, J., and H. Roman, The effect of the mating-type alleles
        on intragenic recombination in yeast, Genetics, 59 (1968)
        33–36.
37. Game, J. C., Radiation-sensitive mutants of yeast, In:
        Molecular Mechanisms for Repair of DNA, P. C. Hanawalt
        and R. B. Setlow (Eds.), Plenum Press, New York, 1975,
        pp. 541–544.
38. Game, J. C., and B. S. Cox, Allelism tests of mutants affecting
        sensitivity to radiation in yeast and a proposed nomen-
        clature, Mutat. Res., 12 (1971) 328–331.
39. Game, J. C., and B. S. Cox, Epistatic interactions between
        four rad loci in yeast, Mutat. Res., 16 (1972) 353–362.
40. Game, J. C., and B. S. Cox, Synergistic interactions between
        RAD mutations in yeast, Mutat. Res., 20 (1973) 35–44.
41. Game, J. C., L. H. Johnston, and R. C. von Borstel, Enhanced
        mitotic recombination in a ligase-defective mutant of the
        yeast Saccharomyces cerevisiae, Proc. Natl. Acad. Sci.
        (U.S.), 76 (1979) 4589–4592.
42. Game, J. C., and R. K. Mortimer, A genetic study of x-ray
        sensitive mutants in yeast, Mutat. Res., 24 (1974) 281–292.
43. Game, J. C., and R. K. Mortimer, personal communication.

44. Game, J. C., T. J. Zamb, R. J. Braun, M. Resnick, and R. M.
       Roth, The role of radiation (rad) genes in meiotic
       recombination in yeast, Genetics, in press.
45. Gocke, E., and T. R. Manney, Expression of radiation-induced
       mutations at the arginine permease (CAN1) locus in
       Saccharomyces cerevisiae, Genetics, 91 (1979) 53–66.
46. Golin, J. E., and M. S. Esposito, Evidence for joint genic
       control of spontaneous mutation and genetic recombination
       during mitosis in Saccharomyces, Mol. Gen. Genet., 150
       (1977) 127–135.
47. Grenson, M., and C. Hou, Ammonia inhibition of the general
       amino acid permease and its suppression in NADPH-specific
       glutamate dehydrogenaseless mutants of Saccharomyces
       cerevisiae, Biochem. Biophys. Res. Commun., 48 (1972)
       749–756.
48. Grenson, M., C. Hou, and M. Crabeel, Multiplicity of the amino
       acid permeases in Saccharomyces cerevisiae. IV. Evidence
       for a general amino acid permease, J. Bacteriol., 103
       (1970) 770–777.
49. Grenson, M., M. Mousset, J. M. Wiame, and J. Bechet,
       Multiplicity of the amino acid permeases in Saccharomyces
       cerevisiae. I. Evidence for a specific arginine-trans-
       porting system, Biochim. Biophys. Acta, 127 (1966) 325–338.
50. Hannan, M. A., P. Duck, and A. Nasim, UV-induced lethal
       sectoring and pure mutant clones in yeast, Mutat. Res.,
       36 (1976) 171–176.
51. Hartwell, L. H., Biochemical genetics of yeast, Ann. Rev.
       Genet., 4 (1970) 373–396.
52. Hartwell, L. H., Genetic control of the cell division cycle in
       yeast. II. Genes controlling DNA replication and its
       initiation, J. Mol. Biol., 59 (1971) 183–194.
53. Hartwell, L. H., Three additional genes required for DNA
       synthesis in Saccharomyces cerevisiae, J. Bacteriol., 115
       (1973) 966–974.
54. Hartwell, L. H., Saccharomyces cerevisiae cell cycle,
       Bacteriol. Rev., 38 (1974) 164–198.
55. Hastings, P. J., S.-K. Quah, and R. C. von Borstel, Spontaneous
       mutation by mutagenic repair of spontaneous lesions in DNA,
       Nature, 264 (1976) 719–722.
56. Haynes, R. H., DNA repair and the genetic control of radio-
       sensitivity in yeast, In: Molecular Mechanisms for Repair
       of DNA, P. C. Hanawalt and R. B. Setlow (Eds.), Plenum
       Press, New York, 1975, pp. 529–540.
57. Hereford, L. M., and L. H. Hartwell, Role of protein synthesis
       in the replication of yeast DNA, Nature New Biol., 244
       (1973) 129–131.
58. Hershfield, M. S., and N. G. Nossal, In vitro characterization
       of a mutator T4 DNA polymerase, Genetics (Suppl.), 73
       (1973) 131–136.

59. Hill, R. F., Ultraviolet-induced lethality and reversion to
     prototrophy in Escherichia coli strains with normal and
     reduced repair ability, Photochem. Photobiol., 4 (1965)
     563-568.
60. Ho, K., Induction of DNA double-strand breaks by X-rays in a
     radiosensitive strain of the yeast Saccharomyces cerevisiae,
     Mutat. Res., 30 (1975) 327-334.
61. Ho, K. S. Y., and R. K. Mortimer, Induction of dominant
     lethality by X-rays in a radiosensitive strain of yeast,
     Mutat. Res., 20 (1973) 45-51.
62. Holliday, R., A mechanism for gene conversion in fungi, Genet.
     Res., 5 (1964) 282-304.
63. Holliday, R., Radiation-sensitive mutants of Ustilago maydis,
     Mutat. Res., 2 (1965) 557-559.
64. Holliday, R., Altered recombination frequencies in radiation-
     sensitive strains of Ustilago, Mutat. Res., 4 (1967)
     275-288.
65. Holliday, R., Biochemical measure of the time and frequency of
     radiation-induced allelic recombination in Ustilago, Nature
     New Biol., 232 (1971) 233-236.
66. Holliday, R., Ustilago maydis, In: Handbook of Genetics,
     R. C. King (Ed.), Vol. 1, Plenum Press, New York, 1974,
     pp. 575-595.
67. Holliday, R., R. E. Halliwell, M. W. Evans, and V. Rowell,
     Genetic characterization of rec-1, a mutant of Ustilago
     maydis defective in repair and recombination, Genet. Res.,
     27 (1976) 413-453.
68. Howard-Flanders, P., DNA repair, Ann. Rev. Biochem., 37 (1968)
     175-200.
69. Howard-Flanders, P., L. Theriot, and J. B. Stedeford, Some
     properties of excision-defective, recombination-defective
     mutants of Escherichia coli K12, J. Bacteriol., 97 (1969)
     1134-1141.
70. James, A. P., and B. J. Kilbey, The timing of UV mutagenesis
     in yeast: A pedigree analysis of induced recessive
     mutation, Genetics, 87 (1977) 237-248.
71. James, A. P., B. J. Kilbey, and G. J. Prefontaine, The timing
     of UV mutagenesis in yeast: Continuing mutation in an
     excision-defective (rad-1) strain, Mol. Gen. Genet., 165
     (1978) 207-212.
72. Johnston, L. H., and J. C. Game, Mutants of yeast with
     depressed DNA synthesis, Mol. Gen. Genet., 161 (1978)
     205-214.
73. Johnston, L. H., and K. A. Nasmyth, Saccharomyces cerevisiae
     cell cycle mutant cdc9 is defective in DNA ligase, Nature
     274 (1978) 891-893.
74. Kato, T., and Y. Shinoura, Isolation and characterization of
     mutants of Escherichia coli deficient in induction of
     mutations by ultraviolet light, Mol. Gen. Genet., 156
     (1977) 121-131.

75. Kilbey, B. J., T. Brychcy, and A. Nasim, Initiation of UV
        mutagenesis in Saccharomyces cerevisiae, Nature, 274 (1978)
        889-891.
76. Kilbey, B. J., and A. P. James, The mutagenic potential of
        unexcised pyrimidine dimers in Saccharomyces cerevisiae
        RAD1-1. Evidence from photoreactivation and pedigree
        analysis, Mutat. Res., 60 (1979) 163-171.
77. Kimball, R. F., The mutagenicity of hydrazine and some of its
        derivatives, Mutat. Res., 39 (1977) 111-126.
78. Kimball, R. F., The relation of repair phenomena to mutation
        induction in bacteria, Mutat. Res., 55 (1978) 85-120.
79. Kimball, R. F., and B. F. Hirsch, Tests for the mutagenic
        action of a number of chemicals on Haemophilus influenzae
        with special emphasis on hydrazine, Mutat. Res., 30 (1975)
        9-20.
80. Kimball, R. F., and B. F. Hirsch, Fixation and loss of
        hydrazine-induced premutational damage in Haemophilus
        influenzae, Mutat. Res., 36 (1976) 39-48.
81. Korch, C. T., and R. Snow, Allelic complementation in the first
        gene for histidine biosynthesis in Saccharomyces cerevisiae.
        I. Characteristics of mutants and genetic mapping of
        alleles, Genetics, 74 (1973) 287-305.
82. Kowalski, S., and W. Laskowski, The effect of three rad genes
        on survival, inter- and intragenic mitotic recombination
        in Saccharomyces, Mol. Gen. Genet., 136 (1975) 75-86.
83. Larimer, F. W., personal communication.
84. Larimer, F. W., D. Ramey, W. Lijinsky, and J. L. Epler, Muta-
        genicity of methylated N-nitrosopiperidines in
        Saccharomyces cerevisiae, Mutat. Res., 57 (1978) 155-161.
85. Laskowski, W., Inaktivierungsversuche mit homozyoten
        Hefestämmen verschiedenen Ploidilgrades, Z. Naturforsch.,
        15b (1960) 495-506.
86. Laskowski, W., Der aα-Effect, eine Korrelation zwischen
        Paarungstypenkonstitution und Strahlenresistenz bei Hefen,
        Zentralbl. Batkeriol. Parasitenkd, Infektionskr. Hyg.
        Abt. I Orig., 184 (1962) 251-258.
87. Lawrence, C. W., and R. Christensen, UV mutagenesis in
        radiation-sensitive strains of yeast, Genetics, 82 (1976)
        207-232.
88. Lawrence, C. W., and R. Christensen, Ultraviolet-induced
        reversion of cyc1 alleles in radiation-sensitive strains
        of yeast. I. rev1 mutant strains, J. Mol. Biol., 122
        (1978) 1-21.
89. Lawrence, C. W., and R. Christensen, Ultraviolet-induced
        reversion of cyc1 alleles in radiation-sensitive strains
        of yeast. II. rev2 mutant strains, Genetics, 90 (1978)
        213-226.

90. Lawrence, C. W., and R. Christensen, Ultraviolet light induced mutagenesis in Saccharomyces cerevisiae, In: DNA Repair Mechanisms, P. C. Hanawalt, E. C. Friedberg, and C. F. Fox (Eds.), Academic Press, New York, 1978, pp. 437-440.

91. Lawrence, C. W., and R. Christensen, Ultraviolet-induced reversion of cyc1 alleles in radiation-sensitive strains of yeast. III. rev3 mutant strains, Genetics, 92 (1979) 397-408.

92. Lawrence, C. W., J. W. Stewart, F. Sherman, and R. Christensen, Specificity and frequency of ultraviolet-induced reversion of an iso-1-cytochrome c ochre mutant in radiation-sensitive strains of yeast, J. Mol. Biol., 85 (1974) 137-162.

93. Lemontt, J. F., Mutants of yeast defective in mutation induced by ultraviolet light, Genetics, 68 (1971) 21-33.

94. Lemontt, J. F., Pathways of ultraviolet mutability in Saccharomyces cerevisiae. II. The effect of rev genes on recombination, Mutat. Res., 13 (1971) 319-326.

95. Lemontt, J. F., Induction of forward mutations in mutationally defective yeast, Mol. Gen. Genet., 119 (1972) 27-42.

96. Lemontt, J. F., Genes controlling ultraviolet mutability in yeast, Genetics (Suppl.), 73 (1973) 153-159.

97. Lemontt, J. F., Induced mutagenesis in Ustilago maydis. I. Isolation and characterization of a radiation-revertible allele of the structural gene for nitrate reductase, Mol. Gen. Genet., 145 (1976) 125-132.

98. Lemontt, J. F., Induced mutagenesis in Ustilago maydis. II. An in vivo biochemical assay, Mol. Gen. Genet., 145 (1976) 133-143.

99. Lemontt, J. F., Mutagenesis of yeast by hydrazine: Dependence upon post-treatment cell division, Mutat. Res., 43 (1977) 165-178.

100. Lemontt, J. F., Pathways of ultraviolet mutability in Saccharomyces cerevisiae. III. Genetic analysis and properties of mutants resistant to ultraviolet-induced forward mutation, Mutat. Res., 43 (1977) 179-204.

101. Lemontt, J. F., Pathways of ultraviolet mutability in Saccharomyces cerevisiae. IV. The relation between canavanine toxicity and ultraviolet mutability to canavanine resistance, Mutat. Res., 43 (1977) 339-355.

102. Lemontt, J. F., Loss of hydrazine-induced mutability in wild-type and excision-repair-defective yeast during post-treatment inhibition of cell division, Mutat. Res., 50 (1978) 57-66.

103. Lemontt, J. F., unpublished data.

104. Lemontt, J. F., D. R. Fugit and V. L. MacKay, Pleiotropic mutations at the TUP1 locus that affect the expression of mating-type-dependent functions in Saccharomyces cerevisiae, Genetics, in press.

105. Lemontt, J. F., and V. L. MacKay, A pleiotropic mutant of
     yeast expressing the mating-specific "shmoo" morphology
     during vegetative growth in the absence of exogenous
     mating hormone (abs.), Genetics (Suppl.), 86 (1977) s38.
106. Livi, G. P., and V. L. MacKay, Mating-type regulation of
     methyl methanesulfonate sensitivity in Saccharomyces
     cerevisiae, Genetics, in press.
107. MacKay, V. L., Mating-type-specific pheromones as mediators
     of sexual conjugation in yeast, In: Molecular Control
     of Proliferation and Differentiation, J. Papaconstantinou
     and W. J. Rutter (Eds.), Academic Press, New York, 1978,
     pp. 243-259.
108. Maloney, D., and S. Fogel, High frequency mitotic conversion
     mutants in yeast (abs.), Genetics (Suppl.), 83 (1976) s47.
109. Manney, T. R., and J. H. Meade, Cell-cell interactions during
     mating in Saccharomyces cerevisiae, In: Microbial Inter-
     actions, Receptors and Recognition, Ser. B, Vol. 3,
     J. L. Reissig (Ed.), Chapman and Hall, London, 1977, pp.
     281-321.
110. Manney, T. R., and R. K. Mortimer, Allelic mapping in yeast
     by x-ray-induced mitotic reversion, Science, 143 (1964)
     581-582.
111. Martin, P., S. Prakash, and L. Prakash, personal communication.
112. McKee, R. H., and C. W. Lawrence, Genetic analysis of gamma
     ray mutagenesis in yeast. I. Reversion in radiation-
     sensitive strains, Genetics, in press.
113. McKee, R. H., and C. W. Lawrence, Genetic analysis of gamma
     ray mutagenesis in yeast. Survival and reversion in
     double mutant strains, Mutat. Res., submitted.
114. McKee, R. H., and C. W. Lawrence, Genetic analysis of gamma
     ray mutagenesis in yeast. II. Allele-specific control
     of mutagenesis, Genetics, in press.
115. Moore, C., and F. Sherman, Role of DNA sequences in genetic
     recombination in the iso-1-cytochrome c gene of yeast.
     I. Discrepancies between physical distance and genetic
     distance determined by five mapping procedures, Genetics,
     79 (1975) 397-418.
116. Moore, C., and F. Sherman, Role of DNA sequences in genetic
     recombination in the iso-1-cytochrome c gene of yeast.
     II. Comparison of mutants altered at the same and nearby
     base pairs, Genetics, 85 (1977) 1-22.
117. Mortimer, R. K., Radiobiological and genetic studies on a
     polyploid series (haploid to hexaploid) of Saccharomyces
     cerevisiae, Radiat. Res., 9 (1958) 312-326.
118. Mortimer, R. K., and D. C. Hawthorne, Yeast genetics, In:
     The Yeasts, Vol. 1, A. H. Rose and J. S. Harrison (Eds.),
     Academic Press, New York, 1969, pp. 385-460.

119.   Mount, D. W., K. B. Low, and S. J. Edmiston, Dominant
        mutants (lex) in Escherichia coli K-12 which affect
        radiation sensitivity and frequency of ultraviolet light-
        induced mutations, J. Bacteriol., 112 (1972) 886–893.
120.   Moustacchi, E., Cytoplasmic and nuclear genetic events induced
        by UV light in strains of Saccharomyces cerevisiae with
        different UV sensitivities, Mutat. Res., 7 (1969) 171–185.
121.   Moustacchi, E., R. Chanet, and M. Heude, Ionizing and ultra-
        violet radiations: Genetic effects and repair in yeast,
        In: Research in Photobiology, A. Castellani (Ed.), Plenum
        Press, New York, 1976, pp. 197–206.
122.   Nakai, S., and S. Matsumoto, Two types of radiation-sensitive
        mutant in yeast, Mutat. Res., 4 (1967) 129–136.
123.   Nakai, S., and R. K. Mortimer, Studies of the genetic mechanism
        of radiation-induced mitotic segregation in yeast, Mol.
        Gen. Genet., 103 (1969) 329–338.
124.   Parker, J. H., and F. Sherman, Fine-structure mapping and
        mutational studies of gene controlling yeast cytochrome c,
        Genetics, 62 (1969) 9–22.
125.   Parry, E. M., and B. S. Cox, The tolerance of aneuploidy in
        yeast, Genet. Res., 16 (1970) 333–340.
126.   Parry, J. M., P. J. Davies, and W. E. Evans, The effects of
        "cell age" upon the lethal effects of physical and
        chemical mutagens in the yeast, Saccharomyces cerevisiae,
        Mol. Gen. Genet., 146 (1976) 27–35.
127.   Parry, J. M., and E. M. Parry, The effects of UV light post-
        treatments on the survival characteristics of 21 UV-
        sensitive mutants of Saccharomyces cerevisiae, Mutat.
        Res., 8 (1969) 545–556.
128.   Patrick, M. H., and R. H. Haynes, Dark recovery phenomena in
        yeast. II. Conditions that modify the recovery process,
        Radiat. Res., 23 (1964) 564–579.
129.   Patrick, M. H., R. H. Haynes, and R. B. Uretz, Dark recovery
        phenomena in yeast. I. Comparative effects with various
        inactivating agents, Radiat. Res., 21 (1964) 144–163.
130.   Prakash, L., Lack of chemically induced mutation in repair-
        deficient mutants of yeast, Genetics, 78 (1974) 1101–1118.
131.   Prakash, L., Repair of pyrimidine dimers in nuclear and mito-
        chondrial DNA of yeast irradiated with low doses of
        ultraviolet light, J. Mol. Biol., 98 (1975) 781–795.
132.   Prakash, L., Effect of genes controlling radiation sensitivity
        on chemically induced mutations in Saccharomyces
        cerevisiae, Genetics 83 (1976) 285–301.
133.   Prakash, L., The relation between repair of DNA and radiation
        and chemical mutagenesis in Saccharomyces cerevisiae,
        Mutat. Res., 41 (1976) 241–248.
134.   Prakash, L., Defective thymine dimer excision in radiation-
        sensitive mutants rad10 and rad16 of Saccharomyces
        cerevisiae, Mol. Gen. Genet., 152 (1977) 125–128.

135. Prakash, L., Repair of pyrimidine dimers in radiation-sensitive
        mutants rad3, rad4, rad6, and rad9 of Saccharomyces
        cerevisiae, Mutat. Res., 45 (1977) 13-20.
136. Prakash, L., D. Hinkle, and S. Prakash, Decreased UV
        mutagenesis in cdc8, a DNA replication mutant of
        Saccharomyces cerevisiae, Mol. Gen. Genet., 172 (1979)
        249-258.
137. Prakash, L., and S. Prakash, Isolation and characterization of
        MMS-sensitive mutants of Saccharomyces cerevisiae,
        Genetics, 86 (1977) 33-55.
138. Prakash, S., and L. Prakash, Increased spontaneous mitotic
        segregation in MMS-sensitive mutants of Saccharomyces
        cerevisiae, Genetics, 87 (1977) 229-236.
139. Quah, S.-K., personal communication.
140. Quah, S.-K., R. C. von Borstel, and P. J. Hastings, Anti-
        mutators in yeast (abs.), Cold Spring Harbor Laboratory
        Meeting on the Molecular Biology of Yeast, 1977, p. 82.
141. Rahn, R. O., N. P. Johnson, A. W. Hsie, J. F. Lemontt, W. E.
        Masker, J. D. Regan, W. C. Dunn, J. D. Hoeschele and
        D. H. Brown, The interaction of platinum compounds with
        the genome: Correlation between DNA binding and biological
        effects, In: The Scientific Basis of Toxicity Assessment,
        H. R. Witschi (Ed.), Elsevier/North Holland, Amsterdam,
        in press.
142. Resnick, M. A., Genetic control of radiation sensitivity in
        Saccharomyces cerevisiae, Genetics 62 (1969) 519-531.
143. Resnick, M. A., Induction of mutations in Saccharomyces
        cerevisiae by ultraviolet light, Mutat. Res., 7 (1969)
        315-332.
144. Resnick, M. A., The induction of molecular and genetic
        recombination in eukaryotic cells, Adv. Radiat. Biol.,
        8 (1978) 175-216.
145. Resnick, M. A., and P. Martin, The repair of double-strand
        breaks in the nuclear DNA of Saccharomyces cerevisiae
        and its genetic control, Mol. Gen. Genet., 143 (1976)
        119-129.
146. Resnick, M. A., and J. K. Setlow, Repair of pyrimidine dimer
        damage induced in yeast by ultraviolet light, J.
        Bacteriol., 109 (1972) 979-986.
147. Reynolds, R. J., Removal of pyrimidine dimers from
        Saccharomyces cerevisiae nuclear DNA under nongrowth
        conditions as detected by a sensitive, enzymatic assay,
        Mutat. Res., 50 (1978) 43-56.
148. Rodarte-Ramon, U.S., Radiation-induced recombination in
        Saccharomyces: The genetic control of recombination in
        mitosis and meiosis, Radiat. Res., 49 (1972) 148-154.
149. Rodarte-Ramon, U. S., and R. K. Mortimer, Radiation-induced
        recombination in Saccharomyces: Isolation and genetic
        study of recombination-deficient mutants, Radiat. Res.,
        49 (1972) 133-147.

150. Roman, H., A system selective for mutations affecting the
     synthesis of adenine in yeast, C. R. Trav. Lab. Carlsberg,
     26 (1956) 299-314.

151. Rose, A. H., and J. S. Harrison (Eds.), The Yeasts, Vol. 1,
     Biology of Yeasts, Academic Press, New York, 1969.

152. Rose, A. H., and J. S. Harrison (Eds.), The Yeasts, Vol. 2,
     Physiology and Biochemistry of Yeasts, Academic Press,
     New York, 1971.

153. Rothstein, R. J., and F. Sherman, Genes affecting the
     expression of cytochrome c in yeast: Genetic mapping
     and genetic interactions, Genetics, in press.

154. Rupp, W. D., and P. Howard-Flanders, Discontinuities in the
     DNA synthesized in an excision-defective strain of
     Escherichia coli following ultraviolet irradiation.
     J. Mol. Biol., 131 (1968) 291-304.

155. Schnaar, R. L., N. Muzyczka, and M. J. Bessman, Utilization
     of aminopurine deoxynucleoside triphosphate by mutator,
     antimutator and wild-type DNA polymerases of bacteriophage
     T4, Genetics (Suppl.), 73 (1973) 137-140.

156. Sherman, F., and C. W. Lawrence, Saccharomyces, In:
     Handbook of Genetics, Vol. 1, R. C. King (Ed.), Plenum
     Press, New York, 1974, pp. 359-393.

157. Sherman, F., and J. W. Stewart, Variation of mutagenic action
     on nonsense mutants at different sites in the iso-1-
     cytochrome c gene of yeast, Genetics, 78 (1974) 97-113.

158. Smith, K. C., and D. H. C. Meun, Repair of radiation-induced
     damage in Escherichia coli. I. Effect of rec mutations
     on postreplication repair of damage due to ultraviolet
     radiation, J. Mol. Biol., 51 (1970) 459-472.

159. Snow, R., Mutants of yeast sensitive to ultraviolet light,
     J. Bacteriol., 94 (1967) 571-575.

160. Snow, R., Recombination in ultraviolet-sensitive strains of
     Saccharomyces cerevisiae, Mutat. Res., 6 (1968) 409-418.

161. Speyer, J. F., Mutagenic DNA polymerase, Biochem. Biophys.
     Res. Commun., 21 (1965) 6-8.

162. Suslova, N. G., and I. A. Zakharov, The gene-controlled
     radiation sensitivity of yeast. VII. Identification of
     the genes for the x-ray sensitivity, Genetika, 6 (1970)
     158-163.

163. Terisima, T., and L. J. Tolmach, Change in x-ray sensitivities
     of HeLa cells during the division cycle, Nature, 190
     (1961) 1210-1211.

164. Unrau, P., R. Wheatcroft, and B. S. Cox, The excision of
     pyrimidine dimers from DNA of ultraviolet irradiated
     yeast, Mol. Gen. Genet., 113 (1971) 359-362.

165. von Borstel, R. C., K. T. Cain, and C. M. Steinberg,
     Inheritance of spontaneous mutability in yeast, Genetics,
     69 (1971) 17-27.

166. von Borstel, R. C., and P. J. Hastings, Mutagenic repair
     pathways in yeast, In: Research in Photobiology,
     A. Castellani (Ed.), Plenum Press, New York, 1976,
     pp. 683–687.
167. von Borstel, R. C., S.-K. Quah, C. M. Steinberg, F. Flury,
     and D. J. C. Gottlieb, Mutants of yeast with enhanced
     spontaneous mutation rates, Genetics (Suppl.), 73 (1973)
     141–151.
168. Waters, R., and E. Moustacchi, The disappearance of ultraviolet
     induced pyrimidine dimers from the nuclear DNA of
     exponential and stationary phase cells of Saccharomyces
     cerevisiae following various post-irradiation treatments,
     Biochim. Biophys. Acta, 353 (1974) 407–419.
169. Waters, R., and E. Moustacchi, The fate of ultraviolet-
     induced pyrimidine dimers in the mitochondrial DNA of
     Saccharomyces cerevisiae following various post-irradiation
     cell treatments, Biochim. Biophys. Acta, 366 (1974)
     241–250.
170. Whelan, W. L., E. Gocke, and T. R. Manney, The CAN1 locus of
     Saccharomyces cerevisiae: Fine-structure analysis and
     forward mutation rates, Genetics, 91 (1970) 35–51.
171. Wickner, R. B., Mutants of Saccharomyces cerevisiae that
     incorporate deoxythymidine-5'-monophosphate into deoxy-
     ribonucleic acid in vivo, J. Bacteriol., 117 (1974)
     252–260.
172. Wildenberg, J., The relation of mitotic recombination to DNA
     replication in yeast pedigrees, Genetics, 66 (1970)
     291–304.
173. Williamson, D. H., Replication of the nuclear genome does not
     require concomitant protein synthesis in yeast, Biochem.
     Biophys. Res. Commun., 52 (1973) 731–740.
174. Witkin, E. M., Radiation-induced mutations and their repair,
     Science, 152 (1966) 1345–1353.
175. Witkin, E. M., Mutation-proof and mutation-prone modes of
     survival in derivatives of Escherichia coli B differing
     in sensitivity to ultraviolet light, Brookhaven Symp.
     Biol., 20 (1967) 17–55.
176. Witkin, E. M., The role of DNA repair and recombination in
     mutagenesis, Proc. XII Int. Congr. Genet., 3 (1969)
     225–245.
177. Witkin, E. M., Ultraviolet-induced mutation and DNA repair,
     Ann. Rev. Genet., 3 (1969) 525–552.
178. Witkin, E. M., Ultraviolet mutagenesis and inducible DNA
     repair in Escherichia coli, Bacteriol. Rev., 40 (1976)
     869–907.
179. Zakharov, I. A., T. N. Kozina, and I. V. Fedorova, Effets
     des mutations vers la sensibilité au rayonnement
     ultraviolet chez la levure, Mutat. Res., 9 (1970) 31–39.

CHAPTER 8

MOLECULAR MECHANISM OF PYRIMIDINE DIMER EXCISION IN Saccharomyces

cerevisiae. I. STUDIES WITH INTACT CELLS AND CELL-FREE SYSTEMS

RICHARD J. REYNOLDS and ERROL C. FRIEDBERG

Laboratory of Experimental Oncology, Department of
Pathology, Stanford University, Stanford, CA 94305
(U.S.A.)

SUMMARY

We have investigated a number of aspects of the excision of
pyrimidine dimers from the DNA of wild-type and UV sensitive mutants
of the yeast Saccharomyces cerevisiae. Our studies show that a
number of rad mutants in the RAD3 group (rad1-2, rad1-11; rad2-2,
rad2-4; rad3-1; rad4-2, rad4-3) that are defective relative to
wild-type strains in pyrimidine dimer excision in vivo, are also
defective in the production of single strand breaks in their DNA
during post-UV incubation. The presence of UV-induced incubation-
independent single-strand breaks prevents definitive conclusions
regarding the role of various RAD loci in the incision process but
provides evidence of a biochemical subdivision in the RAD3 group
loci. Using UV irradiated DNA preincised with dimer-specific
endonuclease activity from Micrococcus luteus, we have also detected
enzymatic activity from extracts of wild-type yeast that catalyzes
the selective excision of thymine-containing pyrmidine dimers.
Normal levels of this activity are present in all mutant strains
thus far examined (rad1-11; rad2-4; rad3-1; rad4-3).

Thus, in Saccharomyces cerevisiae it appears that at least
four of the nine genetic loci governing pyrimidine dimer excision
affect events associated with DNA incision or preincision. This
situation is strikingly analagous to that observed with the numerous
complementation groups in the human disease xeroderma pigmentosum.

INTRODUCTION

For some years now our laboratory has been investigating aspects of the biology and biochemistry of nucleotide excision repair in higher eukaryotes. The availability of cell lines from human patients suffering from xeroderma pigmentosum (XP) (in which there is good evidence for defective nucleotide excision repair) has provided an attractive model for attempting to correlate genetic and biochemical parameters of nucleotide excision repair. Since the early reported observations of defective unscheduled DNA synthesis and defective pyrimidine dimer excision in XP cells in culture, the past decade has witnessed a staggering growth in published cellular and biochemical observations in this disease [1, 5, 9, 28]. While we are far from understanding the details of the molecular biology of pyrimidine dimer excision in normal human cells, or of the defect(s) in excision in XP cells, a number of important observations have emerged. Perhaps the most striking of these is the evidence for the existence of at least seven genetic complementation groups controlling nucleotide excision repair in human cells, many, if not all of which appear to be involved in very early events in pyrimidine dimer excision [1, 5, 9, 28]. The nature of these early events is not yet understood at all, however it is of possible relevance in this regard to note that studies from a number of laboratories have demonstrated the importance of chromatin conformation in determining the sites and possibly the rate of nucleotide excision repair in human cells [4, 29, 30, 34]. Additionally, there is indirect evidence suggesting that defects in the regulation of conformational changes in chromatin may be determinants of defective repair in XP [11, 18].

As a source of biological material from which to isolate both enzymes and possible nonenzyme factors required for nucleotide excision repair, human cells in culture are far from ideal since the logistics of growing sufficient quantities for cell-free studies are formidable. In searching for a biochemically accessible system, the yeast Saccharomyces cerevisiae shows several interesting analogies with the above-mentioned observations in higher eukaryotes. As pointed out in an excellent recent review by Haynes et al. [14], among the simple eukaryotes, S. cerevisiae has been the most extensively studied with respect to DNA repair. Indeed, with increasingly extensive applications of the techniques of genetic engineering and DNA base sequencing, yeast now appears to be one of the most useful model organisms for fundamental studies on eukaryote molecular biology in general. At the time of writing, at least 64 distinct genetic loci affecting UV radiation, ionizing radiation, and methyl methanesulfonate sensitivity are known [14]. These mutants fall into three phenotypic categories which correlate well with three essentially nonoverlapping or epistatic genetic groups [8, 23]. One of these, designated as the RAD3 group (the groups are named as a matter of convenience by a prominent locus

in each group) is of particular interest to us. Members of this
group are sensitive primarily to UV radiation and to nitrogen mustard.
Mutant genes in this group appear to have no effect on meiosis, but
do result in increased levels of mutation above wild-type cells
[14]. At least 9 loci in this group control the excision of
pyrimidine dimers [20-25, 32, 33], a genetic complexity very remi-
niscent of the results of complementation studies in XP.

In this paper we report the results of our early studies on
the molecular biology of pyrimidine dimer excision in S. cerevisiae.
We have carried out a number of studies on intact UV-irradiated
cells in an attempt to determine which mutants in the RAD3 group
are defective in events required for incision of DNA, as distinct
from post-incision dimer excision events. In addition we have
initiated studies with cell-free systems in an attempt to identify
and isolate enzyme activities specifically involved in the excision
of pyrimidine dimers from DNA.

DETECTION OF ENDOGENOUS SINGLE-STRAND BREAKS IN THE DNA OF UV-IRRADIATED S. cerevisiae

The frequently quoted model of the molecular mechanism of
pyrimidine dimer excision involving endonucleolytic incision 5'
with respect to dimers, followed by excision-resynthesis and DNA
ligation, has been derived chiefly from studies with prokaryotes
[13]. However, in its broadest terms this model is thought to have
general applicability to higher organisms as well. While there are
no data of which we are aware that contradict the essential elements
of the model, the large number of mutants in the RAD3 group suggest
a greater complexity of the biochemistry of nucleotide excision
repair in S. cerevisiae than in E. coli. Studies with cell lines
derived from five of the seven known complementation groups in XP
indicate a defect in endonucleolytic incision of DNA in UV
irradiated cells in vivo in all five lines [9]. It was thus of
particular interest to survey the numerous excision defective
mutants of the RAD3 group to determine the kinetics and extent of
induction of endogenous single-strand breaks during post-UV
incubation in these strains.

Materials and Methods

Yeast Strains.   All UV-sensitive strains were recovered from
mutagenized cultures of strain S288C (a wild-type haploid strain)
and backcrossed into a related genetic background by Dr. Richard
Snow [31; personal communication].

Growth of Cultures.   Overnight cultures inoculated from YPD
agar plates (1% yeast extract, 2% Bactopeptone, 2% glucose, 2% agar)
were grown in YNB-D liquid medium (0.67% Difco Yeast Nitrogen Base,
2% glucose) at 29°C. Overnight cultures were diluted into fresh
YNB-D medium to a density of 5×10^6 cells/ml, allowed to complete
one cell doubling and were then labeled in medium supplemented with
either [6-^{3}H]uracil (7-10 μCi/ml) or [2-^{14}C]uracil (2 μCi/ml) for
two generations (3 hr). Labeled cells were harvested by centrifugation (500 × g for 5 min at room temperature) and were resuspended
at a density of ∿10^7 cells/ml in 0.067 M potassium phosphate buffer,
pH 7.0, at 0°C.

UV Irradiation and Post-Irradiation Treatment.   Cells in
potassium phosphate buffer were irradiated with a 15-W low-pressure-
mercury germicidal lamp. Incident dose rate was determined with an
IL254 Germicidal-Photometer (International Light, Inc., Newburyport,
Mass.), and the average incident dose rate was calculated as
suggested by Morowitz [17]. Cells were irradiated on ice with
stirring and were kept in the dark or under yellow light emitted
by "gold" fluorescent lamps (Sylvania) during and subsequent to
irradiation.

Immediately following irradiation cells were aerated in
potassium phosphate buffer at 28-30°C. Samples of approximately 10^7
cells each were removed after the desired times of incubation and
cooled to and maintained at 0°C until spheroplast formation. Cells
were converted to spheroplasts by sequential incubations with 2-
mercaptoethanol followed by glusulase (Endo Laboratories, Garden
City, N.Y.) after the method suggested by Cabib [2]. For this
procedure ∿10^7 cells in potassium phosphate buffer were harvested
by centrifugation at 4°C, resuspended in 200 μl of 570 mM 2-
mercaptoethanol, 100 mM Tris-H_2SO_4 (pH 9.3), and incubated for 15 min
at 0°C. Reduced cells were harvested by centrifugation in the cold,
resuspended in 200 μl 2% (v/v) glusulase, 20% (w/v) sorbitol,
10 mM EDTA, 10 mM Tris-H_2SO_4 (pH 9.0), and incubated at 30°C for 30
min. Spheroplasts were cooled to 0°C and harvested by centrifugation
at 4°C. To lyse spheroplasts, they were first resuspended
(∿10^7/100 μl) in 100 mM NaCl, 10 mM EDTA, 50 mM Tris-HCl (pH 7.6)
at 0°C and then quickly lysed by the addition of an equal volume of
1% (w/v) sarkosyl, 20 mM EDTA, 1 M NaOH.

Velocity Sedimentation in Alkaline Sucrose Gradients.   Aliquots
of lysed samples (200 μl) were layered onto 3.9 ml 5-20% alkaline
sucrose gradients (0.5 M NaCl, 0.01 M EDTA, 0.2 M NaOH) formed in
polyallomer ultracentrifuge tubes. Sedimentation was performed in
a Beckman L2-65B ultracentrifuge at 20°C with an SW56 rotor, at
20,000 rpm for 225 or 250 min. Gradients were precalibrated with
respect to molecular weight with T4 and T7 bacteriophage DNA's and
with φX174 and SV40 DNA restriction fragments. Gradients were
fractionated with the aid of a Technicon proportioning pump directly

onto Whatman #17 paper strips as described previously [25]. Paper
strips were washed twice in 5% trichloroacetic acid and twice in
95% ethanol and were air dried. Individual fractions were placed
into vials with a toluene-based liquid scintillation mixture and
radioactivity was measured in a Beckman LS-250 liquid scintillation
spectrometer. Weight-average molecular weights were determined
from the distribution of radioactivity through the gradients as
described previously [25].

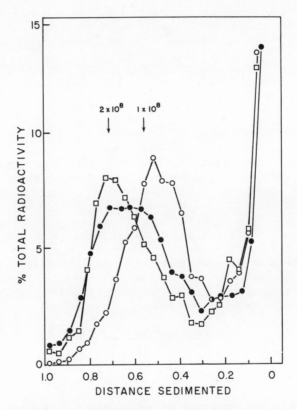

Fig. 1.   Alkaline sucrose gradient profiles of DNA from (☐)
unirradiated RAD cells and from RAD cells irradiated 100 J/m^2 and
aerated in potassium phosphate buffer (pH 7.0) at 28°C for (◯)
1 hr or (●) 24 hr after irradiation. The direction of sedimentation was from right to left and the total acid-precipitable radioactivity recovered from each gradient was 7570, 7780, and 6769 cpm,
respectively.

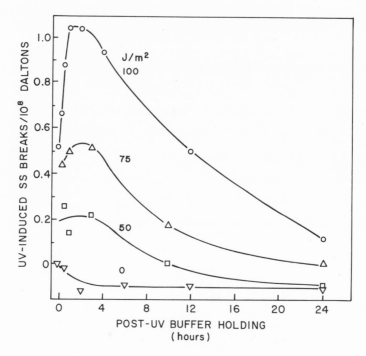

Fig. 2.   Endogenous single strand breaks in nuclear DNA from RAD
cells after UV irradiation. Cells from a log phase culture of
strain S288C (wild-type) prelabeled in potassium phosphate buffer
(pH 7.0) were incubated at 28°C either (▽) without prior UV
irradiation or after irradiation at (☐) 50, (△) 75 or (○)
100 J/m². Cells were converted to spheroplasts by sequential
treatment with 2-mercaptoethanol and glusulase and DNA from lysed
spheroplasts was sedimented in 5-20% alkaline sucrose gradients.
Weight-average molecular weights were calculated from the resulting
distribution of radioactivity through the gradients and single strand
breaks were calculated relative to unirradiated unincubated samples.

Results and Discussion

Sedimentation profiles from a typical experiment are presented
in Fig. 1.   Wild-type cells were either unirradiated, irradiated
at 100 J/m² at 254 nm and incubated for 1 hr at 28°C, or irradiated
and incubated for 24 hr prior to spheroplast formation and sedimentation of DNA. The resulting sedimentation profiles indicated a
reduction in the molecular weight of nuclear DNA at short times
after irradiation, followed by a subsequent increase in molecular
weight at longer times, relative to the unirradiated control.
[Mitochondrial DNA sedimented no further than 30% of the total
distance of the gradients under the sedimentation conditions used
(Reynolds, unpublished data) and did not contribute significantly

to molecular weight values obtained from weight-average calcula-
tions.]   More extensive data from experiments with the wild
haploid strain are presented in Fig. 2.   Clearly the induction of
single-strand breaks and their subsequent disappearance was both
time- and UV dose-dependent, as would be expected for an excision
repair reaction based on the model presented above.   Notice that no
breaks in the nuclear DNA were observed in unirradiated cells.

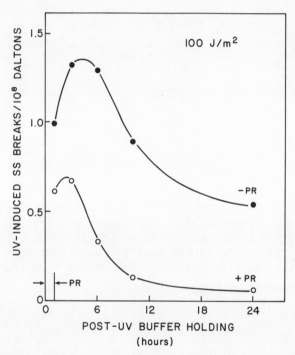

Fig. 3.   Effect of photoreactivating treatment on the appearance
of single strand breaks in the nuclear DNA of UV-irradiated RAD
cells.   Log-phase cells irradiated at 254 nm (100 J/m^2) were
aerated in buffer at 28°C ($\bigcirc$) with or ($\bullet$) without exposure to
PR light (2.3 J/m^2/sec) during the first hour after irradiation
with UV.

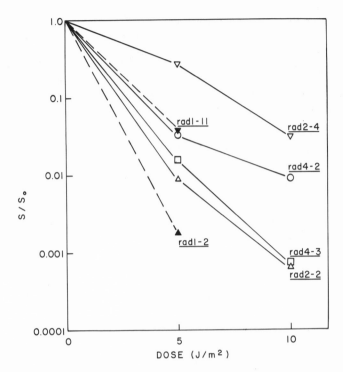

Fig. 4.   UV sensitivity of various <u>rad</u> strains. Log-phase cells
(3-5 x 10[7] cells/ml) in YNB-D liquid medium were diluted in
phosphate buffer, spread on YPD agar plates and irradiated at 254
nm. Macroscopic colonies were counted after 4-5 days of incubation
in the dark at 25°C.   Cultures were the same as those used for
post-UV single-strand DNA break determinations (see Fig. 6).

        The relationship of the UV-induced, incubation-dependent
single-strand breaks observed in wild-type yeast, to the excision
of pyrimidine dimers specifically, was suggested by experiments
under photoreactivating (PR) and non-PR conditions. Prelabeled
cells irradiated at 254 nm (100 J/m^2) were either held in the dark
or exposed to PR light for 1 hr prior to continued incubation in
the dark. The data shown in Fig. 3 demonstrate that exposure to
PR light reduced the number of UV-induced, incubation-dependent
single-strand breaks. Enzymatic PR in yeast is mediated by the
in situ monomerization of pyrimidine dimers (27). In the excision
repair-deficient haploid strain <u>rad4-3</u> this effect can be observed
as a more rapid loss of sites sensitive to a dimer-specific endonuclease when UV irradiated cells are exposed to PR light [25].
The reduction in endogenous single strand DNA breaks by exposure of
UV irradiated cells to PR light (Fig. 3) therefore suggests that the
breaks are related to the presence of pyrimidine dimers specifically.

Having established to our satisfaction that the measurement of endogenous single strand breaks in the DNA of UV irradiated wild-type yeast was both technically reproducible and biologically relevant to the exision of pyrimidine dimers, subsequent studies were performed with a number of mutants in the RAD3 group. At the time of writing, two allelic members of each of three genetic loci (rad1-2, rad1-11; rad2-2, rad2-4; rad4-2, and rad4-3) and a single allele from a fourth locus (rad3-1) have been examined. All of these strains are radiation sensitive [31] (Fig. 4) and are deficient in pyrimidine dimer excision as demonstrated by significantly reduced ability to remove sites in DNA sensitive to a dimer specific endonuclease probe (Fig. 5) (unpublished data).

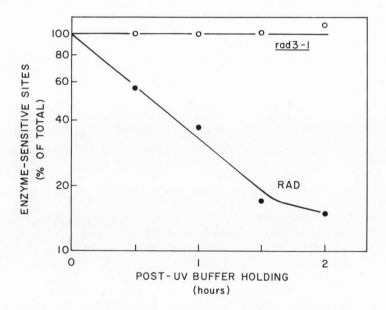

Fig. 5.   Dimer-specific endonuclease sensitive sites in the nuclear DNA of (●) RAD and (○) rad3-1 cells during post-UV holding in buffer. Cells from log phase cultures were irradiated in potassium phosphate buffer (pH 7.0) and then aerated in buffer for various periods of time. The numbers of sites sensitive to M. luteus dimer-specific endonuclease activity were determined as described previously [25].

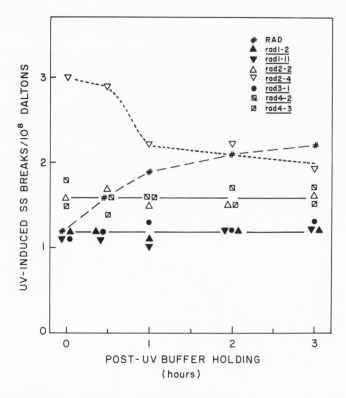

Fig. 6.   UV-induced single strand breaks in the nuclear DNA of
rad and RAD strains of yeast during aeration in buffer at 29°C.
The numbers of breaks were determined relative to unirradiated
unincubated samples as described in Fig. 2.

The results shown in Fig. 6 demonstrate both similarities and
differences between wild-type and mutant strains and within mutants
at different genetic loci.   All strains showed a significant and
reproducible number of single strand breaks in DNA immediately
following irradiation which were apparently incubation-independent
(zero time, Fig. 6).   Whether these very early events represent
enzymatically-catalyzed incisions, photochemical breaks or alkali-
labile sites in DNA is not clear.   As shown in Fig. 6, mutants at
two of the loci thus far investigated (RAD1 and RAD3) showed results
quantitatively identical to the wild-type strain.   However, mutants
at the other two loci (RAD2 and RAD4) expressed a larger number of
strand breaks immediately following irradiation.   The exact nature
of the substrate sites involved in this early reaction is being
investigated further.

At times beyond the zero time, the number of incubation-
dependent single-strand DNA breaks continued to increase in the
wild-type strain but not in any of the mutants examined. Independent
studies quoted above have demonstrated a relationship between
incubation-dependent single-strand breaks in DNA and the presence
of pyrimidine dimers. Thus, irrespective of the mechanism of origin
of the very early breaks in DNA observed in both wild-type and
mutant strains, the absence of incubation-dependent breaks in DNA
suggests that the mutants thus far examined are defective to some
extent in incision-related events during pyrimidine dimer excision.
Until the nature of the zero time increase in strand breaks is
clearly understood we are reluctant to make more definitive conclusions about the nature of the biochemical defect in these mutants.

STUDIES WITH CELL-FREE EXTRACTS

Pyrimidine Dimer-Specific DNA Incising Activity

We have made a number of preliminary attempts to demonstrate
an activity in cell-free preparations of S. cerevisiae that would
catalyze the selective incision of UV-irradiated DNA or chromatin.
Thus far we have not been successful in this endeavor. The results
of our in vivo studies described above, which demonstrate that
multiple genetic loci are apparently involved in the incision of
nuclear DNA in UV-irradiated cells, together with the results of
our direct, though as yet somewhat limited, experience with cell-
free systems, suggests that the yeast equivalent of the endonuclease
activity coded by the uvrA, B and C genes of E. coli may be at
least as difficult to identify and isolate as has been the case
with that prokaryote. Further studies are in progress in this area.

Pyrimidine Dimer Excising Activity

Nuclease activity that catalyzes the selective excision of
pyrimidine dimers can be measured independent of a dimer-specific
incising activity by using as a substrate UV-irradiated DNA
previously incised with a dimer-specific endonuclease from another
source [6, 7]. We have exploited this experimental approach using
the dimer-specific endonuclease from M. luteus. An inherent
assumption in this approach is that the incisions catalyzed by the
endonuclease probe are chemically the same as those created by the
putative yeast activity. Thus far, the only well characterized
dimer-specific endonuclease activities from any biological source
are those from M. luteus [3, 15, 19] and from phage T4-infected
E. coli [10, 35]. Until recently, evidence suggested that both
enzymes catalyze cleavage of phophodiester bonds 5' with respect
to dimers, leaving 3'OH and 5'P termini. More recent studies [12]

suggest a more complex mechanism of action of both enzymes. The
details of this postulated mechanism are not germane to the present
discussion, since irrespective of the precise mechanism of DNA
incision, both enzymes leave a substrate in which excision of the
dimer must be effected by a 5'→3' exonuclease activity. Using a
preincised DNA substrate we have detected such dimer excising
activity in extracts of S. cerevisiae.

Preparation of Cell-Free Lysates.   Overnight cultures
inoculated from YPD agar (1% yeast extract, 2% Bactopeptone, 2%
glucose, 2% Bactoagar) were grown in YPD medium. Overnight cultures
were diluted into fresh YPD liquid medium, grown to mid-log phase
($\sim$6 × 10^7 cells/ml) and then harvested by centrifugation. Cells
were washed once with 0.1 M Tris-HCl (pH 7.6) and once with 0.02 M
Tris-HCl (pH 7.6). Washed cells from 150 ml cultures were then
resuspended in 2 ml of 0.02 M Tris-HCl (pH 7.6) and shaken by hand
in a scintillation vial with 0.5 mm diameter glass beads for
intervals of 30 sec for a total of 4 min. Disruption was normally
95-99% complete as judged by cell refractility under a phase contrast
microscope. The lysate was harvested by aspiration and the beads
washed 2-3 times with 1 ml of 0.02 M Tris-HCl (pH 7.6). The
original lysate was combined with the washes and clarified by
centrifugation at 10,000 × g for 15 min at 4°C. The supernatant was
made 10% with respect to glycerol and stored at 4°C.

Preparation of Pre-Incised UV Irradiated DNA.   DNA was purified
from E. coli 15T⁻ grown in a minimal medium supplemented with
250 µg/ml deoxyadenosine and 10 µCi/ml [methyl-^{3}H]thymidine (final
concentration of 4 µg/ml thymidine). After treatment with Proteinase
K, and successive extractions with buffered phenol and chloroform:
isoamyl alcohol (24:1, v/v) the DNA was dialyzed against 100 mM
NaCl, 10 mM EDTA, 10 mM Tris-HCl (pH 7.6). The dialyzed DNA was
irradiated at 254 nm with a dose sufficient to convert ca. 1% of
the total thymine residues into thymine-containing pyrimidine dimers.
DNA was preincised by incubation with M. luteus UV endonuclease
prepared by a modification of the method of Carrier and Setlow [3].
The preparation used corresponded to their fraction II. Prenicked
DNA was repurified as above and dialyzed against 1 mM EDTA, 10 mM
Tris-HCl (pH 7.6).

Measurement of Thymine Dimer Excision.   Standard reactions
contained 12-18 µg preincised DNA (1-1.5 × 10^5 cpm), 10% glycerol,
10 mM MgCl$_2$, and 20 mM Tris-HCl (pH 7.6). Incubations were at 30°C
for varying periods of time. Following incubation samples were
treated with proteinase K and extracted once with buffer-equilibrated
phenol and once with chloroform:isoamyl alcohol (24:1, v/v) prior
to separation of acid-precipitable DNA from the acid-soluble
fraction. The percent of radioactivity present as thymine-containing
pyrimidine dimers in the acid-precipitable fraction was determined as
described by Reynolds et al. [26]. The fraction of radioactivity

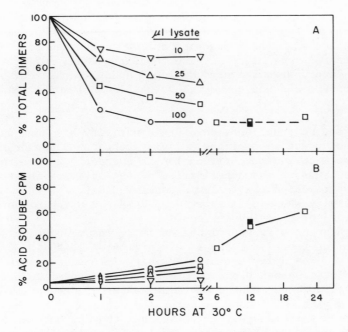

Fig. 7. Loss of thymine-containing pyrimidine dimers (A) and
appearance of [^{3}H] in acid-soluble form during incubation of UV-
irradiated preincised DNA with RAD (S288C) lysate: (A) 100% = 1%
of thymine in thymine-containing pyrimidine dimers; (B) 100%
radioactivity is ∿2 × 10^5 cpm. Preincised DNA (66 μg/reaction) in
a final volume of 300 μl was incubated at 30°C in the presence of
10% (v/v) glycerol, 3 mM MgCl$_2$, 20 mM Tris-HCl (pH 7.6), and various
amounts of clarified yeast lysate. Reactions were terminated by
the addition of EDTA to a final concentration of 20 mM and by
freezing the samples at -20°C. Thymine dimer contents in acid-
precipitable DNA and radioactivity in acid-soluble fractions of the
same incubation mixtures were determined as described under
Materials and Methods.

released into the acid-soluble phase was measured directly by liquid
scintillation spectrometry. Dimer excising activity was defined
as activity catalyzing a reduction in the thymine dimer content of
acid-precipitable DNA relative to appropriate controls, i.e., no
enzyme present and zero time incubations with enzyme.

Results and Discussion

Typical reaction kinetics for thymine dimer excision during
incubation with yeast lysates are presented in Fig. 7A). With
increasing amounts of lysate, increasing numbers of dimers were

selectively released from preincised DNA. The specificity of the
reaction was revealed by a comparison of the percent activity in
dimers released with the precent of the DNA converted to acid-
soluble material. At higher lysate concentrations, 90% of the
thymine in dimers were released during 2 hr of incubation, but only
about 10% of the DNA was converted to acid-soluble material
(Fig. 7B).

Thus far, no fractionation of this activity has been performed
and we cannot state whether the activity represents one or more
enzymes. Work on enzyme purification is currently in progress.
However, preliminary characterization of the activity in crude
extracts has revealed the following observations:
1. The activity was not stimulated by 2 mM ATP using either
    undialyzed or dialyzed lysates.
2. In the absence of glycerol the activity was mildly labile at
    30°C in the reaction buffer. Glycerol (10%) stabilizes the
    activity. The dimer excising activity in crude lysates was
    stable for long periods at 0°C in the presence of 10% glycerol
    (no detectable decrease in activity after 47 days storage) or
    at -20°C with or without glycerol (no detectable decrease in
    activity after 47 days). Freezing and thawing however increased
    nonspecific degradative activity in the clarified lysate.
3. The dimer excising activity has a requirement for divalent
    cation and no activity was observed in the presence of EDTA.
    Optimal activity was observed in the presence of 10 mM Mg^{2+}
    (Fig. 8). The effect of other divalent cations has not yet
    been tested.
4. The activity was present at apparently normal levels in four
    different mutants of the RAD3 group thus far investigated
    (rad1-11, rad2-4, rad3-1 and rad4-3). (Fig. 9).

CONCLUSIONS

Our results to date support our hopes that studies on the
yeast S. cerevisiae will yield significant information on the
molecular mechanism(s) of nucleotide excision repair in eukaryotes
in general. The data on UV sensitivity, loss of sites sensitive to
dimer-specific endonuclease activity, endogenous production of
single strand breaks and measurement of dimer excising nuclease
activity in vitro, are all consistent with the general mode of
pyrimidine dimer excision discussed in the Introduction. Transient,
UV radiation-dependent single-strand breaks were detectable in the
nuclear DNA of wild-type yeast cells during post UV incubation at
28-30°C. Both the photoreactivability of these breaks in wild-type
strains and their absence in the DNA of a number of excision
defective strains suggest that they reflect events associated with
pyrimidine dimer excision. The presence of UV radiation-dependent
but incubation-independent single-strand DNA breaks (or alkali

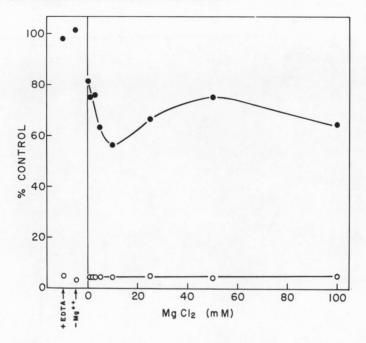

Fig. 8. Dependence of dimer excising activity in clarified RAD
(S288C) lysate on divalent cation concentration. UV irradiated
preincised DNA (ca. 20 µg/reaction) was incubated with 50 µl of
clarified RAD lysate (ca. 7 mg protein/ml as determined by the
method of Lowry et al. [16]) in the presence of 10% (v/v) glycerol,
20 mM Tris-HCl (pH 7.6), and various concentrations of $MgCl_2$ for
30 min at 30°C. Thymine dimer contents in acid-precipitable DNA
and acid-soluble fractions were determined as described under
Material and Methods. The control value (= 100%) for the percentage
of thymine in thymine-containing pyrimidine dimers (●) was 0.835%
of the total radioactivity. The control value (= 100%) for the
percentages of radioactivity in acid-soluble material (○) was
determined separately by measuring the total radioactivity in 10 µl
just prior to acid-precipitation. Total radioactivity per sample
was ∿1.9 × 10^5 cpm. Each point represents the average of two
parallel determinations.

labile sites) in both wild-type and mutant strains currently prevents
any definitive conclusions concerning DNA incision defects in the
various rad mutants examined. Nonetheless, the demonstration that
lysates of strains mutant in the RAD1, RAD2, RAD3, and RAD4 genes
excised thymine dimers normally from preincised DNA supports the
conclusion that these gene products are all concerned with early
events in nucleotide excision repair.

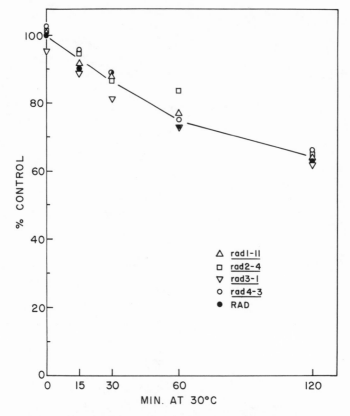

Fig. 9.   Dimer excising activity in RAD and rad clarified lysates.
Reaction conditions were as described in Fig. 8.   All lysates
contained similar numbers of cell equivalents (2×10^9 cell
equivalent/ml) and similar protein concentrations (7-8 mg/ml).
100% = 1.06% of the total thymine present as thymine-containing
pyrimidine dimers.

        Our studies demonstrate that biochemical complexity for
nucleotide excision repair is common to both lower (yeast) and
higher (human) eukaryotes.   At the present time we can only speculate
on the meaning of this complexity.   Judging from the difficulty we
have so far experienced in identifying a DNA incising activity in
cell free extracts, this enzyme (presumably an endonuclease) may
consist of multiple subunits or may constitute a component of a
multi-enzyme repair complex, either of which could be very labile
in cell-free extracts.   In addition or alternatively, the
accessibility to repair enzymes of sites of base damage in DNA
organized into chromosomes may require specific biochemical events
unique to eukaryotes.   Hopefully further studies both with intact

cells and with extracts of S. cerevisiae will provide definitive
answers to some of these speculations in the not too distant future.

ACKNOWLEDGMENTS

Studies at Stanford University were supported by research
grants CA 12428 from the USPHS and NP 174 from the American Cancer
Society, as well as by contract 79EV70032 from the U.S. Department
of Energy. E.C.F. is the recipient of Research Career Development
Award CA 71005 from the USPHS. R.J.R. was supported by a grant
from the Bank of America-Gianinni Foundation and by Tumor Biology
Training Grant 09151 from the USPHS.

Early phases of this study were completed while R.J.R was a
predoctoral trainee with Dr. R. B. Setlow at the University of
Tennessee-Oak Ridge Graduate School of Biomedical Sciences, Biology
Division, Oak Ridge National Laboratory, Oak Ridge, Tenn. At that
time R.J.R was supported by grant GM1974 from the USPHS and research
was sponsored by the U.S. Department of Energy (formerly the U.S.
Energy Research and Development Administration) under contract with
the Union Carbide Corporation.

REFERENCES

1. Arlett, C. F., and A. R. Lehmann, Human disorders showing
        increased sensitivity to the induction of genetic damage,
        Ann. Rev. Genet., 12 (1978) 95–115.
2. Cabib, E., Yeast spheroplasts, In: Methods in Enzymology, Vol.
        22, W. B. Jakoby (Ed.), Academic Press, New York, 1971,
        pp. 120–122.
3. Carrier, W. L., and R. B. Setlow, Endonuclease from Micrococcus
        luteus which has activity toward ultraviolet-irradiated
        deoxyribonucleic acid: purification and properties, J.
        Bacteriol., 102 (1970) 178–186.
4. Cleaver, J. E., Nucleosome structure controls rates of excision
        repair in DNA of human cells, Nature, 270 (1977) 451–453.
5. Cleaver, J. E., and D. Bootsma, Xeroderma pigmentosum:
        biochemical and genetic characteristics, Ann. Rev. Genet.,
        9 (1975) 19–38.
6. Cook, K., E. C. Friedberg, H. Slor, and J. E. Cleaver,
        Excision of thymine dimers from specifically incised DNA
        by extracts of xeroderma pigmentosum cells, Nature, 256
        (1975) 235–236.
7. Cook, K. H., and E. C. Friedberg, Multiple thymine dimer
        excising nuclease activities in extracts of human KB cells,
        Biochemistry 17 (1978) 850–857.
8. Cox, B., and J. Game, Repair systems in Saccharomyces, Mutat.
        Res., 26 (1974) 257–264.

9. Friedberg, E. C., U. K. Ehmann, and J. I. Williams, Human
    diseases associated with defective DNA repair, In: Advances
    in Radiation Biology, Vol. 8, J. T. Lett and H. Adler
    (Eds.), Academic Press, New York, 1979, in press.
10. Friedberg, E. C., and J. J. King, Dark repair of ultraviolet-
    irradiated deoxyribonucleic acid by bacteriophage T4:
    purification and characterization of a dimer-specific phage-
    induced endonuclease, J. Bacteriol., 106 (1971) 500-507.
11. Friedberg, E. C., J. M. Rudé, K. H. Cook, U. K. Ehmann,
    K. Mortelmans, J. E. Cleaver, and H. Slor, Excision repair
    in mammalian cells and the current status of xeroderma
    pigmentosum, In: DNA Repair Processes, W. W. Nichols and
    D. G. Murphy (Eds.), Symposia Specialists, Miami, 1977,
    pp. 21-36.
12. Grossman, L., S. Riazudden, W. Haseltine, and C. Lindan,
    Nucleotide excision repair of damaged DNA, Cold Spring
    Harbor Symp. Quant. Biol., 43, (1979) 947-955.
13. Hanawalt, P. C., P. K. Cooper, A. K. Ganesan, and C. A. Smith,
    DNA repair in bacteria and mammalian cells, Ann. Rev.
    Biochem. 48 (1979) 783-836.
14. Haynes, R. H., B. J. Barclay, F. Eckhardt, O. Landman, B. Kunz,
    and J. G. Little, Genetic control of DNA repair in yeast,
    In: Proceedings of the XIV International Congress on
    Genetics, Moscow, in press.
15. Kaplan, J. C., S. R. Kushner, and L. Grossman, Enzymatic repair
    of DNA.   I. Purification of two enzymes involved in the
    excision of thymine dimers from ultraviolet-irradiated
    DNA, Proc. Natl. Acad. Sci. (U.S.), 63 (1969) 144-151.
16. Lowry, O. H., N. J. Rosebrough, A. L. Farr, R. J. Randall,
    Protein measurement with the Folin phenol reagent, J.
    Biol. Chem., 193 (1951) 265-275.
17. Morowitz, H. J., Absorption effects in volume irradiation of
    microorganisms, Science, 111 (1950) 229-230.
18. Mortelmans, K., E. C. Friedberg, H. Slor, G. Thomas, and J. E.
    Cleaver, Defective thymine dimer excision by cell-free
    extracts of xeroderma pigmentosum cells, Proc. Natl. Acad.
    Sci. (U.S.), 73 (1976) 2757-2761.
19. Nakaryama, H., S. Okubo, and Y. Takagi, Repair of ultraviolet-
    damaged DNA in Micrococcus lysodeikticus. I. An endo-
    nuclease specific for ultraviolet-irradiated DNA, Biochim.
    Biophys. Acta, 228 (1971) 67-82.
20. Prakash, L., Repair of pyrimidine dimers in nuclear and
    mitochondrial DNA of yeast irradiated with low doses of
    ultraviolet light, J. Mol. Biol., 98 (1975) 781-795.
21. Prakash, L., Repair of pyrimidine dimers in radiation-sensitive
    mutants rad3, rad4, rad6 and rad9 of Saccharomyces
    cerevisiae, Mutat. Res., 45 (1977) 13-20.
22. Prakash, L., Defective thymine dimer excision in radiation-
    sensitive mutants rad10 and rad16 of Saccharomyces
    cerevisiae, Mol. Gen. Genet., 152 (1977) 125-128.

23. Prakash, L., and S. Prakash, Pathways of DNA repair in yeast, In: DNA Repair Mechanisms, P. C. Hanawalt, E. C. Friedberg, and C. F. Fox (Eds.), Academic Press, New York, 1978, pp. 413-416.

24. Resnick, M. A., and J. K. Setlow, Repair of pyrimidine dimer damage induced in yeast by ultraviolet light, J. Bacteriol., 109 (1972) 979-986.

25. Reynolds, R. J., Removal of pyrimidine dimers from Saccharomyces cerevisiae nuclear DNA under nongrowth conditions as detected by a sensitive, enzymatic assay, Mutat. Res., 50 (1978) 43-56.

26. Reynolds, R. J., K. H. Cook, and E. C. Friedberg, The measurement of thymine-containing pyrimidine dimers in DNA by one-dimensional thin-layer chromatography, In: Handbook of DNA Repair Techniques, E. C. Friedberg and P. C. Hanawalt (Eds.), Marcel Dekker, New York, in press.

27. Setlow, J. K., The effects of ultraviolet radiation and photoreactivation, In: Comprehensive Biochemistry, Vol. 27, M. Florkin and E. H. Stotz (Eds.), Elsevier, Amsterdam, 1967, pp. 157-209.

28. Setlow, R. B., Repair deficient human disorders and cancer, Nature, 271 (1978) 713-717.

29. Smerdon, M. J., and M. W. Lieberman, Nucleosome rearrangement in human chromatin during UV-induced DNA repair synthesis, Proc. Natl. Acad. Sci. (U.S.), 75 (1978) 4238-4241.

30. Smerdon, M. J., T. D. Tlsty, and M. W. Lieberman, Distribution of ultraviolet-induced DNA repair synthesis in nuclease sensitive and resistant regions in human chromatin, Biochemistry, 17 (1978) 2377-2386.

31. Snow, R., Mutants of yeast sensitive to ultraviolet light, J. Bacteriol., 94 (1967) 571-575.

32. Unrau, P., R. Wheatcroft, and B. S. Cox, The excision of pyrimidine dimers from DNA of ultraviolet irradiated yeast, Mol. Gen. Genet., 113 (1971) 359-362.

33. Waters, R., and E. Moustacchi, The disappearance of ultraviolet-induced pyrimidine dimers from the nuclear DNA of exponential and stationary phase cells of Saccharomyces cerevisiae following various post-irradiation treatments, Biochim. Biophys. Acta, 353 (1974) 407-419.

34. Williams, J. I., and E. C. Friedberg, DNA excision repair in chromatin after ultraviolet irradiation of human fibroblasts in culture, Biochemistry, 18 (1979) 3965-3972.

35. Yasuda, S., and M. Sekiguchi, T4 endonuclease involved repair of DNA, Proc. Natl. Acad. Sci. (U.S.), 67 (1970) 1839-1845.

CHAPTER 9

GENETIC ANALYSIS OF ERROR-PRONE REPAIR SYSTEMS IN

Saccharomyces cerevisiae

LOUISE PRAKASH[1] and SATYA PRAKASH[2]

[1]Department of Radiation Biology and Biophysics,
School of Medicine, and [2]Department of Biology,
University of Rochester, Rochester, New York 14627
(U.S.A.)

SUMMARY

The manner in which ultraviolet induced mutagenesis occurs in
yeast is discussed and compared with ultraviolet mutagenesis in
Escherichia coli.   In both excision proficient and excision
deficient strains of Escherichia coli, mutations arise as the
square of the ultraviolet dose whereas in yeast, mutations arise
as the square of the dose only in excision proficient strains. In
excision defective yeast strains, mutations induced by ultraviolet
arise with linear kinetics. Ultraviolet irradiation of excision
proficient haploid or diploid yeast during G1 results in fixation
of mutation in both DNA strands prior to DNA replication, whereas
in excision defective strains, the frequency of two strand
mutations is very low, and the frequency of one strand mutations
and mutations appearing in the second post irradiation mitotic
division is increased. All of these results in yeast can be
explained by error prone excision repair of two closely spaced
dimers in opposite DNA strands in excision proficient strains and
occasional error prone filling of postreplication gaps, which are
not usually overlapping daughter strand gaps, in excision defective
yeast. The dependence of UV mutagenesis on functional RAD6, REV3,
CDC8 and MMS3 gene functions is discussed. The MMS3 function
appears to be required for UV mutagenesis in a/α diploids but is
dispensible in a/a or α/α diploids and in haploids, suggesting that
differences exist between error prone repair processes in haploids,
a/a, α/α diploids vs. a/α diploids.

141

Alkylating agent induced mutations in yeast depend on functional RAD6, RAD9, RAD51 and RAD52 genes. Different alleles of the RAD52 locus differ in their effects on ethyl methanesulfonate induced mutations of different sites within the same gene. Misreplication of O^6-alkyl guanine probably does not account for most of the mutations induced by alkylating agents in yeast: instead, they probably result from RAD6-dependent error prone repair of gaps opposite O^6-alkyl guanine. Error prone repair pathways for repair of radiation damage differ in some respects from error prone repair of damage induced by chemical agents.

INTRODUCTION

Cells exposed to DNA damaging agents can respond in a variety of ways to potentially lethal or mutagenic alterations in their genome. The way in which DNA damage is modified depends on the genetic constitution of the organism as well as the post-exposure conditions. Conversion of lethal to nonlethal lesions can occur in an error-free way, in which case, no mutations are produced, or in an error-prone manner, which generates mutations.

Specific steps involved in repair of damage induced by different agents may vary, but, many steps are shared. For example, although ultraviolet light (UV) irradiation, gamma-ray irradiation, and methyl methanesulfonate (MMS) treatment all produce single-strand breaks in DNA, the mechanism by which the breaks arise is different for each agent. Absence of exonucleolytic activity or repair synthesis or ligase activity during excision repair of UV induced pyrimidine dimers will result in single-strand breaks; gamma-ray irradiation can induce DNA strand breaks directly; alternatively, they can also arise indirectly following excision of modified bases. In the case of DNA alkylated with MMS, breaks can arise by apurinic (AP) endonucleases acting at AP sites generated either by spontaneous depurination or specific excision of certain alkylated bases. The ability to repair single-strand breaks in DNA will thus be required for repair of damage induced by all three agents.

REPAIR OF UV-INDUCED DAMAGE AND MUTAGENESIS

By far the most characterized damaging agent is UV, and our knowledge of repair of UV damage comes from studies in Escherichia coli and the yeast, Saccharomyces cerevisiae. Since yeast can be maintained as stable haploids or diploids and has a typical higher eukaryotic cell cycle, one can examine various repair processes during different stages of the cell cycle and in cells of different ploidy. Recent work from our laboratory indicates that different repair processes may operate in haploids and diploids.

In yeast [1, 28, 52, 65] as in E. coli [3, 19, 25, 61], excision deficient strains yield mutants at doses which are nonmutagenic in excision-proficient strains. However, the number of loci known to be involved in excision of UV induced pyrimidine dimers is larger in yeast than in E. coli, where uvrA, uvrB and uvrC products function as a complex in endonucleolytic nicking at the site of a dimer [57] and uvrD plays a role in some later step of the excision repair process [58]. In yeast, a mutation at any one of the following nine loci, RAD1 [40, 59, 60], RAD2 [53], RAD3, RAD4 [42], RAD10, RAD16 [43], RAD7, RAD14 and MMS19 [46] results in retention of dimers in the DNA. It is not known which loci are the structural genes for UV endonuclease and it is likely that some of the gene products play an indirect role in dimer excision [43, 46]. A mutation at each of these loci results in enhanced UV induced mutations. Thus, in both E. coli and yeast, an unexcised dimer is more mutagenic than an excised dimer. In both organisms, photo-reactivation can substantially reduce the yield of mutations.

There is a great deal of evidence from E. coli that most lesions are repaired in an error-free manner and that the potentially mutagenic lesions are a rare class of the total damage induced by UV [2, 33, 64]. A commonly held view of mutagenesis in E. coli is that lesions which occur in close enough proximity so as to block constitutive error-free repair, induce a system of repair, designated SOS repair, which can take care of otherwise irreparable damage [51, 62-64]. This induced SOS repair is lexA+, recA+ and polC+ dependent and probably occurs because of incorporation of bases opposite noncoding lesions due to inhibition of editing function of polymerase III [4, 5]. It has been suggested that the lesion responsible for inducing this repair system is an overlapping daughter strand gap (ODSG) [56]; this lesion cannot be repaired by conventional postreplication recombination repair [54]. An ODSG arises when DNA containing unexcised dimers in close proximity to each other, on opposite strands, replicates. In excision proficient strains, mutations can also arise prior to DNA replication when excision of one of two closely spaced dimers on opposite strands exposes the other dimer on the other strand. In such a case, error-prone excision repair could take place, as suggested by Sedgwick [56]. The requirements of two dimers for induction of SOS repair and mutagenesis can explain the dose-squared kinetics observed in excision-proficient and excision-deficient strains of E. coli. Other interpretations of the observed data have also been proposed [16, 64]. Studies on the loss of photoreversibility of mutations can provide information on when and how mutational lesions become fixed. Experiments with uvrA⁻ E. coli on loss of photoreversibility kinetics have been interpreted as error-prone repair occurring only in the first replication after UV and not in subsequent rounds of DNA replication [8].

Somewhat different conclusions have been reached from studies in yeast in which mutations were monitored for several cell generations following UV irradiation of RAD+/RAD+ diploids. For these experiments, a system of a high mutation frequency associated with high survival was necessary; the system used measured the frequency of recessive lethal mutations in diploid yeast exposed to UV irradiation [22]. Diploid RAD+/RAD+ cells in G1 were UV-irradiated and placed at different locations on solid media so that individual cells could be monitored microscopically for one or two post-irradiation divisions and then physically separated from each other. Clones derived from the isolated cells were transferred to media where meiosis could take place; meiotic products were identified and characterized genetically so that the genetic constitution of the original irradiated diploid cell could be determined. At doses resulting in 90% survival, two-strand mutations occur with twice the frequency as one-strand mutations; and virtually all mutations arise by the first round of DNA replication. Different results are obtained when similar experiments are carried out in the excision-defective rad1-1 mutant [23]. The frequency of two-strand mutations falls to about 0 in the excision-defective strain compared to 0.168 in the RAD+ strain; the frequency of delayed mutations, i.e., occurring in the second cell division, rises from 0 in the RAD+ strain to 0.122 in the rad1-1 mutant. Similar results were obtained in another excision defective mutant, rad2-20 [11], using a different mutational system. Experiments in the rad2-20 mutant were carried out in stationary haploid cells using a forward nonselective system, that of scoring white adex ade2 double auxotrophs arising after UV irradiation of the red pigmented ade2 cells. In the RAD+ strain, pure mutant clones occurred with 10X the frequency as sectored clones, suggesting that the UV-induced mutations are fixed in both DNA strands prior to replication. In the excision-defective rad2-20 mutant, pure clones and sectored clones were equally frequent. All of these results suggest that excision ability is required for two-strand mutagenesis. In excision-proficient strains of yeast, repair of closely spaced dimers on opposite DNA strands may be mutagenic, excision of one dimer on one strand may result in the dimer on the complementary strand, near the first dimer, being exposed. Such a lesion could not be repaired by conventional error-free repair, and error-prone repair activity may be required. Such a mechanism of UV mutagenesis in excision proficient strains of yeast also explains the occurrence of two strand mutations. There is no evidence in yeast to indicate whether the error-prone repair activity is inducible or constitutive.

In the excision-defective strains of yeast, mutations must arise in a different way. Two-strand mutations are not observed, and delayed mutations are frequent. Error-prone post-replication repair could account for the mutagenesis observed in excision-defective strains. Gaps could be filled in opposite the dimer with some mistakes being made.

Another difference between E. coli and yeast is apparent when one considers the kinetics of mutation induction in yeast. In RAD+ haploid [24] or diploid [30] yeast, UV-induced revertants at the arg4-17 site arise as the square of the dose. In the excision-defective rad1-1 mutant, however, they arise in proportion to the first power of the dose [24]. In E. coli on the other hand, mutations at a trp ochre allele arise as the square of the dose in both uvr+ and uvr- strains [8, 9]. Induced reversion at two other ochre alleles, ade2-1 and lys2-1, also occur with linear kinetics in the excision defective rad2-20 mutant of yeast [12]. This holds only for low doses, of up to $0.9 \, J/m^2$. At higher doses, a departure from linearity, to almost $(dose)^4$ was observed for both site and suppressor revertants [12]. Linear kinetics of mutation induction in excision defective yeast are compatible with error prone filling in of some post-replication gaps which are not necessarily ODSGs.

GENETIC CONTROL OF UV-INDUCED MUTATIONS

Several mutations exist in yeast which result in a substantial decrease in the UV mutability of many loci. These include mutations in the RAD6, REV3, CDC8 and MMS3 loci. Survival following UV irradiation in rad6-1 rev3-1, rad6-1 cdc8-3, and rad6-1 mms3-1 strains indicate that all four genes, RAD6, REV3, CDC8, and MMS3 are involved in the same repair pathway. Mutants at each of these four genes were isolated by different methods. The rad6-1 mutant, an amber allele, was obtained by screening for UV sensitive strains among the survivors of EMS and UV treated cells [7]; rev3 mutants were obtained by screening for strains which showed a great reduction of UV-induced reversion of the highly UV-revertible ochre allele, arg4-17 [34]; cdc8 mutants were isolated as mutants temperature sensitive for growth and shown to be temperature-sensitive for DNA synthesis [17]; the mms3 mutant was obtained by screening for clones sensitive to MMS [45]. Mutants at these four loci, although they are phenotypically different, do share a common property, that of reducing UV-induced reversions at many loci. The rad6-1 mutant shows pleiotropic effects: marked sensitivity to the lethal effects of UV, X-rays, MMS, and trimethoprim [7, 14] and numerous other chemical mutagens such as ethyl methanesulfonate (EMS) and N-methyl-N'-nitro-N-nitrosoguanidine (MNNG) and HNO_2 [39]. Although UV induced mutations are greatly reduced, rad6-1 mutants are spontaneous mutators [18]. Premeiotic DNA synthesis occurs, but sporulation is blocked [47]. In addition, a decrease in meiotic recombination is observed. Homologous genetic recombination induced by UV [20] or EMS [47], on the other hand, is not lowered in rad6-1/rad6-1 strains.

UV-induced forward mutations to canavanine resistance and reversion at the his1-1, lys2-1 and arg4-17 loci are greatly reduced in rad6-1 haploids [32]. Diploids homozygous for cyc1-131, an initiation mutant in the structural gene for iso-1-cytochrome c, and rad6-1 show no UV induced mutations even though cyc1-131 reverts with UV in RAD+ strains [28]. Reversion of the ochre allele cyc1-9 is greatly reduced in both haploids and diploids of rad6-1 [32].

In general, rad6 mutants are refractory to UV mutagenesis. Since rad6-1 is a nonsense allele and could be suppressed, the possibility that mutations which appear to be induced in rad6 strains are due to suppression of rad6 always remains. Determining the UV sensitivity of the "induced" revertants does not necessarily provide unambiguous results, since it is possible to have the effect on mutation suppressed without suppressing the component of rad6 which contributes to survival. A second source of "induced" mutations in rad6 strains could be due to spontaneous reversion, since rad6-1 seems to be a spontaneous mutator [18, 50]. The rad6-1 mutation drastically reduces or abolishes UV-induced reversion at all the loci tested which include missense alleles, amber, ochre and frame-shift mutations; and the effect of rad6 manifests itself in both haploids and diploids. The effect of the rad6 gene extends to mutations induced by a wide variety of chemical agents [39] and is not restricted to UV mutagenesis.

Other mutants affecting UV mutability were isolated by Lemontt [34] by screening for a reduction in UV-induced reversion of the highly UV revertible ochre allele, arg4-17. Although spontaneous revertants of arg4-17 consist of both site and suppressor revertants, UV-induced revertants are predominantly locus revertants [24, 34]. Lemontt identified three loci among these mutants: REV1, REV2, and REV3, with three alleles, three alleles and 14 alleles, respectively. At 265 ergs/mm^2, reversion frequencies of the locus for arg4-17 were 1/30 the wild type level in rev1-1 and rev3-1 and 1/3 in rev2-1 haploids. Similar results were obtained in diploids, with the greatest reduction in rev1-1/rev1-1 and rev3-1/rev3-1; rev2-1/rev2-1 showed the least effect. Both the rev1-1 and rev3-1 mutants also decrease UV reversion of another ochre suppressible allele, lys1-1, and of the missense allele arg4-6, whereas rev2-1 strains have less of an effect on lys1-1 and none on arg4-6. The yield of UV-induced auxotrophs in prototrophic rev strains is reduced to 4% the wild type level in rev1-1 and rev3-1 and to 64% the wild type level in rev2-1 strains; for ade1 or ade2 auxotrophs, the yield is reduced to 2%, 19%, and 88% the wild type level in rev3-1, rev1-1 and rev2-1 strains respectively [36]. Since neither meiotic nor UV or x-ray-induced mitotic recombination is lowered in strains homozygous for rev mutations, Lemontt concluded that UV mutagenesis may not require recombinational events [35].

Diploids homozygous for rad6-1 show UV induced recombination but no mutability. In addition, rad52 homozygous diploids are defective in all kinds of recombination - UV and x-ray-induced mitotic, as well as meiotic [49], yet UV induced mutations occur to near normal (RAD+) levels [28]. All these results suggest that if recombination plays any role in UV mutagenesis in yeast, it is probably a very minor one.

Further evidence for allele-specific control of UV induced reversion comes from studies with mutants in the CYC1 gene, the structural gene for iso-1-cytochrome c of yeast. In diploids homozygous for rev1-1 or rev1-3, no decrease in UV induced reversion was seen for cyc1-115, a proline missense mutant at residue 14; cyc1-131, a missense mutant containing GUG instead of the normal AUG initiation codon; and for three frameshift mutants, cyc1-183, cyc1-239, and cyc1-331, with +A at position 10, -G at position 4 and -A at position 2, respectively [29]. The REV1+ function was required for reversion at 11 other sites in the CYC1 gene, which included three other initiation mutants, cyc1-13, cyc1-51 and cyc1-133, with AUPy or AUA; CUG and AGG, respectively; three ochre mutants, three amber mutants, another proline missense mutant, cyc1-6, at position 12, and one frameshift mutant.

The rev2-1 mutation, on the other hand, affects reversion of only certain highly revertible ochre alleles, a result in agreement with the earlier observation of Lemontt [34, 36]. No effect of rev2-1 occurred for reversion of any of the other 10 alleles tested [30]. Of the three ochre alleles tested, REV2+ was required only for reversion of cyc1-91 and not cyc1-72 or cyc1-17. The REV2+ product is apparently required for mutation of arg4-17 and cyc1-91, two highly revertible ochre alleles, and not for any of the amber, missense, or frameshift mutations tested so far.

The REV3+ function shows a broader spectrum of alleles for which its function is required for UV induced reversions. As in the case of rev1, which was not required for reversion of cyc1-115 or cyc1-131, rev3 is also apparently dispensible for reversion of these two sites. The decrease in UV mutability of these loci is only about 50% in rev3 strains [31]. All other alleles of cyc1 examined, which include one ochre allele, one amber allele, three missense alleles, and four frameshift alleles, required REV3+ for reversion [31]. Thus, the three REV loci are required at different sites and to different extents for UV mutability: REV2+ acts mainly at highly revertible ochre alleles, REV1+ is somewhat broader in its spectrum, being required for mutation of all amber and ochre alleles, but only some missense and frameshift alleles. REV3+ shows that same mutational spectrum as REV1+, but in addition, is required for reversion of all the frameshift sites tested.

In order to determine whether gene functions required for DNA synthesis also play a role in mutagenic repair of UV damage in yeast, we examined UV induced mutations in cdc mutants which affect DNA synthesis [44]. Mutations at the CDC4 and CDC7 loci, which block initiation of DNA synthesis, and a mutation at the CDC21 locus, the structural gene for thymidylate synthetase, did not lower UV-induced reversions. Mutations at the CDC8 locus did reduce UV induced reversion at all loci tested. The cdc8 mutation shows cessation of DNA synthesis upon incubation at the restrictive temperature and is classified as an elongation mutant. UV induced reversion of two ochre alleles, arg4-17 and lys2-1, and two nonsuppressible alleles, tyr1 and ura1, was lowered in cdc8-1 mutants [44]. At comparable levels of survival, the frequency of UV induced reversion of arg4-17 in cdc8-1 haploids was 1/8 the level obtained in CDC+ haploids. Two other alleles, cdc8-2 and cdc8-3, behaved in a similar manner. The CDC8+ function is probably involved in excision repair as well as in RAD6-dependent repair since double mutants of cdc8 rad1 appear to have about the same UV sensitivity as rad1 single mutants, which are more sensitive than cdc8 mutants [44]. Mutants at the rad1 locus, as mentioned above, show enhanced UV induced mutation frequencies whereas rad51 mutants do not alter mutation frequency. Since double mutants of cdc8 rad1 and cdc8 rad51 show the characteristic low UV induced reversion frequencies observed in cdc8 single mutants [44], the CDC8+ gene probably plays a direct role in error prone repair. Although the product of CDC8 is not known, experiments with purified DNA polymerases I and II from CDC+ and cdc8 strains suggest that CDC8+ is not the structural gene for either DNA polymerase I or II [44].

Error-prone repair in yeast does not appear to be a major repair pathway contributing to survival following UV irradiation, since cdc8 mutants are not particularly UV-sensitive but show a great reduction in UV-induced reversion at all loci tested. The rad6 mutants, which show low or no UV induced reversion, are quite UV sensitive. The enhanced UV sensitivity of rad6, therefore, very likely derives from its largely error free role in repair.

Thus far, our discussion on repair of UV damage and its genetic control has not dealt with the problem of susceptibility to lethal effects and ability to repair as a function of cell cycle and ploidy. The ability of a haploid cell to repair DNA damage induced by ionizing radiation depends on whether one or two copies of the genomes are present, as manifested by the resistant tail observed after exposure of haploids to x-rays or gamma-rays. This tail is correlated with the fraction of budded cells in the population, representing cells that have replicated their DNA. For UV-induced mutations, we have found that the mms3-1 mutation shows a differential effect on mutability in haploids and a/α diploids. The mutant was found among MMS-sensitive mutants isolated by Prakash and Prakash [45] and is not allelic to any rad mutants. It shows sensitivity to UV, gamma-rays, and EMS as well. No effect on UV-induced reversion of ochre suppressible sites arg4-17 and lys2-1, or the missense allele his1-7, is observed in mms3-1 haploids. A significant lowering of reversion of these same alleles occurs

following UV irradiation of a/α mms3-1/mms3-1 diploids. In either
a/a or α/α mms3-1/mms3-1 diploids, wild type (MMS+) levels of
revertibility of arg4-17 are restored; mms3-1, MMS+, mms3-1/mms3-1
a/a or α/α or MMS+/MMS+ a/a or α/α diploids, and a/α MMS+/MMS+
diploids all show high UV revertibility. The only genotype among
these which shows low reversion is a/α mms3-1/mms3-1 [47]. The
mms3-1 mutant belongs in the same epistatic group as rad6. The
MMS3+ function appears to be required for UV mutagenesis in a/α
diploids but is dispensible in haploids and a/a or α/α diploids.
This suggests that differences do exist between error prone repair
processes in haploids, a/a, α/α diploids vs. a/α diploids.

CHEMICAL MUTAGENESIS IN YEAST AND ITS DEPENDENCE
ON FUNCTIONAL REPAIR

Although the RAD6+, REV3+, CDC8+, and MMS3+ gene products are
required for UV mutagenesis, they are not all required for chemical
mutagenesis, which, in yeast, is dependent on a functional repair
system [39]. A class of chemical mutagens studied and used extensively is the alkylating agents, such as EMS and MNNG. For a long
time, the mutagenicity of alkylating agents was thought to result
from errors made during replication of alkylated DNA [10, 13].
Alkylated bases were believed to be miscoding and cause misincorporation; therefore, mutations induced by such agents were thought
to be independent of cellular repair mechanisms. The predominant
lesion found in DNA after treatment of either whole cells or
purified DNA with alkylating agents is 7-alkyl guanine (7-alk G)
[26, 27]. Other minor reaction products are formed, the proportion
of each type of product varies with the different agents. The idea
of 7-alk G being the mutagenic lesion was abandoned when the
mutagenic potency of various alkylating agents was compared and
great differences were observed [27]. EMS is highly mutagenic in
many systems whereas MMS is not, yet, both form 7-alk G as the
major lesion in DNA. Loveless [37] suggested that the mutagenic
potency and carcinogenic potency of a chemical agent and the amount
of O^6-alkyl guanine (O^6-alk G) produced in the DNA by the agent
were correlated. The earlier ideas were modified to replace 7-alk
G with O^6-alk G as the mutagenic lesion responsible for replication
errors. The mutagenicity of the various agents could be explained
by the amount of O^6-alk G formed in the DNA. Another aspect of
mutagenicity of the potent alkylating agents is that they also tend
to be highly specific in the type of alteration they produce:
there is preferential induction of GC to AT transitions only by the
agents which also are producers of large amounts of O^6-alk G
relative to 7-alk G. Mutagenic specificity was demonstrated in the
iso-1-cytochrome c system in yeast where mutants with defined
alterations existed [48]. EMS, diethyl sulfate (DES), and MNNG
were found preferentially to revert cyc1-131, which requires a GC
to AT transition to yield true revertants, whereas MMS and dimethyl

sulfate (DMS) showed no preferential reversion. It was then
suggested that both mutagenic potency as well as mutagenic
specificity might be accounted for by 0^6-alk G in the DNA. Confirming data on specificity of EMS and MNNG induced mutations comes
from work in E. coli where a forward mutational system was employed
[6]. Specific base changes in mutants of the lacI gene were
determined in a total of 321 amber mutants and 370 ochre mutants
induced by EMS, and 303 amber and 215 ochre mutants induced by MNNG.
Over 97% of the induced mutants are due to GC to AT transitions.

In vitro experiments utilizing synthetic polymers of 0^6-methyl-
deoxyguanylic acid (m^6dG) as templates of Micrococcus luteus RNA
polymerase show misincorporation of UMP in the product [38]. While
both poly(dC, dG) and poly(dC, m^6dG) lead to misincorporation of
UMP when the preferred substrate CTP is absent, only poly(dC,
m^6dG) causes misincorporation in the presence of CTP. Since CTP
does not inhibit incorporation of UMP, C is probably not normally
paired with 0^6-methyl G [15].

These ideas on the mechanism of alkylation mutagenesis
occurring by misreplication were reinforced by studies in E. coli
where it was found that the recA function, known to be required for
UV and ionizing radiation induced mutations, was not required for
mutations induced by MNNG and EMS [21, 25]. Contrasting results
were obtained in yeast where the effect of a wide variety of
chemical mutagens was found to be decreased in the presence of a
mutation at either the RAD6+ or RAD9+ locus [39]. This work was
carried out in stationary phase diploids homozygous for either
rad6-1 or rad9-1 and cyc1-131, an allele which reverts well with
both radiation and chemical agents [48]. A functional RAD6+ or
RAD9+ gene is required for induction of mutations at cyc1-131 when
any of the following agents is used: EMS, DES, MMS, DMS, nitrogen
mustard, nitroquinoline oxide, MNNG, β-propiolactone, and tritium
decay following incorporation of ^{3}H-uracil. In each of these cases,
there was no induction of even a low level of mutations. A dose-
response curve for survival and mutation following MNNG treatment
is given in Figure 1, as a representative example of the response
obtained with several mutagens. Even at doses where survival is
still high in rad6 and rad9 strains, very few, if any, mutations
are induced by MNNG. It was concluded that a functional repair
system was required for chemical mutagenesis to occur. Two mutagens
which responded somewhat differently were nitrous acid and nitroso-
imidazolidone (NIL). At nonlethal doses of either NIL or HNO_2,
mutations were induced in both rad6-1/rad6-1 and rad9-1/rad9-1, to
the same extent or more than in the RAD+/RAD+ strains, but as the
dose increased and survival decreased, mutation frequencies also
decreased below the wild type level in both strains.

A study of the effect of various rad genes on chemically
induced mutations at cyc1-131 showed that revl, rev2, or rev3

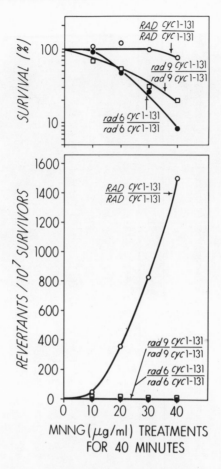

Fig. 1.   Survival and cycl-131/cycl-131 dose-response curves for
(○) RAD+/RAD+, LC-0, (●) rad6-1/rad6-1, LC-6, and (□) rad9-1/
rad9-1, LC-9 treated with MNNG. Reproduced from Prakash [39] with
permission.

strains had no effect on EMS induced mutations and that the only
other strain with a pronounced effect on reducing EMS induced
reversion was rad52-1 [41], a member of the group of genes believed
to be involved in recombination. Four other alleles of the RAD52+
locus and another member of this epistatic group, rad51, were
studied for their effect on EMS induced reversion of both cycl-131
and cycl-115. Results are presented in Table 1. Although both
sites are EMS-revertible, cycl-115 is more mutable with EMS than is
cycl-131. Allele specific effects are observed both for the site
at which reversion is being measured as well as with different
alleles of the RAD locus. A rad51-1/rad51-1 diploid shows marginal
reduction of EMS reversion of cycl-131 but there is a drastic

TABLE 1

FREQUENCY OF INDUCED CYC1 MUTATIONS (EXPRESSED AS REVERTANTS PER 10^7 SURVIVORS) IN RAD+ AND rad DIPLOID YEAST TREATED FOR VARYING TIMES WITH 1% EMS

Strains	Frequency (revertants/10^7 survivors)[a] cyc1-131 → CYC1				Frequency (revertants/10^7 survivors)[a] cyc1-115 → CYC1			
	0.5 hr	1.0 hr	1.5 hr	2.0 hr	0.5 hr	1.0 hr	1.5 hr	2.0 hr
RAD+/RAD+	173 (93)	366 (87)	640 (83)	861 (83)	722 (99)	1391 (100)	2413 (83)	3284 (81)
rad51-1/rad51-1	100 (76)	225 (51)	323 (35)	395 (30)	0 (56)	1 (39)	70 (24)	101 (22)
rad52-1/rad52-1	24 (83)	33 (51)	29 (26)	2 (13)	18 (41)	35 (18)	58 (7)	42 (0.4)
rad52-3/rad52-3	15 (79)	22 (40)	4 (24)	24 (16)	27 (67)	90 (41)	112 (24)	149 (18)
rad52-4/rad52-4	15 (90)	11 (82)	8 (69)	10 (44)	62 (78)	61 (49)	71 (40)	41 (26)
rad52-5/rad52-5	42 (100)	47 (100)	24 (100)	20 (100)	135 (100)	229 (79)	303 (100)	333 (81)
rad52-6/rad52-6	36 (93)	41 (93)	46 (88)	68 (85)	291 (89)	638 (72)	956 (59)	1282 (53)

[a] Numbers in parentheses represent percent survival. Reversion frequencies are expressed as number of revertants obtained after treating cells with 1% EMS for times shown minus those that occurred spontaneously. In most experiments, spontaneous reversion frequencies were less than 1 per 10^7 cells.

reduction of EMS reversion of cycl-115. The rad52 alleles also show differential effects: rad52-1, rad52-3, and rad52-4 reduce EMS reversion of both cycl-131 and cycl-115 to about the same extent. These three alleles are also the most sensitive of the five alleles to the lethal effects of EMS. Both rad52-5 and rad52-6, on the other hand, are less sensitive and both show a greater reduction of EMS reversion of cycl-131 compared to cycl-115, just the opposite result obtained with rad51-1. Different alleles of the same rad gene therefore differ in their effects on EMS induced mutations of different sites in the genome.

Recent work on EMS- and MNNG-induced mutagenesis in E. coli using higher doses than used in the earlier work also suggests the existence of lexA+-dependent error-prone repair for MNNG and EMS damage. In lexA− mutants, the frequency of MNNG induced mutations rises at low doses, presumably because misreplication, which is independent of lexA+, occurs [55]. As the MNNG dose increases, mutation frequency in the lexA− mutants levels off and remains constant whereas mutations continue to rise in lexA+ strains.

From our work in yeast, we conclude that (1) error-prone repair is required for chemical mutagenesis in yeast and RAD6+, RAD9+, RAD51+ and RAD52+ play a role in this repair, at least at the sites examined; (2) misreplication of O^6-alkyl guanine cannot account for most of the mutations induced by alkylating agents, since rad6 mutants show no alkylation induced mutations at the cycl-131 site; if misreplication does occur, then we have to postulate the requirement for the RAD6+ function for this misrepli-cation; (3) error-prone repair pathways for repair of radiation damage differ in some respects from error prone repair of damage induced by chemical agents, e.g., rev3 has no effect on EMS-induced mutations but affects UV mutability; rad51 and rad52 have no effect on UV mutability but lower EMS mutability. Any model of alkylation mutagenesis in yeast must incorporate the immutability towards EMS and MNNG of rad6 strains and the specificity of these agents for inducing GC to AT transitions. Alkylation induced mutations in yeast may arise during repair of AP sites on one DNA strand when the opposite DNA strand has an unexcised O^6 alkyl guanine and overlaps the gap formed during excision of the AP site. During the repair process requiring RAD6+ and various other gene products, thymine is inserted opposite to O^6 alkyl guanine. Thus, O^6 alkyl guanine will be mutagenic when replicated by the repair complex.

ACKNOWLEDGEMENTS

LP was supported in part by PHS Career Development Award K04 GM-00004. This investigation was supported in part by NIH Grant GM 19261 and in part by the U.S. Department of Energy at the

University of Rochester Department of Radiation Biology and
Biophysics. This paper has been assigned Report No. UR-3490-1666.

REFERENCES

1. Averbeck, D., W. Laskowski, F. Eckardt, and E. Lehmann-Brauns,
    Four radiation sensitive mutants of Saccharomyces.
    Survival after UV- and X ray-irradiation as well as UV-
    induced reversion rates from isoleucine-valine dependence
    to independence, Mol. Gen. Genet., 107 (1970) 117-127.
2. Bridges, B. A., Recent advances in basic mutation research,
    Mutat. Res., 44 (1977) 149-163.
3. Bridges, B. A., R. E. Dennis, and R. J. Munson, Differential
    induction and repair of ultraviolet damage leading to true
    reversions and external suppressor mutations of an ochre
    codon in Escherichia coli B/r WP2, Genetics 57 (1967)
    897-908.
4. Bridges, B. A., R. P. Mottershead, and S. G. Sedgwick,
    Mutagenic DNA repair in Escherichia coli. III. Requirements
    for a function of DNA polymerase III in ultraviolet light
    mutagenesis, Mol. Gen. Genet., 144 (1976) 53-58.
5. Caillet-Fauquet, P., M. Defais and M. Radman, Molecular
    mechanisms of induced mutagenesis. Replication in vivo of
    bacteriophage ϕX174 single-stranded, ultraviolet light-
    irradiated DNA in intact and irradiated host cells,
    J. Mol. Biol., 117 (1977) 95-112.
6. Coulondre, C. and J. H. Miller, Genetic studies of the lac
    repressor. IV. Mutagenic specificity in the lacI gene of
    Escherichia coli, J. Mol. Biol., 117 (1977) 577-606.
7. Cox, B. S. and J. M. Parry, The isolation, genetics and
    survival characteristics of ultraviolet-light sensitive
    mutants in yeast, Mutat. Res., 6 (1968) 37-55.
8. Doubleday, O. P., B. A. Bridges, and M. H. L. Green, Mutagenic
    DNA repair in Escherichia coli. II. Factors affecting
    loss of photoreversibility of UV induced mutations, Mol.
    Gen. Genet., 140 (1975) 221-230.
9. Doudney, C. O., Complexity of the ultraviolet mutation
    frequency response curve in Escherichia coli B/r
    SOS induction, one-lesion and two-lesion mutagenesis,
    J. Bacteriol., 128 (1976) 815-826.
10. Drake, J. W., and R. H. Baltz, The biochemistry of mutagenesis,
    Ann. Rev. Biochem., 45 (1976) 11-37.
11. Eckardt, F., and R. H. Haynes, Induction of pure and sectored
    mutant clones in excision-proficient and deficient strains
    of yeast, Mutat. Res., 43 (1977) 327-338.
12. Eckardt, F. and R. H. Haynes, Kinetics of mutation induction
    by ultraviolet light in excision-deficient yeast, Genetics,
    85 (1977) 225-247.

13. Freese, E., and E. B. Freese, Mutagenic and inactivating DNA
    alterations, Radia. Res. Suppl., 6 (1966) 97–140.
14. Game, J. C., J. G. Little, and R. H. Haynes, Yeast mutants
    sensitive to trimethoprim, Mutat. Res., 28 (1975) 175–182.
15. Gerchman, L. L., and D. B. Ludlum, The properties of O^6-methyl
    guanine in templates for RNA polymerase, Biochim. Biophys.
    Acta, 308 (1973) 310–316.
16. Green, M. H. L., On the possible immunity of newly synthesized
    DNA to error-prone repair, Mutat. Res., 44 (1977) 161–163.
17. Hartwell, L. H., Genetic control of the cell division cycle in
    yeast. II. Genes controlling DNA replication and its
    initiation, J. Mol. Biol., 59 (1971) 183–194.
18. Hastings, P. J., S.-K. Quah, and R. C. von Borstel, Spontaneous
    mutation by mutagenic repair of spontaneous lesions in
    DNA, Nature 264 (1976) 719–722.
19. Hill, R. F., Ultraviolet-induced lethality and reversion to
    prototrophy in Escherichia coli strains with normal and
    reduced dark repair ability, Photochem. Photobiol., 4
    (1965) 563–568.
20. Hunnable, E. G., and B. S. Cox, The genetic control of dark
    recombination in yeast, Mutat. Res., 13 (1971) 297–309.
21. Ishii, Y., and S. Kondo, Comparative analysis of deletion and
    base-change mutabilities of Escherichia coli B strains
    differing in DNA repair capacity (wild-type, uvrA-, polA-,
    recA-) by various mutagens, Mutat. Res., 27 (1975) 27–44.
22. James, A. P. and B. J. Kilbey, The timing of UV mutagenesis
    in yeast: a pedigree analysis of induced recessive
    mutation, Genetics 87 (1977) 237–248.
23. James, A. P., B. J. Kilbey, and G. J. Prefontaine, The timing
    of UV mutagenesis in yeast: continuing mutation in an
    excision defective (rad1-1) strain, Mol. Gen. Genet., 165
    (1978) 207–212.
24. Kilbey, B. J., T. Brychcy, and A. Nasim, Initiation of UV
    mutagenesis in Saccharomyces cerevisiae, Nature, 274 (1978)
    889–891.
25. Kondo, S., H. Ichikawa, K. Iwo, and T. Kato, Base-change
    mutagenesis and phophage induction in strains of
    Escherichia coli with different DNA repair capacities,
    Genetics, 66 (1970) 187–217.
26. Lawley, P. D., Alkylation of nucleic acids and mutagenesis,
    In: Molecular and Environmental Aspects of Mutagenesis,
    L. Prakash, F. Sherman, M. W. Miller, C. W. Lawrence,
    and H. W. Taber, Eds., Charles C Thomas, Springfield, Ill.,
    1974, pp. 17–33.
27. Lawley, P. D., Some chemical aspects of dose-response relation-
    ships in alkylation mutagenesis, Mutat. Res., 23 (1974)
    283–295.
28. Lawrence, C. W., and R. Christensen, UV mutagenesis in
    radiation sensitive strains of yeast, Genetics, 82 (1976)
    207–232.

29. Lawrence, C. W., and R. Christensen, Ultraviolet-induced
      reversion of cyc1 alleles in radiation-sensitive strains
      of yeast: I. rev1 mutant strains, J. Mol. Biol., 122
      (1978) 1-21.
30. Lawrence, C. W., and R. Christensen, Ultraviolet-induced
      reversion of cyc1 alleles in radiation-sensitive strains
      of yeast. II. rev2 mutant strains, Genetics, 90 (1978)
      213-226.
31. Lawrence, C. W., and R. Christensen, Ultraviolet-induced
      reversion of cyc1 alleles in radiation-sensitive strains
      of yeast. III. rev3 mutant strains, Genetics 92 (1979)
      397-408.
32. Lawrence, C. W., J. W. Stewart, F. Sherman, and R. Christensen,
      Specificity and frequency of ultraviolet-induced reversion
      of an iso-1-cytochrome c ochre mutant in radiation-
      sensitive strains of yeast, J. Mol. Biol., 85 (1974)
      137-162.
33. Lehmann, A. R., and B. A. Bridges, DNA repair, Essays Biochem.,
      13 (1977) 71-119.
34. Lemontt, J., Mutants of yeast defective in mutation induced
      by ultraviolet light, Genetics, 68 (1971) 21-33.
35. Lemontt, J., Pathways of ultraviolet mutability in Saccharomyces
      cerevisiae. II. The effect of rev genes on recombination,
      Mutat. Res., 13 (1971) 319-326.
36. Lemontt, J., Induction of forward mutations in mutationally
      defective yeast, Mol. Gen. Genet., 119 (1972) 27-42.
37. Loveless, A., Possible relevance of 0^6 alkylation of deoxy-
      guanosine to the mutagenicity and carcinogenicity of
      nitrosamines and nitrosamides, Nature, 223 (1969) 206-207.
38. Mehta, J. R., and D. B. Ludlum, Synthesis and properties of
      0^6-methyl-deoxyguanylic acid and its copolymers with
      deoxycytidylic acid, Biochim. Biophys. Acta, 521 (1978)
      770-778.
39. Prakash, L., Lack of chemically induced mutation in repair-
      deficient mutants of yeast, Genetics, 78 (1974) 1101-1118.
40. Prakash, L., Repair of pyrimidine dimers in nuclear and
      mitochondrial DNA of yeast irradiated with low doses of
      ultraviolet light, J. Mol. Biol., 98 (1975) 781-795.
41. Prakash, L., Effect of genes controlling radiation sensitivity
      on chemically-induced mutations in Saccharomyces cerevisiae,
      Genetics, 83 (1976) 285-301.
42. Prakash, L., Repair of pyrimidine dimers in radiation-
      sensitive mutants rad3, rad4, rad6 and rad9 of Saccharomyces
      cerevisiae, Mutat. Res., 45 (1977) 13-20.
43. Prakash, L., Defective thymine dimer excision in radiation-
      sensitive mutants rad10 and rad16 of Saccharomyces
      cerevisiae, Mol. Gen. Genet., 152 (1977) 125-128.
44. Prakash, L., D. Hinkle, and S. Prakash, Decreased UV mutagenesis
      in cdc8, a DNA replication mutant of Saccharomyces
      cerevisiae, Mol. Gen. Genet., 172 (1979) 249-258.

45. Prakash, L. and S. Prakash, Isolation and characterization of
         MMS-sensitive mutants of Saccharomyces cerevisiae, Genetics,
         86 (1977) 33-55.
46. Prakash, L. and S. Prakash, Three additional genes involved
         in pyrimidine dimer removal in Saccharomyces cerevisiae:
         RAD7, RAD14 and MMS19, Mol. Gen. Genet., (1979) in press.
47. Prakash, L., and S. Prakash, unpublished results.
48. Prakash, L., and F. Sherman, Mutagenic specificity: reversion
         of iso-1-cytochrome c mutants of yeast, J. Mol. Biol.,
         79 (1973) 65-82.
49. Prakash, S., L. Prakash, W. Burke, and B. Montelone, Effects
         of the RAD52 gene on recombination in Saccharomyces
         cerevisiae, Genetics, in press (1979).
50. Quah, S.-K., personal communication, University of Alberta.
51. Radman, M., Phenomenology of an inducible mutagenic DNA repair
         pathway in Escherichia coli: SOS repair hypothesis, In:
         Molecular and Environmental Aspects of Mutagenesis,
         L. Prakash, F. Sherman, M. W. Miller, C. W. Lawrence, and
         H. W. Taber, Charles C Thomas, Springfield, Ill., 1974,
         pp. 128-142.
52. Resnick, M. A., Induction of mutations in Saccharomyces
         cerevisiae by ultraviolet light, Mutat. Res., 7 (1969)
         315-332.
53. Resnick, M. A., and J. K. Setlow, Repair of pyrimidine dimer
         damage induced in yeast by ultraviolet light, J. Bacteriol.,
         109 (1972) 979-986.
54. Rupp, W. D., C. E. Wilde, III, D. L. Reno, and P. Howard-
         Flanders, Exchanges between DNA strands in ultraviolet-
         irradiated Escherichia coli, J. Mol. Biol., 61 (1971)
         25-44.
55. Schendel, P. F., M. Defais, P. Jeggo, L. Samson, and J. Cairns,
         Pathways of mutagenesis and repair in E. coli exposed to
         low levels of simple alkylating agents, J. Bacteriol.,
         135 (1978) 466-475.
56. Sedgwick, S. G., Misrepair of overlapping daughter strand
         gaps as a possible mechanism for UV induced mutagenesis
         in uvr strains of Escherichia coli: a general model for
         induced mutagenesis by misrepair (SOS repair) of closely
         spaced lesions, Mutat. Res., 41 (1976) 185-200.
57. Seeberg, E., Reconstitution of an Escherichia coli repair
         endonuclease activity from the separated uvrA+ and
         uvrB+/uvrC+ gene products, Proc. Natl. Acad. Sci. (U.S.),
         75 (1978) 2569-2573.
58. Smith, K. C., D. A. Youngs, E. van der Schueren, K. M. Carlson,
         and N. J. Sargentini, Excision repair and mutagenesis are
         complex processes, In: DNA Repair Mechanisms, P. C.
         Hanawalt, E. C. Friedberg, and C. F. Fox, eds., Academic
         Press, New York, Vol. 9, 1978, pp. 247-250.

59. Unrau, P., R. Wheatcroft, and B. S. Cox, The excision of
       pyrimidine dimers from DNA of ultraviolet irradiated yeast,
       Mol. Gen. Genet., 113 (1971) 359–362.
60. Waters, R. and E. Moustacchi, The disappearance of ultraviolet-
       induced pyrimidine dimers from the nuclear DNA of exponen-
       tial and stationary phase cells of Saccharomyces cerevisiae
       following various post-irradiation treatments, Biochim.
       Biophys. Acta, 353 (1974) 407–419.
61. Witkin, E. M., Radiation-induced mutations and their repair,
       Science, 152 (1966) 1345–1353.
62. Witkin, E., Elevated mutability of polA and uvrA polA
       derivatives of Escherichia coli B/r at sublethal doses of
       ultraviolet light: evidence for an inducible error-prone
       repair system ("SOS repair") and its anomalous expression
       in these strains, Genetics, 79 (1975) 199–213.
63. Witkin, E. and D. L. George, Ultraviolet mutagenesis in polA
       and uvrA polA derivatives of Escherichia coli B/r:
       Evidence for an inducible error-prone repair system,
       Genetics, 73 (1973) 91–108.
64. Witkin, E. M., Ultraviolet mutagenesis and inducible DNA
       repair in Escherichia coli, Bacteriol. Rev., 40 (1976)
       869–907.
65. Zakharov, I. A., T. N. Kozina, and I. V. Fedorova, Effets
       des mutations vers las sensibilité rayonnement ultraviolet
       chez la levure, Mutat. Res., 9 (1970) 31–39.

CHAPTER 10

DNA REPAIR AND MUTAGEN INTERACTION IN SACCHAROMYCES:

THEORETICAL CONSIDERATIONS

R. C. VON BORSTEL and P. J. HASTINGS

Department of Genetics, The University of Alberta
Edmonton, Alberta, Canada   T6G 2E9

SUMMARY

DNA repair pathways have been identified in the yeast Saccharomyces cerevisiae. One or more of these pathways are mutagenic, i.e.,
induce mutations during the process of repair of lesions in DNA.
Some types of lesions in DNA require components of more than one
pathway for repair.

When more than one mutagen is used in an experiment, they can
interact in a variety of ways: additively, synergistically, epistatically (dominantly), or antagonistically. These are the result
of the way in which mutagens cause effects on DNA repair systems or
on metabolic activation or detoxification systems.

Preliminary rules are presented for interpreting the interactions of mutagens. Mutation yield will be additive or more than
additive (1) if the agents compete for a nonmutagenic repair system,
(2) if one of them inhibits a nonmutagenic repair system, (3) if one
inactivates a metabolic inactivation system, (4) if one induces a
metabolic activation system. The converse situations all reduce
mutation yield.

Four pathways or systems have been identified in the yeast
Saccharomyces cerevisiae which are associated with repair of lesions
induced by ultraviolet radiation. Three pathways have been identified
by genetic methodology, namely, by assigning each radiation-sensitive
mutant to an epistasis group [1, 4, 5, 7]. The epistasis groups are
called the RAD3, RAD51, and RAD18 pathways. The initial steps have
been identified by (1) synergistic interaction with the presumed

initial step in another epistasis group, (2) dominance of phenotype over other members of the same epistasis group, and (3) a mutator phenotype which, because of channelling of lesions into a mutagenic repair pathway, is expected for a mutant of the gene encoding the enzyme which catalyzes the initial step of a nonmutagenic repair pathway [10]. The fourth system is the photorepair system, PHR1 [30].

EPISTASIS GROUPS

The RAD3 Epistasis Group

The RAD3 epistasis group comprises the mutants rad1, rad2, rad3, rad4, rad7, rad10, rad14, rad16, and mms19 [27]; it is regarded as a nonmutagenic (error-free) repair pathway. The mutant rad3 is a strong mutator, and rad1 is a weak mutator. Consequently, the mutator evidence is consistent with other evidence which suggested that rad3 blocked the first step, with rad1 perhaps blocking the second step. None of the mutants on this pathway are sensitive to ionizing radiation.

The RAD3 pathway is the excision-repair pathway. It is known that this pathway is responsible for excision of thymine dimers. Presumably it is this pathway which is active during liquid-holding recovery, where dimers are excised from nongrowing cells over a 24-hr period, since rad3 strains do not exhibit liquid-holding recovery for lesions induced by ultraviolet radiation [23, 35]. Nevertheless, a strain has been found which is not sensitive to ultraviolet radiation but exhibits no liquid-holding recovery [34]. It is possible that this strain carries a mutation which controls a late step or a branch of the excision-repair pathway.

The RAD3 pathway is not restricted to removal of thymine dimers. For example, it also removes monoadducts of furocoumarins and, 20 times less efficiently, furocoumarins which form crosslinks between the two strands of DNA. The furocoumarins bind to thymine both as monoadducts and as crosslinks. Also, most of the mutant strains of the RAD3 pathway exhibit decreased survival and enhanced mutagenesis after exposure to formaldehyde [2] or nitroquinoline oxide [24], indicating that the RAD3 system is active in removing lesions induced by certain other classes of chemical mutagens.

The RAD51 Epistasis Group

The RAD51 epistasis group is a minor system for repair of lesions induced by ultraviolet radiation, but it is the most important pathway for repair of lesions induced by γ-radiation [7]. It

is regarded as a nonmutagenic repair pathway, but steps of this
pathway are needed for mutagenic repair of lesions induced by ethyl
methanesulfonate [25]. The RAD51 epistasis group comprises rad50,
rad51 (mut5), rad52, rad54, rad55, rad56, and rad57. The mutant rad6
is a member of this epistasis group for repair of lesions induced by
ionizing radiation, but a member of the RAD18 epistasis group for
repair of lesions induced by ultraviolet radiation. All but two
members of the RAD51 epistasis group are mutators.

The RAD51 pathway is the double-strand break repair pathway.
It repairs direct double-strand breaks from radiation [11, 20, 31],
from close single lesions [3], from crosslinks [12], and possibly
from post-replication gaps across nonreplicating lesions [20]. It
appears that RAD51 repair involves recombination between sisters in
the G2 period of the cell cycle, and between homologs in a/α diploids
[8, 11, 18, 19, 31].

The RAD18 Epistasis Group

The RAD18 epistasis group is generally regarded as a mutagenic
(error-prone) repair pathway. This group comprises rad6 (for repair
of lesions induced by ultraviolet radiation), rad8, rad9, rad18,
rev1, rev2 (rad5), rev3 (ant2) [15-17], and cdc8 [28]. It has been
suggested that this system is involved in gap-filling such as post-
replication gaps, and gaps produced in base-excision repair [20].
Mutation may result from polymerization across nonreplicating lesions
during this gap-filling.

The mutants rad18, rad6, and rev2 (rad5) are mutators, and all
alleles of rev3 so far examined are antimutators [29]. The mutant
rad6-1 appears to be a mutator for certain lesions and an antimutator
for others. The mutator activity of some steps has been used as
evidence for a second, and hypothetical, mutagenic repair pathway
[10, 33].

The PHR1 System

The PHR1 pathway is a single step and is the photorecovery
system. The enzyme for the photorecovery has been isolated and
purified [21], and a photorecovery mutant, phr1, has been identified
[30].

Other Repair Systems

Mutant strains sensitive to methyl methanesulfonate have been
isolated, and many of these are not sensitive to either ionizing or
nonionizing radiation [26]. Similarly, mutator strains have been

isolated which are sensitive to methyl methanesulfonate and/or
ionizing and/or nonionizing radiation and/or neither radiations, or
not sensitive to any mutagen so far tested [10, 22]. This implies
that lesions induced by methyl methanesulfonate are being repaired
by the known radiation repair systems, and by a system which was not
identified by the rad phenotype. It is also possible that further
systems remain to be discovered.

REASSORTMENT OF COMPONENTS OF DNA REPAIR PATHWAYS

The pathways described above have been defined by mass action,
i.e., survival data, with UV and ionizing radiations. It is now
clear that for other repair purposes the same steps are assorted
differently, and it may well be that the steps operate in different
combinations for a minority of events occurring in response to
radiation.

Even with radiations, an ambiguity is apparent in assigning
genes to pathways, as described above for rad6, which gives a different result with UV and γ-rays.

Two more examples of this are now apparent: First, Prakash
[24, 25] has shown that EMS mutagenesis requires both the RAD51 and
the RAD18 systems to be intact. We suggest that the interpretation
of this should be that the premutational lesions caused by EMS are
double-strand breaks (perhaps from close single-strand lesions), and
that repair of double-strand breaks by recombination sometimes
involves a gap-filling, and hence mutagenic, process. It is possible
that a mutational endpoint for recombination repair applies in other
situations, but is not seen because other processes cause a higher
proportion of the mutations. Thus, the RAD51 system should not be
regarded as error-free. A second example concerns the repair of
crosslinks caused by psoralen and 360 nm light. Double-strand breaks
formed during repair of psoralen crosslinks are repaired only in the
presence of functional RAD51 and RAD3 products [12]. Thus these two
steps, which act independently in the repair of UV damage, are part
of a single system for the repair of crosslinks.

The temperature sensitive, cell-division-cycle mutant, cdc9,
encodes mutant DNA ligase [14]. This mutant is also sensitive to
ultraviolet radiation and methyl methanesulfonate when treated at
the same time that the temperature is enhanced [13]. Moreover,
mitotic recombination is enhanced in strains homozygous for cdc9
when the temperature is increased for a short time [6]. It is likely,
therefore, that DNA ligase will be a terminal step in a number of
different repair processes.

Thus it can be seen that the enzymes involved in repair of DNA act not so much as pathways but rather as systems which can be reassorted for different purposes.

In order to examine interactions of mutagens, we shall assume that most induced lesions in DNA are repaired via one or more non-mutagenic repair pathways and one or more mutagenic repair pathways.

LEVELS OF INTERACTIONS OF MUTAGENS

In DNA repair systems, a mutagen can have several positive or negative effects with respect to the action of a second mutagen. These include (1) the induction of a mutagenic or a nonmutagenic repair pathway, (2) the inactivation of a repair system by attack by a mutagen on a repair protein or on a gene which must be transcribed to produce a repair protein, (3) the allosteric inhibition of an enzyme involved in a process, or (4) the competition of the two muta-genic lesions for the same pathway, which may lead to a saturation.

There is an exact corollary for the effect of mutagens on repair systems, and that is their action on detoxification systems which activate or inactivate premutagens and mutagens. These include (1) the induction of a detoxification system leading either to the acti-vation or to the inactivation of a mutagen, (2) the inactivation of a system, (3) the inhibition of a system, and (4) the competition of two agents for the same detoxification system.

With 2^{15} possibilities for positive and negative effects for any two mutagens from these causes alone, the predictability of the behavior of two mutagens vanishes. Nevertheless, some preliminary rules may be formulated which can be used as a guide to interpreting the interaction of two mutagens when antagonistic, dominant, additive, or synergistic effects are demonstrated (Table 1).

Interactions Increasing Yield of Mutations

If a second mutagen simply adds more lesions as a substrate for repair, the effect of these extra lesions will be additive. This additive relationship will not always be seen, since the slope of the response curve may be increasing. This will give an apparent synergistic interaction, which we call pseudo-synergistic. Such an interaction can be seen with two doses of the same mutagen under appropriate circumstances [9].

Many of the types of interaction in Table 1 do not merely alter the number of lesions formed, but rather, alter the proportion of the lesions which lead to mutation by inhibiting or inactivating nonmutagenic repair, or by inducing mutagenic repair. In this case,

TABLE 1

PROCESSES THAT LEAD TO ENHANCED OR REDUCED MUTATION YIELD;
DETOXIFICATION SYSTEMS AND REPAIR SYSTEMS LEAD TO THE SAME RESULTS

	Detoxification Systems	
	Agent Inactivation	Agent Activation
	Repair Systems	
	Nonmutagenic	Mutagenic
Reduced mutation yield	Induction	Competition Inhibition System Inactivation
Enhanced mutation yield	Competition Inhibition System Inactivation	Induction

an increase in mutation will be seen as a synergistic interaction.
Change in the number of lesions also leads to a change in the proportion of repair which is mutagenic if some pathways become saturated so that they accept no more lesions. This competition is
expected to give a synergistic increase in mutation yield.

Interactions Decreasing Yield of Mutations

There are two types of negative interaction to be considered.
One possibility is that the two agents together give less mutation
than either alone – an antagonistic interaction. This could be
caused by mutation resulting from different mutagenic repair pathways for the two agents, which mutually inhibit of inactivate the
mutagenic process used by the other. A similar mutual interference
with detoxification enzymes activating two premutagens could occur.
The other style of negative interaction is the dominance or epistasis
of one agent over the other, so that the effect of adding the second
mutagen is not seen. This interaction can be explained if one agent
inhibits or represses (prevents induction of) a mutagenic repair
process handling lesions produced by a second agent.

Similar antagonistic or dominant effects could, however, stem
from causes more remote from the mutagenic process. If, for example,
two agents together produce a more marked inhibition of cell

duplication and division processes than either alone, less mutation
would occur. We routinely see that the point on the mutation induction curve at which mutation yield per survivor starts to decline is
the dose at which cell division is inhibited [32]. It would appear
that less mutation occurs when there is more time for repair, perhaps
by avoiding the formation of postreplication gaps opposite lesions.
(It should also be noted that mutation yield would be less than
additive if one agent is markedly more toxic than the other. This
should not be seen, however, if one measures mutation per survivor.)

There are more possibilities for less than additive interaction
which do not apply to direct acting mutagens, namely any interference
with a system activating a premutagen.

GENERAL CONCLUSIONS

On the basis of our present knowledge of repair, we would expect
additive and synergistic interactions to be more common than interactions which are less than additive. Perhaps the most obvious
reason for this is that we know of more error-free than mutagenic
modes of repair, so that there are more points at which the accurate
repair systems could be attacked. A more important consideration is
that it is not to be expected that lesion-containing cells which have
reduced mutagenic repair capacity will survive, since we see mutagenic repair as a last resort in situations in which all homologous
template has been lost, so that only cells which can proceed to
replicate without template (i.e., mutagenically) will be able to
survive.

We cannot, at present, estimate whether the occurrence of inducible repair systems is more likely to cause an increased or a
decreased interaction in mutagen combinations, since both mutagenic
and nonmutagenic repair systems have been shown to be inducible in
different organisms.

REFERENCES

1. Brendel, M., and R. H. Haynes, Interactions among genes
        controlling sensitivity to radiation and alkylation in
        yeast, Mol. Gen. Genet., 125 (1973) 197-216.
2. Chanet, R., C. Izard, and E. Moustacchi, Genetic effects of
        formaldehyde in yeast. II. Influence of ploidy and of
        mutations affecting radiosensitivity on its lethal effect,
        Mutat. Res., 35 (1976) 29-38.
3. Chlebowicz, E., and W. J. Jachymczyk, Repair of MMS-induced DNA
        double-strand breaks in haploid cells of Saccharomyces
        cerevisiae, which requires the presence of a duplicate
        genome, Mol. Gen. Genet., 167 (1979) 279-286.

4. Game, J. C., A study of radiation-sensitive mutants in yeast,
    D. Phil. Thesis, Oxford, 1971.
5. Game, J. C., and B. S. Cox, Synergistic interaction between RAD
    mutations in yeast, Mutat. Res., 20 (1973) 35-44.
6. Game, J. C., L. H. Johnston, and R. C. von Borstel, Enhanced
    mitotic recombination in a ligase-defective mutant of the
    yeast Saccharomyces cerevisiae, Proc. Natl. Acad. Sci.
    (U.S.), 76 (1979) 4589-4592.
7. Game, J. C., and R. K. Mortimer, A genetic study of x-ray
    sensitive mutants in yeast, Mutat. Res., 24 (1974) 281-292.
8. Hannan, M. A., and A. Nasim, Caffeine enhancement of radiation
    killing in different strains of Saccharomyces cerevisiae,
    Mol. Gen. Genet., 158 (1977) 111-116.
9. Hastings, P. J., Unpublished data.
10. Hastings, P. J., S.-K. Quah, and R. C. von Borstel, Spontaneous
    mutation by mutagenic repair of spontaneous lesions in DNA,
    Nature, 264 (1976) 719-722.
11. Ho, K., Induction of DNA double-strand breaks by x-rays in a
    radio-sensitive strain of the yeast Saccharomyces cerevisiae,
    Mutat. Res., 30 (1975) 327-334.
12. Jachymczyk, W. J., and R. C. von Borstel, Unpublished data.
13. Johnston, L. H., The DNA repair capability of cdc9, the
    Saccharomyces cerevisiae mutant defective in DNA ligase,
    Mol. Gen. Genet., 170 (1979) 89-92.
14. Johnston, L. H., and K. A. Nasmyth, Saccharomyces cerevisiae
    cell cycle mutant cdc9 is defective in DNA ligase, Nature,
    274 (1978) 891-893.
15. Lawrence, C. W., and R. Christensen, UV mutagenesis in radiation
    sensitive strains of yeast, Genetics, 82 (1976) 207-232.
16. Lemontt, J. F., Mutants of yeast defective in mutation induced
    by ultraviolet light, Genetics, 68 (1971) 21-33.
17. Lemontt, J. F., Genetic and physiological factors affecting
    repair and mutagenesis in yeast, This volume, p. 85.
18. Morrison, D. P., Repair parameters in mutator mutants of
    Saccharomyces cerevisiae, Ph.D. Thesis, University of
    Alberta, 1978, 172 pages.
19. Morrison, D. P., S.-K. Quah, and P. J. Hastings, Expression in
    diploids of the mutator phenotype of some mutator mutants
    of Saccharomyces cerevisiae, Can. J. Genet. Cytol., in
    press.
20. Mowat, M. R. A., Repair of γ-ray induced DNA strand breaks in
    radiation sensitive mutants of yeast, Ph.D. Thesis,
    University of Alberta, 1979.
21. Muhammed, A., Studies on the yeast photoreactivating enzyme.
    I. A method for the large scale purification and some
    properties of the enzyme, J. Biol. Chem., 241 (1966)
    516-523.
22. Nasim, A., and Brychcy, T., Cross sensitivity of mutator strains
    to physical and chemical mutagens, Can. J. Genet. Cytol.,
    21 (1979) 129-137.

23. Parry, J. M., and E. M. Parry, The effect of UV-light post-
     treatments on the survival characteristics of 21 UV-sensi-
     tive mutants of Saccharomyces cerevisiae, Mutat. Res., 8
     (1969) 345-356.
24. Prakash, L., Lack of chemically induced mutation in repair-
     deficient mutants of yeast, Genetics, 78 (1974) 1101-1118.
25. Prakash, L., Effect of genes controlling radiation sensitivity
     on chemically-induced mutations in Saccharomyces cerevisiae,
     Genetics, 83 (1976) 285-301.
26. Prakash, L., and S. Prakash, Isolation and characterization of
     MMS-sensitive mutants of Saccharomyces cerevisiae, Genetics,
     86 (1977) 33-55.
27. Prakash, L., and S. Prakash, Three additional genes involved in
     pyrimidine dimer removal in Saccharomyces cerevisiae: RAD7,
     RAD14 and MMS19, Mol. Gen. Genet., submitted
28. Prakash, L., and S. Prakash, Genetic analysis of error-prone
     repair systems in Saccharomyces cerevisiae, This volume,
     p. 141.
29. Quah, S.-K., Unpublished data.
30. Resnick, M. A., Genetic control of radiation sensitivity in
     Saccharomyces cerevisiae, Genetics, 62 (1969) 519-531.
31. Resnick, M. A., The repair of double-strand breaks in chromo-
     somal DNA of yeast, In: Molecular Mechanisms for Repair of
     DNA, Part B, P. C. Hanawalt and R. B. Setlow, Eds., Plenum
     Press, New York, 1975, pp. 549-556.
32. von Borstel, R. C., Unpublished data.
33. von Borstel, R. C., and P. J. Hastings, Mutagenic repair path-
     ways in yeast, In: Research in Photobiology, A. Castellani,
     Ed., Plenum Press, London, 1977, pp. 683-687.
34. von Borstel, R. C., and E. Moustacchi, Unpublished data.
35. Zuk, J., D. Zaborowska, and Z. Swietlinska, Comparison of
     sensitivity and liquid holding recovery in rad mutants of
     Saccharomyces cerevisiae inactivated by UV and DEB,
     Mol. Gen. Genet. 166 (1978) 91-96.

CHAPTER 11

REPAIR AND MUTAGENESIS IN LOWER EUKARYOTES:

A SUMMARY AND PERSPECTIVE

HERMAN E. BROCKMAN

Department of Biological Sciences, Illinois State
University, Normal, Illinois   61761 (U.S.A.)

The impetus for the research reviewed in the session "Repair
and Mutagenesis in Lower Eukaryotes" came in part from related
research in Escherichia coli and other prokaryotes. Mutants that
are more sensitive than wild type to the killing activity of a mutagen (mutagen-sensitive strains) were reported in Neurospora crassa
and Saccharomyces cerevisiae in 1967—three years after the first
reports of the enzymatic removal of thymine dimers from DNA (nucleotide excision repair) in E. coli by Setlow and Carrier and by Boyce
and Howard-Flanders, two years after Clark and Margulies reported
results with recombination-deficient mutants of E. coli that indicated an association between recombination and DNA repair, and in
the same year that Witkin proposed that UV-induced DNA lesions in
E. coli were repaired by mutation-proof and mutation-prone pathways.
The early investigators of DNA repair in eukaryotes were interested
in whether the repair mechanisms being elucidated in prokaryotes
would occur in eukaryotes, and they also suspected that the mechanisms for repair would be more complex in eukaryotes than in prokaryotes. The lower eukaryotes S. cerevisiae and N. crassa became
the objects of a great deal of the research on DNA repair in eukaryotes. It was thought that the increase in complexity of the DNA
repair mechanisms would be less for the lower eukaryotes than for
higher eukaryotes and, therefore, that these mechanisms would be
somewhat simpler to elucidate in yeast and Neurospora than in higher
eukaryotes. Both of these lower eukaryotes generally have the advantage of ease-of-handling of prokaryotic microbes, and there is
a large body of literature on their genetics and biochemistry.
Moreover, the structures in which radiation or chemicals cause
lesions—and in which those lesions may be repaired—are eukaryotic
chromosomes, which undergo mitosis and meiosis. Therefore, researchers on DNA repair in Neurospora and yeast thought that the

mechanisms of repair they were elucidating might be applicable, at least in a general way, to higher eukaryotes, including humans.

The session was organized into three papers on N. crassa followed by three papers on S. cerevisiae. In the first of each group of three papers, the isolation and the genetic and biochemical characterization of presumptive repair-deficient mutants were reviewed: in N. crassa by A. L. Schroeder and L. D. Olson, and in S. cerevisiae by J. F. Lemontt. Various techniques have been used in these two microbes to select for mutants that might be defective in some step of a DNA repair pathway. Most commonly the mutants have been selected as being sensitive to the killing activity of a mutagen, but mutants also have been selected as being defective in some aspect of DNA metabolism such as genetic recombination or DNA replication, as being resistant to an agent's mutagenic activity, or as having a greater spontaneous mutation rate than that found in wild type. Attempts to "saturate the genome" with these mutants have been much more extensive in yeast than in Neurospora. For example, Lemontt reports that 65-70 loci (by complementation analysis) are represented among mutagen-sensitive mutants of yeast. Not all of the genes identified by the various selective techniques function in DNA repair directly, and the mutants often are pleiotropic. Nevertheless, the number of cistrons in yeast that function in DNA repair and related DNA phenomena is very large—probably more than 100. The characteristics of many repair-deficient mutants of these two lower eukaryotes are similar, but not identical, to those of the repair-deficient mutants of E. coli. All of the repair-deficient mutants to data are due to nuclear mutations despite efforts by Schroeder and Olson to isolate cytoplasmic mutants controlling UV sensitivity in N. crassa.

Through various genetic and biochemical studies, many of these mutants have been assigned to DNA repair "pathways." In these two lower eukaryotes, there is a nucleotide excision-repair (relatively mutation-proof) pathway, which can be demonstrated biochemically. There also appears to be a post replication-repair (mutation-prone) pathway. The two pathways are similar, but not identical, to these pathways in E. coli. Some mutants appear to reside in one or more other repair pathways, which may be unique to eukaryotes. Lemontt also reviewed the research in yeast showing that physiological functions such as "cell age," DNA replication, and the regulatory state of the mating-type locus also affect DNA repair and, therefore, mutagenesis.

In the second of each group of three papers, a major aspect of the biochemistry of DNA repair was reviewed: by M. J. Fraser, T. Y.-K. Chow, and E. Käfer on nucleases and their role in DNA repair in wild-type and mutant strains of N. crassa, and by R. J. Reynolds and E. C. Friedberg on the molecular mechanisms of pyrimidine dimer

excision in wild-type and UV-sensitive mutant strains of S.
cerevisiae. The nuh mutants of N. crassa were selected by the criterion that they secrete less than a wild-type amount of alkaline
DNAse. Some of the nuh mutants are sensitive to a broad spectrum
of mutagens. Two of the UV-sensitive mutants of N. crassa isolated
previously also have the nuh phenotype, but other repair-deficient
mutants of N. crassa do not have this phenotype. Fraser et al.
suggest that five nucleases with markedly different properties are
derived by different routes of proteolysis from a single inactive
precursor polypeptide. One of these nucleases appears to be involved in DNA repair. Two repair-deficient mutants of Neurospora,
uvs-3 and nuh-4, which appear to be allelic and which may be defective in a mutation-prone repair pathway, may have a lesion in pro-
tease(s) that affect the amount of the nuclease or may have a lesion
in some function that regulates the protease(s).

    Reynolds and Friedberg initiated their studies in yeast because
of their interest in nucleotide excision in higher eukaryotes. The
results from studies on cell lines from humans with xeroderma pigmentosum (XP) indicate the existence of seven complementation groups
that function in nucleotide excision repair—most or all of which
are involved in very early steps in this repair pathway. They decided to use yeast as a biochemically accessible system in which to
study nucleotide excision repair, in part because at least nine loci
within the RAD3 group of mutants control the excision of pyrimidine
dimers—a genetic complexity similar to that observed in the studies on XP. They have concluded that at least four of the nine
genetic loci that function in pyrimidine dimer excision in S.
cerevisiae are associated with the early step(s) of DNA incision or
preincision. Thus, the early steps of nucleotide excision repair
are complex in both yeast and humans.

    In the last of each group of these papers, aspects of mutation
induction in certain repair-deficient mutants were reviewed. F. J.
de Serres summarized the effects of seven repair-deficient genes on
mutation induction at the ad-3 region of N. crassa, and L. Prakash
and S. Prakash reviewed UV and alkylating agent mutagenesis via
mutation-prone pathways in S. cerevisiae. A number of features of
the ad-3 system of N. crassa make it useful for the detection of
effects of repair-deficient genes on mutation induction by physical
and chemical agents. Because the system detects forward mutation
at two cistrons by a direct method that does not eliminate leaky
mutants, a wide spectrum of genetic alterations is recovered. By
use of a heterokaryon, a diploid-like condition is established, and
multilocus deletions in the ad-3 region, which act as recessive
lethals, are also recovered. Quantitative and qualitative differences have been found in the ad-3 mutants induced in a repair-
sufficient strain and repair-deficient mutants. For example, the
uvs-2 and upr-1 strains are sensitive to the killing and mutagenic
activities of UV, and among UV-induced ad-3B mutants, the ratio of

frameshift to base-pair substitution mutants is greater in the uvs-2 or upr-1 strain than in the repair-sufficient strain. Studies with heterokaryons have shown that with certain agents such as methyl methanesulfonate (MMS) the ratio of multilocus deletions to intra-cistronic mutations is greater in the uvs-2 strain than in the uvs-2$^+$ strain. Therefore, the lesions induced in DNA by an agent such as UV or MMS may be processed differently, quantitatively and qualti-tatively, in the uvs-2 strain than in the uvs-2$^+$ strain.

Prakash and Prakash reviewed the literature on how the extensive collection of relatively well-characterized repair-deficient mutants of yeast has been used to elucidate the genetic control of mutation induction by UV and certain alkylating agents. In the case of UV, they conclude that all of the results in yeast can be explained by these models: in excision repair-sufficient strains, closely spaced pyrimidine dimers in opposite DNA strands are repaired by a mutation-prone excision repair pathway; whereas in excision repair-deficient strains, postreplication gaps, which are not usually overlapping daughter-strand gaps, occasionally are filled in via an error-prone pathway. Evidences that stage of the cell cycle and conditions of ploidy also affect repair ability were discussed. Prakash and Prakash suggest that ethyl methanesulfonate (EMS)-induced mutants in yeast arise from mutation-prone repair of gaps opposite 0^6-alkyl guanine rather than from misreplication of 0^6-alkyl guanine. The interesting results on allele-specific control of UV-induced rever-sion also were reviewed by Prakash and Prakash, as well as by Lemontt.

It is clear that a great deal of information on DNA repair and mutagenesis has resulted from studies on S. cerevisiae and N. crassa in the 12 years since the first reports of mutagen-sensitive mutants in these two lower eukaryotes. The expectations that the character-istics of repair-deficient mutants and the features of DNA repair pathways would be similar, but not identical, to those of bacteria have been realized—as has the prediction that repair in these lower eukaryotes would be more complex than repair in bacteria. The question of the degree of similarity between DNA repair in lower eukaryotes and higher eukaryotes, including humans, is still largely unanswered because of the incompleteness of our understanding of the complex repair mechanisms in eukaryotes.

Each investigator using Neurospora or yeast in this area of research undoubtedly has a list of "important" experiments to do. In Neurospora, the example of the yeast investigators in attempting to saturate the map with repair-deficient mutants, and in assigning these mutants to repair pathways, needs to be followed. Part of the characterization of repair-deficient mutants is determining their relative sensitivity or resistance, compared to a repair-sufficient strain, to the killing and mutagenic activities of various physical and chemical mutagens. In this part of the characterization of these mutants, a "standard set" of mutagens would be very useful, not only in Neurospora and yeast, but in prokaryotes and higher eukaryotes as well. My suggested "standard set" is UV, x-ray, MMS, EMS, and N-ethyl-N-nitrosourea (monofunctional alkylating agents with increasing ratios of 0-6 to N-7 alkylations of guanine); 6-N-hydroxylamino purine (a highly mutagenic base analog in N. crassa); mitomycin C (a crosslinking agent); and ICR-170 (for eukaryotes) and ICR-191 (for prokaryotes), acridine nitrogen mustards that are frameshift mutagens. The question of the degree of dominance or recessiveness of the repair-deficient mutant alleles relative to their wild-type alleles can be studied in diploids of yeast and in heterokaryons of Neurospora. Results of such studies can suggest the relative risk, if any, of heterozygotes for repair-deficient genes in the human population. Little is known in the lower eukaryotes about the effect of repair-deficient genes on the clastogenic activity of mutagenic agents; further use of the ad-3 system of N. crassa should increase our knowledge in this area. S. cerevisiae is ideally suited for repair studies involving both aneuploidy and euploidy, and for studies on the effect of repair-deficient mutants on meiotic and mitotic recombination.

Recent discoveries on the organization of nucleotide sequences in eukaryotic DNA and on the nucleosome organization of chromatin permit us to begin to have more precise molecular models for the structures (chromosomes) that are being damaged by mutagenic agents and repaired by complex enzymatic "pathways." On the other hand, other findings from many fields of study lead most of us, I suspect, to think that we understand only a small fraction of what happens during DNA repair and mutagenesis in yeast and Neurospora. Many aspects of the cell must be important in determining whether a lesion occurs in a eukaryotic chromosome and whether, and how, it becomes a mutation. The organization of nucleotide sequences and of histones and other proteins in the eukaryotic chromosome may determine where, within a sequence of nucleotides, lesions can be produced by a given agent—as well as the type(s) of lesion(s) that can be found at a given location. This complex organization of the eukaryotic chromosome also may determine the efficiency and the type of repair that can occur at lesions at different locations. S. cerevisiae and N. crassa, standing on a scale of complexity between the prokaryotes and the higher eukaryotes, will continue to be used extensively in studies on DNA repair and mutagenesis.

CHAPTER 12

ISOLATION AND CHARACTERIZATION OF REPAIR-DEFICIENT MUTANTS OF

Drosophila melanogaster

P. DENNIS SMITH, RONALD D. SNYDER,[*] and
RUTH L. DUSENBERY

Department of Biology, Emory University, Atlanta, GA
        (U.S.A.)

SUMMARY

   Mutagen-sensitive mutants of Drosophila melanogaster are being
utilized to determine the number and function of genes which
control various aspects of DNA metabolism including replication,
repair and recombination and to define the relationship of each of
these functions to mutation production.

   Nineteen loci which confer enhanced sensitivity to killing by
methyl methanesulfonate have been detected on the X and second
chromosomes. These loci can be grouped into five separate classes
on the basis of cross-sensitivity to methyl methanesulfonate, x-ray,
UV and nitrogen mustard. Some loci affect both somatic and meiotic
functions, as assayed by mutagen sensitivity and recombination
deficiency, while others affect only somatic functions.

   Genetic methods have been employed to determine whether these
mutants, which are able to survive in the absence of mutagen
treatment, represent loci which have dispensable functions or leaky
alleles of loci which have indispensable cellular functions. In
several cases, both leaky and null alleles have been identified,
indicating that at least some of these loci represent apparently
dispensable cellular functions.

---

   [*]Present address: Biology Division, Oak Ridge National
Laboratory, Oak Ridge, TN 37830 (U.S.A.)

The mutagen sensitivity of doubly-mutant mus strains is being employed to assign mutants to common pathways for DNA repair in order to corroborate data obtained from biochemical studies and to explore whether a genetic ordering of metabolic steps in each repair pathway is possible. These data may be used in conjunction with the effects on the frequency and nature of mutations produced by various agents in each of the mutant strains to identify which of these pathways involve error-free or error-prone repair processes.

INTRODUCTION

The isolation and characterization of mutagen-sensitive bacterial and fungal strains has provided considerable insight into the genetic control of DNA metabolism in unicellular organisms [12, 24, 31]. These studies have indicated that genetic recombination, DNA replication, DNA repair, and mutation production share common enzymatic steps and exhibit complex overlapping controls [7, 23]. Genetic studies of both prokaryotic and lower eukaryotic organisms indicate a multiplicity of DNA repair systems which may exhibit strong effects on mutation production [8, 14, 15, 22, 30]. The isolation and characterization of mutagen-sensitive mutants of Drosophila offer the promise of understanding the genetic controls of DNA repair and mutagenesis in a multicellular animal system. In this report, we review the isolation of such mutants and discuss certain pertinent features of the complex phenotypes exhibited by these strains.

ISOLATION OF mus MUTANTS

Procedures for the specific detection of mutagen-sensitive (mus) mutants have been developed in our laboratory for the isolation of both X-chromosomal and autosomal mutant strains [25, 27, 29]. These procedures have two essential features: mus strains are detected on the basis of enhanced sensitivity to killing by a mutagenic agent applied during the developmental cycle (the majority of the mus strains isolated in our laboratory and elsewhere [4] were initially detected as methyl methanesulfonate-sensitive strains) and the mus mutants were detected as conditional mutants, defined as inviable in the presence of the mutagenic agent but viable in its absence. Although these genetic procedures specifically identify mutagen-sensitive mutants, it should be noted that, since the mutagenic agents may be toxic to other cellular systems, such mutants are not necessarily DNA repair-deficient.

Table 1 summarizes data from our laboratory describing the frequency of isolation of X and second chromosome methyl methane-sulfonate (MMS)-sensitive mutant strains [27, 29]. For comparative purposes, isolation data for 13 MMS-sensitive X-chromosomal mutants

TABLE 1

ISOLATION OF MUTAGEN–SENSITIVE MUTANTS

Chromosome	Number of mutagenized chromosomes tested	Number of mus strains	Frequency of mus strains
X	28,341	52	1.83×10^{-3}
II	4,039	5	1.24×10^{-3}
X (Davis)	6,850	13	1.90×10^{-3}

detected in Dr. J. B. Boyd's laboratory are included and indicate
a similarity in isolation frequency in both laboratories [4].
Since these initial studies, a number of additional X-linked mus
strains have been isolated or detected in other laboratories [11,
17] and, at present, nearly 100 X chromosome mus strains have been
identified. From a sample of mutagenized autosomal stocks received
from J. B. Boyd, we have isolated three additional MMS-sensitive
second chromosome strains.

Complementation and recombination analyses of the X chromosome
mutants have identified 12 loci which control MMS sensitivity
(Table 2).   Each mus locus has been assigned a number designating
chromosomal location and allele identification (see reference 27
for nomenclatural scheme). Two of these mutagen-sensitive loci were
originally identified as meiotic mutants and have retained their mei
designation [1]. There appears to be no unusual regional distribution of loci along the chromosome and, with the possible exception
of mus 104 and mei-41, no extremely tight linkage of separate loci.
Multiple alleles have been identified at seven of the loci.
Complementation analysis of the eight second chromosome mutants has
identified seven complementation groups tentatively designated mus
201-mus 207. Only mus 201 is represented by more than a single
allele.

These studies raise the question of how many mus loci exist in
the Drosophila genome? Although we are employing the general term,
"mus locus," the majority of studies to date have focused on MMS-
sensitive loci which may, in fact, represent only a subset of
potential mus loci. On the basis of our current criterion for
designating MMS sensitivity and multiple allelism, we assume that
we have approached saturation for possible sex chromosome loci.
Since the frequency of isolation of second chromosome MMS loci in
our laboratory is similar to that of the X, which represents 20% of

TABLE 2

LOCATION OF X CHROMOSOME mus LOCI

mus mutant	Genetic locus
101	44.8
102	0.5
103	36–44
104	53
105	14.8
106	36–44
107	33–36
108	10.8
109	30.2[a]
111	27[a]
mei-9	6
mei-41	53.8

[a]Data of Mason [17].

the entire genome, we anticipate the identification of as many as 60 separable MMS loci in the entire genome. This estimate of 60 potential MMS-sensitive loci compares favorably with yeast studies, where approximately 40 MMS-sensitive loci have already been identified [13, 19, 20].

MUTAGEN SENSITIVITY

The mus mutants can be classified into specific groups on the basis of their mutagen sensitivity phenotypes. Most of the mutant strains have been examined for sensitivity to at least three additional mutagenic agents: x-ray, UV, and nitrogen mustard (HN2). These data, outlined in Table 3, indicate five separable patterns of sensitivity. Nine of the 18 mutants display sensitivity to all four agents. Seven of the remaining nine display sensitivity to MMS and at least one additional agent, while one mutant appears to be sensitive to MMS alone. The majority of mutants on the X

TABLE 3

PATTERNS OF MUTAGEN SENSITIVITY

Mutant	Sensitivity[a]			
	MMS	x–Ray	UV	HN2
103	+	–	–	–
102	+	+	–	–
105	+	+	–	–
106	+	+	–	–
204	+	–	+	–
205	+	–	+	–
206	+	–	+	+
207	+	–	+	+
101	+	+	+	+
104	+	+	+	+
107	+	+	+	+
109	+	+	+	+
mei–9	+	+	+	+
mei–41	+	+	+	+
201	+	+	+	+
202	+	+	+	+
203	+	+	+	+
108	+	0	0	0
111[b]	+	0	0	+

[a]Sensitivity: + = sensitive; – = not sensitive; 0 = not tested.

[b]Data of Mason [17].

chromosome appear sensitive either to MMS and x–ray or to a wide variety of mutagenic compounds. Preliminary studies of mutants more recently detected on the second chromosome suggest several additional patterns of mutagen sensitivity. Several conclusions can be drawn from these studies. Firstly, with the exception of mus 103, all fully tested mutants exhibit sensitivity to at least one radiation mutagen. This observation suggests that these mutants are not simply sensitive to exogenously applied chemical mutagens on the basis of defects in cellular transport mechanisms. Secondly, the variations in patterns observed suggest that mutants in

different steps in repair functions have been identified. Lastly,
although the patterns of sensitivity do not allow conclusions
concerning defects in specific enzymatic repair steps, the
observations permit various working hypotheses concerning potential
repair deficiencies.

RECOMBINATION DEFICIENCY

The allelism of our original X-linked MMS-sensitive mutant
[26] with the recombination-deficient meiotic mutant, mei-41 [1],
provided strong support for the hypothesis that mutagen sensitivity
and recombination deficiency exhibit overlapping genetic controls
in Drosophila. Since this observation, a large proportion of the
X-linked mus mutants have been shown to exhibit female infertility,
abnormal meiotic chromosome segregation behavior and alterations in
meiotic recombination [4, 27, 29]. These studies and more recent
observations on the effects of mus loci on mitotic chromosome
stability are reviewed by Baker [2, 3].

Unlike the X chromosome loci, chromosome II mus mutants do not
exhibit strong alterations of meiocyte functions. Table 4 summarizes
our observations on female fertility, nondisjunction and recombination proficiency of these mutants. Of the seven complementation
groups identified, only two, mus 203 and mus 204, can be classified
as affecting meiotic functions, and in both cases, the effects are
considerably weaker than those observed for X-linked meiotic mutants.
In contrast, chromosome II mus mutants are not distinguished from
X-linked mutants on the basis of levels of mutagen sensitivity since
they span a similar sensitivity range. The mus 201^{D1} mutants are as
sensitive to killing by MMS (D_{37} = 0.02%) [27] as are mei9^a mutants
(0.02%, Table 6), yet they exhibit no appreciable alteration in
meiocyte function (Table 4) characteristic of the X-linked mei
mutants. From this initial sample of X and second chromosome mus
loci, we conclude that there is not a strong correlation between
somatic mutagen sensitivity and meiotic dysfunction.

mus GENE FUNCTION

The detection procedures employed in the isolation of the mus
mutants relied upon at least partial viability of the mutant strain
in the absence of mutagen treatment. Such a methodology implies
that the locus identified specifies a dispensable gene function, an
indispensable gene function represented by leaky alleles or a gene
function which may be substituted by alternate loci. The determination of the indispensability or relative leakiness of specific
loci is an important consideration for the interpretation of data
from a variety of in vivo and in vitro experiments, particularly
double mutant experiments designed to provide genetic evidence for
specific DNA repair pathways.

TABLE 4

EFFECTS OF CHROMOSOME II mus MUTANTS ON MEIOCYTE FUNCTION[a]

Mutant	Female infertility	Nondisjunction	Recombination deficiency
201^{D1}	−	−	−
201^{A1}	−	0	0
202^{A1}	+	−	0
203^{A1}	+	+	−
204^{A1}	+	+	(+)
205^{A1}	(+)	−	−
206^{A1}	−	0	0
207^{A1}	−	0	0

[a] + = exhibits mutant phenotype; (+) = exhibits mutant phenotype weakly; − = does not exhibit mutant phenotype; 0 = not tested.

Two experimental approaches are being employed to examine this question. In one experiment, the embryonic lethality of homozygous mus strains is determined in the absence of mutagen treatment. Table 5 summarizes lethality studies for a number of homozygous mei-9 alleles. These data indicate that the Oregon-R, y and w control strains exhibit high levels of hatchability while the various mei-9 alleles exhibit severe reductions. Although a large percentage of this embryonic inviability may be attributed to aneuploid effects derived from meiotic nondisjunction, the role of the mei-9^{+} gene product in normal embryonic cellular metabolism is not well defined. A second approach focuses on the leakiness of specific mutant alleles for repair of mutagen damage.   Leaky alleles (hypomorphs) can be identified as those which are more mutagen sensitive when in heterozygous combination with a deficiency for the locus than when homozyous. Null alleles (amorphs) are expected to exhibit the same level of mutagen sensitivity in the homozygous or heterozygous deficiency configuration. Results of such a hypomorphism test are presented in Table 6 for the mei-9 alleles examined for viability. The mei-9^{AT1} is a null mutation; mei-9^{AT2} and mei-9^{AT3} represent examples of leaky alleles. A third response is exhibited by the mei-9^{a} allele. In this case, the mei-9^{a} allele in

TABLE 5

EMBRYONIC LETHALITY OF mei-9 ALLELES

Genotype	Eggs examined	Frequency of hatching $\pm$ S.D.
Oregon-R	362	0.92 $\pm$ 0.05
w	582	0.77 $\pm$ 0.13
y	544	0.70 $\pm$ 0.18
y mei-9^a	383	0.19 $\pm$ 0.03
w mei-9^{AT1}	367	0.20 $\pm$ 0.07
y mei-9^{AT1}	407	0.27 $\pm$ 0.05
w mei-9^{AT2}	619	0.16 $\pm$ 0.05
w mei-9^{AT3}	386	0.18 $\pm$ 0.09

homozygous condition appears more sensitive to killing by MMS than the deficiency heterozygote. This antimorphic response, originally identified in clonal studies of mitotic cell functions [16] suggests that the mei-9^a allele specifies a gene product which is more inhibitory to repair than the complete absence of gene function. The viability and hypomorphism test results suggest that the mei-9$^+$ locus specifies a gene product which is partially dispensable. Apparent dispensability may be the result of multiple cellular functions which can provide at least partial substitution for absence of mei-9$^+$ activity.

DOUBLE MUTANT ANALYSIS

Examination of the mutagen sensitivity of doubly mutant mus strains has provided genetic evidence for the notion of alternate repair functions. Analysis of rad multiple mutants in yeast has suggested the existence of three pathways for the repair of UV and x-ray damage [13]. These genetic studies have been important not only in permitting the assignment of individual rad mutants to specific pathways of repair but also in suggesting a genetic ordering of certain metabolic steps in the repair sequence [9]. Nine mutagen-sensitive yeast strains have been assigned by such genetic analysis to a single epistasis group and biochemical studies have confirmed that each mutant is defective in excision repair of pyrimidine

TABLE 6

RELATIVE GENE FUNCTION OF mei-9 ALLELES

Mutant	MMS LD_{37}	$\dfrac{LD_{37}\ \text{Deficiency Heterozygote}}{LD_{37}\ \text{Homozygote}}$	Interpretation
y mei-9^a/y mei-9^a	0.020%	1.45	Antimorphic
y mei-9^a/deficiency	0.029%		
w mei-9^{AT1}/w mei-9^{AT1}	0.063%	0.92	Amorphic
w mei-9^{AT1}/deficiency	0.058%		
w mei-9^{AT2}/w mei-9^{AT2}	0.074%	0.73	Hypomorphic
w mei-9^{AT2}/deficiency	0.054%		
w mei-9^{AT3}/w mei-9^{AT3}	0.086%	0.38	Hypomorphic
w mei-9^{AT3}/deficiency	0.033%		

dimers [27]. In addition, the observation that a mutant may belong
to two separate epistasis groups suggests that repair pathways may
exhibit branch-points which involve overlapping gene functions [13].
Recent studies of the pol A, uvr and alk mutants of E. coli have
provided evidence for such a branched pathway for excision repair of
alkylation and UV damage [32].

Current studies in our laboratory are focused on the extension
of this genetic methodology to the multicellular Drosophila system.
Double mutant studies are best performed with null alleles for the
loci under study in order to eliminate interactions between two
leaky mutants within the same pathway. In the absence of known
nonsense mutations, we are relying on two methods for identifying
null alleles. One technique, described above for a series of mei-9
alleles, employs deficiency analysis to identify alleles with no
apparent gene function. In the absence of a known deficiency for
the locus in question, the most sensitive allele from a series of
multiple alleles is employed.

Because a high proportion of the X-linked mus mutants affect
female meiotic processes and embryonic viability in the absence of
mutagen treatment, double mutant analysis of homozygous strains is
impractical for the more severely affected mutants. In these cases,
determinations of the mutagen sensitivity of multiple mutant strains
is made on individuals derived from repair-proficient females. Our
studies on embryonic lethality as well as comparisons of mutagen
sensitivities of single mus mutants derived from repair-proficient
versus repair-deficient females [10] suggest that maternally derived
mus^+ gene products are important during early stages of the developmental cycle. In view of this maternal effect on mutagen
sensitivity, comparisons of relative survival of single versus
double mutant mus strains should be made on individuals collected
during later periods of postembryonic development.

From preliminary studies, several examples of double mutant
interactions are of particular interest (Table 7). The $mei-9^a$
$mei-41^{A3}$ double mutant appears to exhibit an additive interaction
suggesting that these gene products act on different substrates in
independent pathways. This interaction agrees with biochemical
data which places mei-9 in an excision pathway and mei-41 in a
postreplication pathway [5, 6]. In combination with $mus-105^{A1}$, the
$mei-9^a$ allele exhibits a strongly synergistic interaction. This
observation suggests that the mus 105 and mei-9 loci function in
different repair pathways. To date, however, no in vitro repair
defect has been associated with the mus 105 locus. The mus 101,
mus 105 and mei-41 mutants exhibit a striking interaction in the
absence of mutagen treatment. No double mutant combination of
these three loci can be constructed. Such synthetic lethality has
been observed for certain E. coli double mutants involving the

TABLE 7

DOUBLE MUTANT RELATIONSHIPS

Double mutant	Relationship
mei-9^a mei-41^{A3}	Additive
mei-9^a mus 105^{A1}	Synergistic
mus 101^{A1} mus 105^{A1} mus 101^{A1} mei-41^{A3} mus 105^{A1} mei-41^{A3}	Lethal
mei-9^a mus 205^{A1}	Epistatic

pol A gene [18]. Since these mutants cannot be constructed even in the absence of mutagen treatment, these data suggest that these loci provide important functions for normal cellular metabolism. Finally, the mei-9^a mus 205^{A1} double mutant appears to exhibit an epistatic interaction suggesting that mus 205 is defective in excision repair ability. These initial studies of double mutant combinations indicate that the range of interactions observed with yeast mutants are also observed in the Drosophila system.

From these double mutant studies, we hope to classify mus mutants to specific epistasis groups in order to understand the genetic basis of DNA repair pathways in Drosophila. Examination of mutation production in mutants defective in specific repair pathways should outline the role of each pathway in providing error-free or error-prone repair functions. Such investigations, in conjunction with in vitro DNA repair studies, should provide insight into the control of DNA repair and mutagenesis in a complex multicellular organism.

ACKNOWLEDGEMENTS

The studies reported in this paper were supported by P.H.S. grant ES-01101. P.D.S. is a recipient of P.H.S. Research Career Development Award GM-70758. R.L.D. is a recipient of P.H.S. Young

Investigator Award ES-02037. The authors wish to express their appreciation to Drs. J. B. Boyd, J. Mason and B. S. Baker for communicating unpublished data referred to in portions of the manuscript.

REFERENCES

1. Baker, B. S., and A. T. C. Carpenter, Genetic analysis of sex
        chromosomal meiotic mutants in Drosophila melanogaster,
        Genetics, 71 (1972) 255-286.
2. Baker, B. S., A. T. C. Carpenter, and P. Ripoll, The utiliza-
        tion during mitotic cell division of loci controlling
        meiotic recombination and disjunction in Drosophila
        melanogaster, Genetics, 90 (1978) 531-578.
3. Baker, B. S., and D. A. Smith, The effects of mutagen-sensitive
        mutants of Drosophila melanogaster in non-mutagenized cells,
        Genetics, in press.
4. Boyd, J. B., M. D. Golino, T. D. Nguyen, and M. M. Green,
        Isolation and characterization of X-linked mutants of
        Drosophila melanogaster which are sensitive to mutagens,
        Genetics, 84 (1976) 485-506.
5. Boyd, J. B., M. D. Golino, and R. B. Setlow, The mei-9^a mutant
        of Drosophila melanogaster increases mutagen sensitivity a
        and decreases excision repair, Genetics, 84 (1976) 527-544.
6. Boyd, J. B., and R. B. Setlow, Characterization of postrepli-
        cation repair in mutagen sensitive strains of Drosophila
        melanogaster, Genetics, 84 (1976) 507-526.
7. Clark, A. J., and M. R. Volkert, A new classification of path-
        ways repairing pyrimidine dimer damage in DNA. In: DNA
        Repair Mechanisms, P. C. Hanawalt, E. C. Friedberg, and
        C. F. Fox (Eds.), Academic Press, New York, 1978, pp. 57-
        57-72.
8. de Serres, F. J., Mutation induction in repair-deficient strains
        of Neurospora, This volume , p. 75.
9. Game, J. C., and B. S. Cox, Epistatic interactions between four
        rad loci in yeast, Mutat. Res., 16 (1972) 353-362.
10. Graf, U., and F. E. Würgler, Mutagen sensitive mutants in
        Drosophila: relative MMS sensitivity and maternal effects,
        Mutat. Res., 52 (1978) 381-394.
11. Graf, U., E. Vogel, U. P. Biber, and F. E. Würgler, Genetic
        control of mutagen sensitivity in Drosophila melanogaster.
        A new allele at the mei-9 locus on the X-chromosome,
        Mutat. Res., 59 (1979) 129-133.
12. Haynes, R. H., DNA repair and the genetic control of radiosen-
        sitivity in yeast. In: Molecular Mechanisms for Repair
        of DNA, Part B, P. C. Hanawalt and R. B. Setlow (Eds.),
        Plenum Press, New York-London, 1975, pp. 529-540.

13. Haynes, R. H., Workshop summary: DNA repair in lower eukaryote
       eukaryotes. In: DNA Repair Mechanisms, P. C. Hanawalt,
       E. C. Friedberg, and C. F. Fox (Eds.), Academic Press, New
       York, 1978, pp. 405-411.
14. Kimball, R. F., Relationship between repair processes and
       mutation induction in bacteria, This volume, p. 1.
15. Lawrence, C., and R. B. Christensen, Ultraviolet light induced
       mutagenesis in Saccharomyces cerevisiae. In: DNA Repair
       Mechanisms, P. C. Hanawalt, E. C. Friedberg, and C. F. Fox
       (Eds.), Academic Press, New York, pp. 437-440.
16. Lawlor, T., personal communication.
17. Mason, J., personal communication.
18. Morimyo, M., and Y. Shimazu, Evidence that gene uvrB is
       indispensable for a polymerase-I deficient strain of
       E. coli, Molec. Gen. Genet., 147 (1976) 243-250.
19. Prakash, L., The relation between repair of DNA and radiation
       and chemical mutagenesis in Saccharomyces cerevisiae.
       Mutat. Res., 41 (1976) 241-248.
20. Prakash, L. and S. Prakash, Isolation and characterization of
       MMS-sensitive mutants of Saccharomyces cerevisiae.
       Genetics, 86 (1977) 33-55.
21. Prakash, L. and S. Prakash, Pathways of DNA repair in yeast.
       In: DNA Repair Mechanisms, P. C. Hanawalt, E. C. Friedberg
       and C. F. Fox (Eds.), Academic Press, New York, 1978,
       pp. 413-416.
22. Prakash, L., and S. Prakash, Genetic analysis of error-prone
       repair systems in Saccharomyces cerevisiae, This volume, 141.
23. Samson, L., and J. Cairns, A new pathway of DNA repair in
       Escherichia coli, Nature, 267 (1977) 281-282.
24. Smith, K. C., Multiple pathways of DNA repair in bacteria and
       their role in mutagenesis, Photochem. Photobiol., 28 (1978)
       121-129.
25. Smith, P. D., Mutagen sensitivity of Drosophila melanogaster.
       I. Isolation and preliminary characterization of a methyl
       methanesulfonate-sensitive strain, Mutat. Res., 20 (1973)
       215-220.
26. Smith, P. D., and C. G. Shear, X-ray and ultraviolet light
       sensitivities of a methyl methanesulfonate-sensitive strain
       of Drosophila melanogaster, In: Mechanisms in Recombina-
       tion, R. F. Grell (Ed.), Plenum Press, New York-London,
       1974, pp. 399-403.
27. Smith, P. D., Mutagen sensitivity of Drosophila melanogaster.
       III. X-linked loci governing sensitivity to methyl
       methanesulfonate, Molec. Gen. Genet., 149 (1976) 73-85.
28. Snyder, R. D., unpublished data.
29. Snyder, R. D. and P. D. Smith, in preparation.
30. Witkin, E. M., Ultraviolet mutagenesis and inducible DNA repair
       in Escherichia coli, Bacteriol. Rev., 40 (1976) 869-907.

31. Yamamoto, Y., M. Katsuki, M. Sekiguchi, and N. Otsuji,
      Escherichia coli gene that controls sensitivity to
      alkylating agents, J. Bacteriol., 135 (1978) 144-152.
32. Yamamoto, Y., and M. Sekiguchi, Pathways for repair of DNA
      damaged by alkylating agent in Escherichia coli, Molec.
      Gen. Genet., 171 (1979) 251-256.

CHAPTER 13

EFFECTS OF RECOMBINATION-DEFICIENT AND REPAIR-DEFICIENT LOCI ON

MEIOTIC AND MITOTIC CHROMOSOME BEHAVIOR IN DROSOPHILA MELANOGASTER

BRUCE S. BAKER, MAURIZIO GATTI, ADELAIDE T. C. CARPENTER,
SERGIO PIMPINELLI, and DAVID A. SMITH

Biology Department, University of California
San Diego, La Jolla, California 92093 (U.S.A.)
and
Instituto de Genetica, Faculta di Scienze
Citta Universitaria 00185, Roma, Italy

SUMMARY

The results of recent genetic and cytological studies on recombination-defective and repair-defective mutants of Drosophila
melanogaster are summarized. These studies show that there is substantial overlap between the functions used in various aspects of
DNA metabolism in Drosophila. Most loci first identified by either
recombination-defective or mutagen-sensitive mutants have been shown
also to function in nonmutagenized mitotic cells where their action
is necessary to maintain the integrity of the genome: mutants at
particular loci produce elevated frequencies of chromosome breakage,
mitotic exchange, mutation, and/or chromosome loss.

Genetic studies of meiotic recombination show that many of the
loci identified by recombination-defective mutants restrict where
along the chromosome arms exchange may occur. Recent EM studies
suggest that the products of at least some of these loci are components of recombination nodules. Region-specific control of DNA
metabolism is also indicated by the finding of nonrandom patterns
of chromosome breakage in some mutagen-sensitive mutants.

Recombination-defective mutants at two loci have been studied
for their effects on sister chromatid exchanges (SCEs) and x-ray
induced aberrations. Mutants at both loci are defective in steps
necessary for the production of symmetrical chromatid interchanges
but have little effect on SCEs.

INTRODUCTION

Chromosomes, when considered as cellular organelles, have evolved not only to allow the orderly expression of the genome but also to undergo with extreme precision the complex series of changes necessary for their regular inheritance during meiotic and mitotic cell divisions. The interests of our laboratories are in the control and integration of the various processes affecting chromosomes (e.g., recombination, replication, condensation, movement, repair, etc.) which together comprise the chromosome cycle. There are two levels at which the control of any of the processes that comprise the chromosome cycle may be exerted: (1) on the expression of the loci controlling these processes and the activities of their products, and (2) by the ability of chromosomes, or regions of chromosomes, to serve as substrates for these processes. Chromosomes exhibit morphological and functional differentiation along their lengths and to some degree these regional specializations have arisen as a consequence of evolutionary demands for precise inheritance. It has long been evident that regional differentiations modulate the response of segments of chromosomes to the cell's metabolic machinery; constitutive heterochromatin lacks meiotic recombination, euchromatic and heterochromatic segments of the genome exhibit different (allocyclic) times of replication, centromeres exhibit kinetic activity, and so on. Thus, an understanding of the chromosome cycle must include a description of the mechanism of each process, whether each given process is restricted to specific portions of the genome, and, if so, a description of the cause of the restriction.

The approach we have taken to investigate the processes that govern chromosome behavior during cell division is to isolate and analyze mutants that disrupt various aspects of the chromosome cycle. In Drosophila melanogaster a systematic approach of this type began with the isolation of meiotic mutants — mutants defective in processes necessary for recombination and/or chromosome segregation during the meiotic divisions [32, 42]. As the result of several screens for meiotic mutants in Drosophila [1, 25, 31, 34, 42, 43] there are now known over 40 mutants, representing at least 29 loci. Initial studies of these mutants focused on the genetical characterization of the defective meioses they produce with the aim of inferring the roles of their wild-type alleles in insuring normal meiotic divisions. One result of these studies was to identify a number of recombination-defective mutants, mutants whose primary meiotic lesions are in a process necessary for recombination along the chromosome. These studies, as well as studies on meiotic mutants in other organisms, have been recently reviewed [2, 4, 33, 44].

In the past few years two other approaches have been utilized to isolate mutants in Drosophila that are defective in processes necessary for a normal chromosome cycle. Firstly, a number of mutants hypersensitive to killing by mutagens — mutagen-sensitive

mutants — have been isolated [8, 26, 35, 38, 47, 48, 51]. As these
mutants identify loci that may specify products necessary for the
repair of mutagen damage, many of these mutants have been assayed
biochemically for the normality of several repair pathways [9-11, 37].
These mutants have also been investigated for their effects on sensitivity to a variety of mutagens and carcinogens [3, 5, 8-11, 26, 38,
47-52]. Secondly, we [7] have isolated temperature-sensitive-lethal
mutants that are defective in events necessary for the regular behavior of chromosomes during mitotic cell division. Together these
three types of mutant screens have identified a broad range of functions necessary for normal chromosome behavior in Drosophila.

     Our recent work on these mutants, which we review briefly below,
has focused on two broad topics. One major area of interest has
been in defining the domains of action and nature of the loci identified by these mutants. Here we have asked: (1) whether the functions utilized for meiotic recombination and segregation are also
utilized during mitotic cell division; (2) whether loci that function in the repair of exogenous mutagen damage are also involved in
chromosomal metabolism in nonmutagenized cells; and (3) whether
extant meiotic and mutagen sensitive mutants are leaky alleles at
loci that specify essential cellular functions or represent loci that
are dispensable for viability (the screening procedures used requires
such mutants to be homozygous viable). The second area of interest
has been in utilizing these mutants to investigate the nature of the
events involved in generating two classical endpoints of chromosomal
metabolism: recombinant chromosomes during meiosis and the production of chromosome aberrations by mutagen damage.

        DOMAINS OF ACTION OF MUTAGEN-SENSITIVE AND MEIOTIC MUTANTS

             Meiotic Recombination and DNA Repair

     Some enzymatic steps in DNA repair and recombination are under
common genic control in prokaryotes (for reviews see [20, 27, 40]).
It is thus not surprising that mutant alleles of at least two recombination defective loci (mei-9, mei-41) which were isolated on the
basis of defective meioses also confer hypersensitivity to a variety
of mutagens [3, 5, 8, 10, 26, 47, 48, 50]. Moreover, alleles at both
of these loci have been isolated by screens for mutagen-sensitive
mutants [35, 48]. That the mei-9 and mei-41 alleles isolated on the
basis of mutagen sensitivity cause the same types of defects as the
original alleles is suggested by the fact that they produce elevated
frequencies of nondisjunction during female meiosis [35, 48]; nondisjunction is increased in all recombination-defective mutants in
Drosophila, and, with but one exception [34], this has been shown to
be solely the consequence of the misbehavior of nonexchange bivalents
which are produced in elevated frequencies by these mutants [1, 4,
16, 18, 39, 41]. The occurrence of nondisjunction does not, however,

show that a mutant is defective in recombination; lesions in later
stages of the meiotic process are known that disrupt segregation but
not exchange (for reviews see [2, 4]). Thus we have directly examined meiotic recombination in the presence of four mei-9 alleles
isolated as mutagen-sensitive mutants. The results (Table 1) show
that all four alleles drastically reduce meiotic recombination.
Moreover, the reduction in recombination is nearly uniform in all
regions in these mutants, as it is in the presence of mei-9 alleles
isolated as meiotic mutants [1, 18]. In the centromere region
(pr-cn), recombination in the mutants is not reduced quite as much
relative to the control map distance as it is in the other regions;
however, this nonuniformity may in part be attributable to the fact
that in these control crosses the pr-cn region has less recombination
than in previous control crosses. These data establish that the
types of lesions at the mei-9 locus detected by screens for mutagen-
sensitivity and meiotic abnormalities are the same.

    Further evidence for a common control of meiotic recombination
and DNA repair in Drosophila comes from the observation that mutants
at the mus-101 and mus-102 loci produce elevated frequencies of
nondisjunction from which it has been inferred these mutants reduce
exchange [8, 48].

Roles of Recombination-Defective Loci in
Nonmutagenized Mitotic Cells

    To inquire whether functions that are utilized in normal
meiotic recombination and chromosome segregation are also required
in the chromosome cycle of nonmutagenized mitotic cells we have
examined the effects of meiotic and mutagen-sensitive mutants on
mitotic chromosome stability [3, 5, 6, 21]. Here we restrict our-
selves to the results with recombination-defective meiotic mutants
and mutagen-sensitive mutants; similar studies on disjunction-
defective meiotic mutants are reported elsewhere [5]. Two approaches
— genetical [3, 5, 6] and cytological [21] — have been used to
examine the roles of these loci in nonmutagenized mitotic cells.
The genetic experiments are described first.

    To determine whether recombination-defective and mutagen-sensi-
tive mutants affect chromosome stability, flies were constructed
that carried the mutant of interest and were simultaneously heterozygous for one or more somatic cell markers (mutants that autono-
mously affect the color or morphology of the bristles and/or hairs
of the fly's cuticle). In such flies, effects of mutants that lead
to elevated frequencies of mutation, chromosome breakage, somatic
recombination, chromosome loss and/or nondisjunction are detectable
by increases in the frequency of clones of cells that are homozygous
or hemizygous for the recessive somatic cell marker mutations
(Fig. 1). The clones arising by each of these mechanisms have

TABLE 1

RECOMBINATION ALONG THE LEFT ARM OF CHROMOSOME 2 AND X NONDISJUNCTION
IN CONTROLS AND IN MEI-9 ALLELES ISOLATED AS MUTAGEN-SENSITIVE MUTANTS[a]

	mei-9^AT1	+(AT1 Control)	mei-9^D1	mei-9^D3	mei-9^D4	+(D1-4 Control)
al dp b pr cn	3374	3027	659	1161	1850	431
+ dp b pr cn	43	798	10	40	38	85
+ + b pr cn	159	1822	35	150	130	324
+ + + pr cn	31	253	5	19	8	50
+ + + + cn	11	48	4	6	11	9
al dp b pr +	5	38	1	7	2	9
al dp b + +	22	239	4	17	25	48
al dp + + +	133	1602	18	98	85	237
al + + + +	60	932	11	34	40	123
+ + + + +	5724	4482	1673	2867	3842	762
Doubles	3	228	0	2	2	49
Triples	0	4	0	0	0	0
Total	9565	13,473	2420	4401	6033	2127
Map: al-dp	1.09	13.75	0.87	1.68	1.29	11.00
dp-b	3.07	26.83	2.19	5.68	3.60	28.07
b-pr	0.56	4.30	0.37	0.86	0.58	5.92
pr-cn	0.19	1.13	0.21	0.30	0.22	1.22
Total	4.91	46.01	3.64	8.52	5.69	46.22
Map/Control						
al-dp	0.08	1.0	0.08	0.15	0.12	1.0
dp-b	0.11	1.0	0.08	0.20	0.13	1.0
b-pr	0.13	1.0	0.06	0.14	0.10	1.0
pr-cn	0.17	1.0	0.17	0.25	0.18	1.0
Total	0.11	1.0	0.08	0.18	0.12	1.0
Gametic frequency X-nondisjunction	--	0.0%	25.0%	15.6%	13.3%	0.2%

[a]Crosses are: mei-9-/mei-9-; al dp b pr cn/+ + + + + x +/Y; al dp b pr cn/
al dp b pr cn, with the X chromosomes marked as follows: mei-9^ATI, + (hence
X-exceptional progeny were not recognizable); control ATI, y; mei-9^D1, y^2 sn^3;
mei-9^D3, mei-9^D4, and control -D1, 3, 4, sn^3. For descriptions of the markers used
see Baker and Carpenter [1].

distinguishable properties and thus the source of chromosome instability in any mutant can be identified. For example, somatic recombination produces twin spots whereas mutation and chromosome breakage
produce single spots. The single spots produced by mutation are
euploid and have normal growth characteristics, whereas the clones
produced by breakage are aneuploid and consequently grow poorly and
differentiate short thin bristles when they encompass a bristle-
forming cell.

By using this approach, 12 recombination-defective meiotic
mutants representing seven loci have been examined for effects on
chromosome stability in the cells that produce the wing blade and
the cells that produce the abdominal tergites (the dorsal segments
of the abdomen). The results show that mutants at six of these loci
[mei-9, mei-41, mei-352, mei-W68, mei-S282, and c(3)G] produce
elevated frequencies of mitotic chromosome instability, whereas
mutant alleles at the mei-218 locus do not affect mitotic chromosome
stability. All mutants have comparable effects on mitotic chromosome
stability in males and females. In all cases where more than one
mutant allele at a locus was studied [mei-9, mei-41, mei-W68, c(3)G],
all alleles produced similar patterns of mitotic effects suggesting
that the increased mitotic chromosome instability was being caused
by the absence of the wild-type allele of the locus.

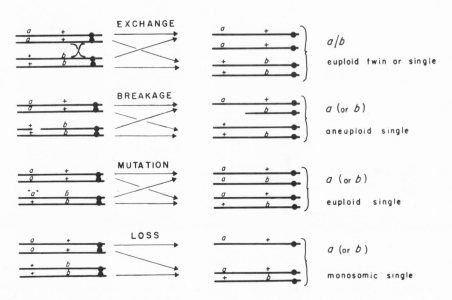

Fig. 1.   Mechanisms by which clones expressing the somatic cell
markers a and b can arise.

The properties of the clones produced by these mutants show
that they cause chromosome instability by a variety of mechanisms.
Most clones produced by mei-41 and mei-9 alleles are aneuploid and
result from chromosome breakage deleting the dominant allele of a
cell marker. A small fraction of the clones produced in the presence
of mutants at these two loci are euploid and probably result from
mitotic recombination. Mutants at the mei-W68 and mei-S282 loci
produce elevated frequencies of mitotic recombination, and, to a
lesser extent, chromosome loss. There was no single predominant
mechanism of clone production by c(3)G alleles or by mei-352.

Taken together, these results show that most functions utilized
during meiotic recombination in Drosophila are also utilized in
somatic cells, where they function in processes requisite for the
stability of mitotic chromosomes. These results are interpreted as
indicating that the functions specified by the wild-type alleles of
these loci act either to prevent discontinuities from occurring in
the genome during somatic cell division or to repair them. If such
discontinuities, which may be either normal intermediates in chromosomal metabolism or spontaneous lesions, are not removed from the
genome, it is suggested that they may initiate a sequence of events
that would culminate in chromosome breakage, mutation, chromosome
loss, mitotic crossing over, or nondisjunction, producing a marked
clone of cells.

In similar experiments, the effects of 13 mutagen-sensitive
mutants, representing seven loci, on the stability of chromosomes in
nonmutagenized somatic cells have been examined [6]. Mutants at
three loci (mus-103, mus-104, and mus-106) do not affect the frequency of clones, whereas mus-101, mus-102, mus-105, and mus-109
alleles cause increases in the frequency of cell marker clones.
Analysis of the size distribution of clones produced by mutants at
the latter four loci suggests that most of the chromosome instability
they produce is the consequence of chromosome breakage; in the
presence of mus-105 and mus-109 alleles a minority of clones arise
via a mechanism (mutation, mitotic recombination, nondisjunction)
that produces euploid clones.

The inferences from these genetic studies have been confirmed
and extended by the cytological examination of the effects of eight
recombination-defective and 12 mutagen-sensitive mutants on the
frequencies and types of spontaneous chromosome aberrations in larval
neuroblast metaphases [21]. Mutants at seven loci (mus-101, mus-103,
mus-104, mus-106, mei-218, mei-251, mei-352) have no detectable
effect on the frequency of spontaneous chromosome aberrations while
mutants at five loci (mei-9, mei-41, mus-102, mus-105, and mus-109)
cause significant increases in the frequency of aberrations. In all
mutants the only aberrations detected were chromatid and isochromatid
breaks. Most breaks detected must have occurred in the cell division
scored, since (1) nearly all isochromatid breaks were associated

with acentric fragments and (2) chromatid breaks must have arisen during or after the preceding S period. Although these two types of breaks are the only frequent aberrations produced by these mutants, very different proportions of chromatid and isochromatid breaks are produced by mutants at different loci (Fig. 2). A third to a half of breaks involve both chromatids in mus-102, mus-105, mus-109, and mei-41 mutants, whereas most of the breaks produced in the presence of mei-9 alleles are single chromatid breaks. For all five loci two mutant alleles were examined and both produced the same patterns of chromatid versus isochromatid breaks [21] (Fig. 2), indicating that the pattern of breaks produced is a property of the locus.

In all mutants the distribution of breaks among chromosomes is random. However, the distributions of breaks along chromosome arms differ strikingly among mutants (Fig. 3). In the presence of mei-9, mus-102, and mei-41 mutants, breaks are approximately equally distributed between heterochromatin and euchromatin. This distribution is also observed when x-ray-induced breaks in wild-type are scored [24]. However, in mus-105 mutants about 80% of breaks occur in euchromatin, whereas in mus-109 about 80% of breaks are heterochromatic. It should be noted that in all mutants roughly 80% of the breaks assigned to heterochromatin seemed to be localized to the heterochromatic-euchromatic junctions.

Together these genetic and cytological studies demonstrate that most loci utilized in meiotic recombination as well as many of the loci utilized in the repair of mutagen damage specify products that are needed to maintain the integrity of chromosomes during mitotic cell division in the absence of exogenous damage. The requirements for these functions in nonmutagenized somatic cells could be for either of two reasons. One possibility is that substantial frequencies of spontaneous lesions are present in somatic cells, and the products of these loci are needed to repair these lesions. If this were the case then the relative rarity of chromosome instability in these mutants (in the most severe mutant examined only 14% of cells had chromosome breaks) could reflect the rarity of such lesions. The second possibility is that these mutants could be alleles of loci that specify essential functions involved in chromosomal metabolism (e.g., DNA replication, chromatin packaging). If the latter possibility be true, then the requirement that meiotic and mutagen-sensitive mutants be viable in order to be detected in the screens that have been employed to date would mean that only leaky alleles at these loci would have been recovered. However, if the first alternative be correct then both leaky and null alleles should have been recoverable.

To inquire whether any of the extant alleles at the mus-101, mus-105, and mus-109 loci are null mutants, the frequencies of cell marker clones in homozygous mus- females and hemizygous mus- (mus-/deficiency) females have been compared [6]. If a mutant is leaky,

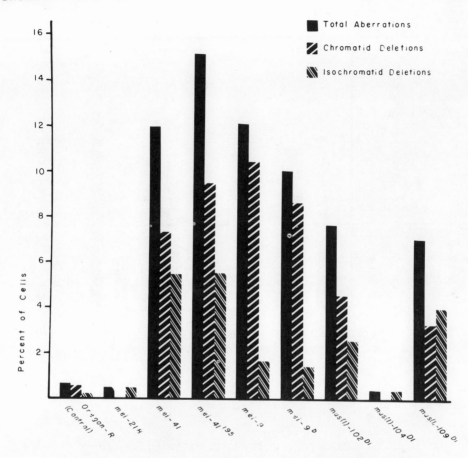

Fig. 2.   Frequencies and types of spontaneous chromosome breaks
observed in larval ganglion metaphase of selected recombination-
defective and mutagen-sensitive mutants.   Data from Gatti [21].

then chromosome instability should be increased in the mus-/defi-
ciency females.   Two alleles at the mus-105 locus and three alleles
at the mus-101 and mus-109 loci were examined in this manner.   In
all cases there was an elevated frequency of mitotic chromosome
instability in mus-/deficiency females as compared to homozygous
mus- females.   Thus these alleles are all leaky mutants.

In this regard it is worth noting that none of the mei-9
alleles tested completely eliminates meiotic recombination suggesting
either that these alleles are leaky or that there is more than one
pathway for meiotic recombination in Drosophila.   The possibilities
are being investigated by Lawlor, who has deficiency-mapped mei-9

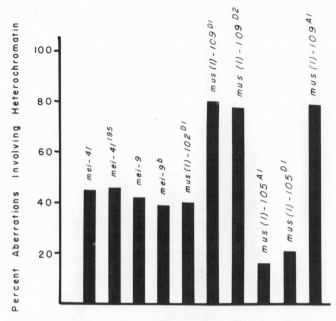

Fig. 3.   Proportions of spontaneous chromosome breaks occurring in heterochromatic regions in larval ganglion metaphase.   Data from Gatti [21].

[29] and is using these deficiences to inquire whether there is residual activity in the mei-9 mutants.

RECOMBINATION, CHROMOSOME ABERRATIONS, AND SISTER CHROMATID EXCHANGES

Recombinant chromosomes that are produced during meiotic (or mitotic) cell division and chromosome aberrations that are produced in response to chromosomal lesions have in common the fact that they are both end products of a complex series of molecular events affecting DNA.   The recombination-defective and repair-defective mutants available in Drosophila provide powerful probes into the processes that lead to these two end points of DNA metabolism.   In this section we summarize some recent studies using these mutants to investigate the control of these two processes.   More detailed consideration of the genetic control of recombination in Drosophila has been given elsewhere [1, 2, 4, 18, 33].

Control of Meiotic Recombination

Meiotic recombination in most, if not all, eukaryotes does not occur with uniform probability throughout the genome.   In Drosophila

there are at least two levels at which constraints on the distribution of meiotic exchange are evident. Firstly, exchanges are distributed nonrandomly along the length of the chromosome arm. In
wild type there is no exchange in the proximal heterochromatin of
each arm, a low frequency of exchange per unit physical length in
the euchromatic regions adjacent to the proximal heterochromatin,
and a relatively high and uniform frequency of exchange per unit
physical length throughout the remainder of the euchromatin [30, 33].
The second level of control is in the relative locations of the
component exchanges in chromosomes with one, two, and three exchanges.
Although this could simply reflect the occurrence of chiasma interference, a deeper analysis by Charles [19] has shown that for chromosomes with a particular number of exchanges the exchange(s) occur
about nodal positions on the chromosome. Thus, in bivalents with
one exchange the exchange occurs in the middle of the arm. When
there are two exchanges, one is near the tip and the other is near
the base of the arm; and in the rare triple exchange bivalents, the
component exchanges are evenly spaced along the arm. An understanding
of the process of recombination in eukaryotes must therefore encompass not only the molecular events of the exchange process itself but
also the factors that control the location of exchange events in the
genome.

    Studies of the frequency and distribution of the residual ex-
change occurring in the presence of recombination-defective mutants
have identified three categories of loci. Mutants at most loci
(e.g., mei-41, mei-218, mei-W68^{L1}, mei-S282) result in nonuniform
reductions in recombination along the chromosome arms relative to
controls; recombination is reduced most severely in distal regions
and progressively less so in regions adjacent to and spanning the
proximal heterochromatin. Mutants at the mei-9 locus reduce recombination uniformly in all regions. In the presence of mei-352 the
frequency of exchange per chromosome arm is unaltered but the distribution of exchange events along the chromosome is altered such
that there are higher frequencies of exchange in regions spanning,
and near, the centromere and lower frequencies of exchange in distal
regions.

    When the distribution of exchange is examined in those mutants
that alter the pattern of recombination, it is found that exchange
is more uniform per unit physical length throughout the euchromatin
than it is in wild type [1, 4, 18, 33, 39]. From these observations
it has been suggested that the wild-type alleles of these loci
(mei-41, mei-218, etc.) specify products that are necessary for both
the occurrence of exchange and the determination of where along the
chromosome exchanges may occur [1]. Thus the nonrandom distribution
of recombination along the euchromatic portions of chromosome arms
observed in wild type would appear to be due to constraints that
are imposed on the locations of exchanges by the products of the
wild-type alleles of these genes.

Recent support for this hypothesis has come from experiments by Sandler and Szauter [45] who inquired whether recombination-defective mutants that relaxed constraints on the location of exchanges along the arms of the major chromosomes also reduced the constraints that normally preclude exchanges between the tiny fourth chromosomes in wild type. Their results showed that in the three mutants of this type examined (mei-218, mei-352. mei-S282) these constraints were indeed relaxed: in the presence of each of these mutants the frequency of recombination on chromosome 4 was elevated. In the presence of mei-9^b, which reduces exchange but does not alter the distribution of exchanges, the frequency of fourth chromosome recombination was not increased. Thus, Sandler and Szauter were able to conclude that the same constraints that were responsible for the nonrandom distribution of recombination on the major chromosomes in wild type were also responsible for the absence of recombination on chromosome 4. Hence it is at least a tenable hypothesis at present to suppose that the nonrandomness in the gross distribution of exchanges along the euchromatic portions of the genome are attributable to constraints imposed by the products of the wild-type alleles of recombination-defective loci.

However, the absence of recombination in the centric heterochromatin in wild type appears to be the result of constraints different from those imposed by these loci. Sandler and Szauter [45] noted that, whereas mei-218, mei-S282 and mei-352 increased recombination in the two euchromatic regions of the fourth chromosome that they examined, these mutants did not permit recombination in the centric heterochromatin of the fourth chromosome. We have shown [17] that this also holds true for the basal heterochromatin of the X chromosome in the presence of six recombination-defective mutants that alter the distribution of exchange (mei-218, mei-218$^{6-7}$, mei-41, mei-41^{195}, mei-352 and mei-251). The regions examined were (1) car-bb, which includes the basal euchromatin and part of the centric heterochromatin and (2) bb-centromere (Dp(1;1)sc^{V1}) which is wholly heterochromatin. For all six mutants substantial frequencies of recombinants in the car-bb interval were recovered, but essentially no recombinants were found in the entirely heterochromatic bb-centromere region. Together, these studies imply that the absence of recombination in the heterochromatin is due to causes different from those that constrain the location of exchanges in the euchromatin.

Some insights into the recombinational roles of loci identified by recombination-defective meiotic mutants have come from recent electron microscope investigations of female meiosis in wild-type [12-14] and in several of these mutants [15]. Examination of meiosis in wild-type D. melanogaster females revealed structures — termed recombination nodules — that are present between paired homologs at pachytene and which parallel exchange events in frequency, location along the chromosome arms, location relative to one another, and in

proportions of arms having zero, one, and two events. These striking
parallels led to the suggestion that recombination nodules mark the
sites of exchange and might indeed contain some or all of the functions necessary to carry out exchange [13, 14]. EM studies of recombination-defective mutants at three loci (mei-218, mei-41, mei-9)
are consistent with this hypothesis [15]. Mutant alleles at the
mei-218 and mei-41 loci reduce the frequency of recombination nodules
to approximately the same extent that they reduce meiotic recombination and they appear to alter the distribution of recombination
nodules along the chromosome arms in the same manner that they alter
the distribution of exchanges. Most strikingly, mutants at both loci
also affect the morphology of recombination nodules. The nature of
these morphological defects has led to the suggestions that the
mei-218[+] locus specifies a major structural component of the recombination nodule and that mei-41[+] specifies a product that is needed
to maintain the stability of recombination nodules. Alleles at the
mei-9 locus have no detectable effect on the frequency, distribution,
or morphology of nodules. Since mei-9 does drastically reduce exchange, these observations provide strong evidence against the
suggestions [28, 36] that recombination nodules arise after exchange
and are simply involved in holding homologs together at the site of
an exchange or in resolving half-chiasmata. It has been argued on
genetic grounds that the product of the mei-9 locus is directly
involved in meiotic exchange [1, 18]; that mutants at this locus
have no detectable effect on recombination nodules is not inconsistent
with either the postulated role of the mei-9[+] product or the hypothesis that the recombination nodule is the structure that houses all
functions necessary for meiotic exchange, since either the absence
of a minor component or the reduced functionality of a nodule component could render nodules nonfunctional without having morpholog-
ically detectable effects.

Genetic Control of Chromosome Aberration Production
and Sister Chromatid Exchanges

One of the many possible fates of a primary lesion in DNA is to
initiate a series of events that culminates in the production of a
chromosome aberration. The existence of mutants that are defective
in processes necessary for the maintenance of chromosomal integrity
provides probes into the processes that are involved in the generation of chromosome aberrations. Our initial experiments along these
lines [22] have focused on the mei-9 and mei-41 loci.

The genetic [3, 5] and cytological [21] characterizations of
mei-9 and mei-41 mutants showed that essentially all aberrations
produced by these mutants in nonmutagenized cells are chromosome
breaks. A small proportion of the clones detected have properties
suggesting that they arise via mitotic recombination; however,
exchanges are not detected cytologically. The latter result is not

surprising since, as pointed out by Gatti [21], in irradiated wild-type cells that have frequencies of breakage (12%) comparable to those observed in the presence of mei-9 and mei-41 mutants, there are only 0.2% of cells with exchanges.

Mutants at the mei-9 and mei-41 loci differ strikingly in the pattern of breakage they produce: mei-9 alleles produce almost exclusively chromatid breaks whereas mei-41 alleles produce comparable frequencies of chromatid and isochromatid breaks. This difference could be either because the wild-type alleles of these loci function at different times during the cell cycle or because the lesions that are the substrates of the wild-type products of these loci have very different probabilities of giving rise to chromatid versus isochromatid breakages.

Insights into the roles of these loci in chromatid interchanges as well as the origin of the different proportions of chromatid and isochromatid breaks produced by these mutants have come from studies of the frequencies and types of chromosome aberrations generated in the presence of these mutants in response to x-rays [22]. Neuroblasts of larvae bearing mei-9 or mei-41 alleles irradiated with 220 R and scored during the subsequent metaphase exhibit about a 10-fold increase in the frequency of chromosome breaks. In mei-9 alleles (mei-9, mei-9^AT1) most breaks are chromatid deletions, whereas in mei-41 alleles (mei-41, mei-41^195) there are equal proportions of chromatid and isochromatid breaks. This strongly suggests that the different patterns of breakage observed in these mutants occur because the lesions (x-ray induced and spontaneous) that are the actual substrates of these loci have very different probabilities, if unrepaired, of producing chromatid and isochromatid breaks.

mei-9 and mei-41 mutants also differ strikingly in their effects on the induction of exchanges by x-rays. At the dose used, there were 1.1 to 1.2 aberrations induced per cell in larvae bearing a mei-41 allele and of these aberrations about 10% were exchanges. In larvae bearing mei-9 alleles, comparable frequencies of total aberrations were induced (1.0-1.3 aberrations per cell) but almost none (0.02%) of these were exchanges. Non-meiotic-mutant-bearing cells irradiated with a high dose of x-rays (1320 R) exhibited 0.7-0.8 aberrations per cell, of which about 25% were exchanges. These data show that the function specified by the mei-9^+ locus is normally necessary for the conversion of a primary x-ray lesion into an exchange. The decreased proportion of exchanges observed in irradiated cells bearing mei-41 alleles suggests that the wild-type function specified by this locus is also utilized in a step necessary for the generation of at least some exchanges. Moreover, when the exchanges detected in the presence of mei-41 alleles are scored as to whether they are symmetrical (X-type) or asymmetrical (U-type), it is found that only 6-12% are symmetrical exchanges, whereas about 30% of x-ray-induced exchanges are symmetrical in non-meiotic mutant controls. This suggests that the $mei-41^+$ product is preferentially utilized in the production of symmetrical exchanges.

In another series of experiments [22], the effects of these $mei-41$ and $mei-9$ alleles on sister chromatid exchange (SCE) have been investigated by using the BUdR-Hoechst 23358 procedure adapted for Drosophila by Gatti et al. [23]. In neuroblasts of larvae bearing either of the $mei-41$ alleles the frequency of SCEs does not differ from that in nonmutant controls. However, in the presence of either of the $mei-9$ alleles examined SCEs occur at only 70% of control rates. Since most, if not all, SCEs in Drosophila appear to be induced by the treatment(s) required to detect them [23], here again $mei-9$ is defective in the conversion of a lesion into an exchange. Thus the wild-type product of the $mei-9$ locus is necessary for the occurrence of at least some SCEs as well as most meiotic exchange and nearly all x-ray-induced exchange.

Meiotic crossing over, symmetrical chromatid interchanges, and SCEs all involve X type physical exchanges of whole chromatids, and, at least superficially, might be expected to be generated by similar, if not identical, sequences of events. Nevertheless these data clearly demonstrate that the two functions examined (those of $mei-9^+$ and $mei-41^+$) are utilized in the production of meiotic exchange and symmetrical chromatid interchanges but not in the generation of most SCEs.

CONCLUSIONS

These genetic and cytological investigations of recombination-defective and repair-defective mutants have shown that there is substantial overlap between the functions used in various aspects of DNA metabolism in Drosophila. All but one ($mei-218$) of the recombination-defective loci examined are necessary for chromosome stability in nonmutagenized mitotic cells. Two of these loci ($mei-9$ and $mei-41$) are also utilized in the repair of damage induced by a wide variety of mutagens. Analogous studies on the loci identified by mutagen-sensitive mutants suggest that at least two of these loci ($mus-101$, $mus-102$) specify functions necessary for meiotic recombination [8, 48], and four of these ($mus-101$, $mus-102$, $mus-105$, $mus-109$) are needed to maintain chromosome integrity in nonmutagenized cells [6, 21]. In two cases ($mei-352$ and $mus-101$ alleles) increased chromosome instability was detected genetically but not cytologically. Thus these mutants increase instability via mechanisms that do not have clear cytological consequences.

The chromosome instability produced by many of these mutants is interpreted to mean that the products of these loci normally function to remove discontinuities from the chromosome which, if unrepaired, can result in chromosome breakage, mutation, mitotic exchange, non-disjunction, or loss. It is at present unclear whether the discontinuities that are the substrates of these loci are the consequence of spontaneous lesions or are instead normal intermediates in DNA metabolism. That all alleles tested at the mus-101, mus-105, and mus-109 loci are leaky is consistent with either view. However, the finding that certain double mutant combinations of these mutants are lethal [49] as well as the isolation of a temperature-sensitive lethal at the mus-101 locus [46] show that several of these loci specify functions that are also involved in essential aspects of normal DNA metabolism.

These recent studies have also helped define the processes that cause meiotic recombination to occur with different probabilities per unit physical length in different segments of the genome and in addition have revealed region-specific controls on chromosomal metabolism in mitotic cells. The constraints that generate nonuniform distributions of meiotic recombination along the euchromatic portions of all chromosome arms appear to be imposed by the functioning of the wild-type alleles of a number of loci, such as mei-218 and mei-41, that control both the frequency and the location of recombination events. Evidence that the products of the mei-218 and mei-41 loci may be components of recombination nodules has led to the suggestion that recombination nodules contain not only most or all of the components necessary to effect exchange but also those that determine the location of exchanges. However, the constraints that preclude exchange in heterochromatic regions appear to be distinct from those that govern the distribution of exchanges in euchromatin; in mutants that relax the constraints on the location of euchromatic exchanges, there is still a complete absence of heterochromatic exchange.

Evidence for region-specific controls of chromosomal metabolism is also provided by the patterns of chromosome breakage detected in mitotic cells of mutants that affect chromosome stability. In alleles at the mus-105 locus most breaks are euchromatic, whereas in mus-109 mutants most breakage is in heterochromatin. Breakage in mus-109 is further restricted, in that approximately 80% of the heterochromatic breaks occur at the heterochromatin-euchromatin junction. In all other mutants examined, breaks are approximately equally distributed between the heterochromatin and the euchromatin, although here too most heterochromatic breaks are localized at the heterochromatin-euchromatin junction. Together, these findings clearly demonstrate that the maintenance of chromosomal integrity in different regions of the genome is under the control of different loci.

Finally, we would like to emphasize the very striking results of the study of the effects of mei-9 and mei-41 mutants on sister chromatid exchange and x-ray-induced chromosome aberrations. These experiments show that the wild-type function of the mei-9 locus, in addition to being essential for meiotic exchange, is also necessary for the production of x-ray-induced exchanges and at least some sister chromatid exchanges. On the other hand, mei-41 alleles reduce the frequencies of meiotic and x-ray induced exchange but have no effect on sister chromatid exchange. Thus these data suggest that chromatid interchanges, but not most SCEs, arise via mechanisms similar to those involved in meiotic recombination.

The extremely wide range of effects of many of the better char-acterized recombination-defective and repair-defective mutants clearly establishes that in Drosophila pathways of DNA metabolism that lead to a great variety of different end points have intermedi-ate steps in common.

ACKNOWLEDGEMENT

This research was supported by U.S. Public Health Service Grants GM 23345 and GM 23338, by the association between Euratom and CNR contract No. 136-74-7 BIOI, and by a grant from Progetto Finalizzato Promozione Qualità dell' Ambiente.

REFERENCES

1. Baker, B. S., and A. T. C. Carpenter, Genetic analysis of sex chromosomal meiotic mutants in Drosophila melanogaster, Genetics, 71 (1972) 255-286.
2. Baker, B. S., A. T. C. Carpenter, M. S. Esposito, R. E. Esposito, and L. Sandler, The genetic control of meiosis, Ann. Rev. Genet., 10 (1976) 53-134.
3. Baker, B. S., J. B. Boyd, A. T. C. Carpenter, M. M. Green, T. D. Nguyen, P. Ripoll, and P. D. Smith, Genetic controls of meiotic recombination and somatic DNA metabolism in Drosophila melanogaster, Proc. Natl. Acad. Sci. (U.S.), 73 (1976) 4140-4144.
4. Baker, B. S., and J. C. Hall, Meiotic mutants: genetic control of meiotic recombination and chromosome segregation, In: The Genetics and Biology of Drosophila, Vol. 1a, M. Ashburner and E. Novitski, Eds., Academic Press, New York - London, 1976, pp. 350-434.
5. Baker, B. S., A. T. C. Carpenter, and P. Ripoll, The utiliza-tion during mitotic cell division of loci controlling meiotic recombination and disjunction in Drosophila melanogaster, Genetics, 90 (1978) 531-578.
6. Baker, B. S., and D. A. Smith, The effects of mutagen-sensitive mutants of Drosophila melanogaster in nonmutagenized cells, Genetics, 92 (1979) 833-847.
7. Baker, B. S., and D. A. Smith, In preparation.

8. Boyd, J. B., M. D. Golino, T. D. Nguyen, and M. M. Green, Isolation and characterization of X-linked mutants of Drosophila melanogaster which are sensitive to mutagens, Genetics, 84 (1976) 485-506.

9. Boyd, J. B., and R. B. Setlow, Characterization of post replication repair in mutagen-sensitive strains of Drosophila melanogaster, Genetics, 84 (1976) 507-526.

10. Boyd, J. B., M. D. Golino, and R. B. Setlow, The mei-9^a mutant of Drosophila melanogaster increases mutagen sensitivity and decreases excision repair, Genetics, 84 (1976) 527-544.

11. Boyd, J. B., P. V. Harris, C. J. Osgood, and K. E. Smith, Biochemical characterization of repair-deficient mutants of Drosophila, This volume, p. 209.

12. Carpenter, A. T. C., Electron microscopy of meiosis of Drosophila melanogaster females. I. Structure, arrangement, and temporal change of the synaptonemal complex in wild-type, Chromosoma, 51 (1975) 157-182.

13. Carpenter, A. T. C., Electron microscopy of meiosis in Drosophila melanogaster females. II. The recombination nodule — a recombination-associated structure at pachytene? Proc. Natl. Acad. Sci. (U.S.), 72 (1975) 3186-3189.

14. Carpenter, A. T. C., Synaptonemal complex and recombination nodules in wild-type Drosophila melanogaster females, Genetics, 92 (1979) 511-541.

15. Carpenter, A. T. C., Recombination nodules and synaptonemal complex in recombination-defective Drosophila melanogaster females, Chromosoma, 75 (1979) 259-292.

16. Carpenter, A. T. C., and B. S. Baker, Genic control of meiosis and some observations on the synaptonemal complex in Drosophila melanogaster, In: Mechanisms in Recombination, R. F. Grell, Ed., Plenum Press, New York, 1974, pp. 365-375.

17. Carpenter, A. T. C., and B. S. Baker, In preparation.

18. Carpenter, A. T. C., and L. Sandler, On recombination-defective meiotic mutants in Drosophila melanogaster, Genetics, 76 (1974) 453-475.

19. Charles, D. R., The spatial distribution of cross-overs in X chromosome tetrads of Drosophila melanogaster, J. Genet., 36 (1938) 103-126.

20. Clark, A. J., Recombination deficient mutants of E. coli and other bacteria, Ann. Rev. Genet., 7 (1973) 67-86.

21. Gatti, M., Genetic control of chromosome breakage and rejoining in Drosophila melanogaster: spontaneous chromosome aberrations in X-linked mutants defective in DNA metabolism, Proc. Natl. Acad. Sci. (U.S.), 76 (1979) 1377-1381.

22. Gatti, M., S. Pimpinelli, and B. S. Baker, Relationships between chromatid interchanges, sister chromatid exchanges and meiotic recombination in Drosophila melanogaster, Proc. Natl. Acad. Sci. (U.S.), (1980), in press.

23. Gatti, M., G. Santini, S. Pimpinelli, and G. Olivieri, Lack of
    spontaneous sister chromatid exchanges in somatic cells of
    Drosophila melanogaster, Genetics, 91 (1979) 255-274.
24. Gatti, M., C. Tanzarella, and G. Olivieri, Analysis of the
    chromosome aberrations induced by x-rays in somatic cells
    of Drosophila melanogaster, Genetics, 77 (1974) 701-719.
25. Gethmann, R. C., Meiosis in male Drosophila melanogaster,
    I. Isolation and characterization of meiotic mutants
    affecting second chromosome disjunction, Genetics, 78
    (1974) 1127-1142.
26. Graf, U., E. Vogel, U. P. Biber, and F. E. Würgler, Genetic
    control of mutagen sensitivity in Drosophila melanogaster.
    A new allele at the mei-9 locus on the X-chromosome,
    Mutat. Res., 59 (1979) 129-133.
27. Hanawalt, P. C., and R. B. Setlow, Molecular Mechanisms for
    Repair of DNA, Plenum Press, New York, 1975, parts A and B.
28. Holliday, R., Recombination and meiosis, Phil. Trans. Roy. Soc.
    (London)B, 277, (1977) 359-370.
29. Lawlor, T. A., Genetic and cytological localization of mei-9,
    Drosophila Inform. Serv., in press.
30. Lefevre, G., Jr., Salivary chromosome bands and the frequency
    of crossing over in Drosophila melanogaster, Genetics, 67
    (1971) 497-513.
31. Lewis, E. B., and W. Gencarella, Claret and nondisjunction in
    Drosophila melanogaster, Genetics (Abstr.) 37 (1952) 600-601.
32. Lindsley, D. L., L. Sandler, B. Nicoletti, and G. Trippa,
    Mutants affecting meiosis in natural populations of
    Drosophila melanogaster, In: Replication and Recombination
    of Genetic Material, W. J. Peacock and R. D. Brock, Eds.,
    Australian Acad. Sci., Canberra, 1968, pp. 253-267.
33. Lindsley, D. L., and L. Sandler, The genetic analysis of
    meiosis in female Drosophila melanogaster, Phil. Trans.
    Roy. Soc. (London)B, 277 (1977) 295-312.
34. Mason, J. M., Orientation disruptor (ord): a recombination-
    defective and disjunction-defective meiotic mutant in
    Drosophila melanogaster, Genetics, 84 (1976) 545-572.
35. Mason, J. M., M. M. Green, K. E. Smith, and J. B. Boyd, Genetic
    analysis of X-linked mutagen-sensitive mutants of Drosophila
    melanogaster, submitted.
36. Moens, P. B., Lateral element cross connections of the synapto-
    nemal complex and their relationship to chiasmata in rat
    spermatocytes, Can. J. Genet. Cytol., 20 (1978) 567-579.
37. Nguyen, T. D., and J. B. Boyd, The mei-9 locus of Drosophila
    melanogaster is deficient in repair replication of DNA,
    Genetics, 83 (1976) s55.
38. Nguyen, T. D., M. M. Green, and J. B. Boyd, Isolation of two
    X-linked mutants in Drosophila melanogaster which are
    sensitive to gamma-rays, Mutat. Res., 49 (1978) 139-143.
39. Parry, D. M., A meiotic mutant affecting recombination in female
    Drosophila melanogaster, Genetics, 73 (1973) 465-486.

40. Radding, C. M., Molecular mechanisms in genetic recombination, Ann. Rev. Genet., 7 (1973) 87-111.
41. Robbins, L. G., Nonexchange alignment: a meiotic process revealed by a synthetic meiotic mutant of Drosophila melanogaster, Mol. Gen. Genet., 110 (1971) 144-166.
42. Sandler, L., D. L. Lindsley, B. Nicoletti, and G. Trippa, Mutants affecting meiosis in natural populations of Drosophila melanogaster, Genetics, 60 (1968) 525-558.
43. Sandler, L., Induction of autosomal meiotic mutants by EMS in D. melanogaster, Drosophila Inform. Serv., 47 (1971) 68.
44. Sandler, L., and D. L. Lindsley, Some observations on the study of the genetic control of meiosis in Drosophila melanogaster, Genetics, 78 (1974) 289-297.
45. Sandler, L., and P. Szauter, The effect of recombination-defective meiotic mutants on fourth-chromosome crossing over in Drosophila melanogaster, Genetics, 90 (1978) 699-712.
46. Smith, D. A., and B. S. Baker, In preparation.
47. Smith, P. D., Mutagen sensitivity of Drosophila melanogaster, I. Isolation and preliminary characterization of a methyl methanesulfonate-sensitive strain, Mutat. Res., 20 (1973) 215-220.
48. Smith, P. D., Mutagen sensitivity of Drosophila melanogaster, III. X-linked loci governing sensitivity to methyl methane-sulfonate, Molec. Gen. Genet., 149 (1976) 73-85.
49. Smith, P. D., Mutagen sensitivity of Drosophila melanogaster, IV. Interactions of X chromosome mutants, In: DNA Repair Mechanisms (ICN-UCLA Symposia on Molecular and Cellular Biology IX), P. C. Hanawalt, E. C. Friedberg, and C. F. Fox, Eds., Academic Press, New York, 1978, pp. 453-456.
50. Smith, P. D., and C. G. Shear, X-ray and ultraviolet light sensitivities of a methyl methanesulfonate-sensitive strain of Drosophila melanogaster, In: Mechanisms in Recombination, R. F. Grell, Ed., Plenum Press, New York, 1974, pp. 399-403.
51. Smith, P. D., R. D. Snyder, and R. L. Dusenbery, Isolation and characterization of repair-deficient mutants of Drosophila melanogaster, This volume.
52. Würgler, F. E., and U. Graf, Mutation induction in repair-deficient strains of Drosophila, This volume.

CHAPTER 14

BIOCHEMICAL CHARACTERIZATION OF REPAIR-DEFICIENT MUTANTS

OF DROSOPHILA

JAMES B. BOYD, PAUL V. HARRIS, CHRISTOPHER J. OSGOOD,
and KAREN E. SMITH

Department of Genetics, University of California
Davis, California 95616 (U.S.A.)

SUMMARY

DNA metabolism is being analyzed in cell cultures derived from
the available mutagen-sensitive stocks. Thus far, mutants occurring
at eleven different genetic loci in Drosophila melanogaster have
been shown to be defective in DNA synthesis or repair. Mutants
associated with the following genetic loci exhibit defects in the
corresponding metabolic functions:

Excision Repair - mei-9, mus(2)201, mus(2)205, mus(3)308
Postreplication Repair - mei-41, mus(1)101, mus(1)104,
                         mus(2)205, mus(3)302, mus(3)310,
                         mus(3)311
DNA Synthesis - mus(1)101, mus(1)104, mus(2)205, mus(3)307,
                mus(3)308

The pleiotropic effect of several of these mutants indicates that
their wild type alleles normally participate in more than one of
these processes. Since mutants in at least three of these classes
[mei-9, mei-41, mus(1)101] also alter meiotic recombination, their
biochemical analysis in the more plentiful somatic cells can
potentially reveal the function of the normal alleles in the rare
meiotic tissues. A survey of the mutant properties is presented
in Table 3.

The existence of a photorepair system has been documented in
Drosophila, although no genetic blocks in that process have been
identified. Identification of an AP-endonuclease activity suggests
that Drosophila may possess a base excision mechanism. A technical

advance is also described which will permit biochemical analysis of
stocks in which homozygous females are sterile.

INTRODUCTION

The preceding papers have clearly established the genetic
advantages of Drosophila as a model organism for the analysis of
DNA metabolism in multicellular eukaryotes. Baker [1] has high-
lighted our capacity to analyze chromosome stability, exchange, and
segregation, both in the germ line and in somatic cells. The results
of such studies provide essential information for assessing the
biological significance of parallel biochemical studies. The
powerful selection techniques described by Smith [27] have permitted
the acquisition of a variety of mutants that are either deficient
in meiotic recombination or are sensitive to chemical mutagens.
An analogous mutant collection in bacteria has been instrumental in
the analysis of DNA metabolism in prokaryotes [18]. Those studies
have made it clear that repair, recombination, and synthesis of
DNA are highly coordinated activities which share common functions.
In the studies reported here, emphasis has been placed on the
biochemical characterization of DNA repair in the available mutants.
Because of the integrated nature of DNA metabolism, however,
analysis of DNA repair potentially illuminates aspects of DNA
recombination and synthesis as well. The fidelity of these
processes, of course, has a strong bearing on the mutation rate
[30] and thus on the theme of this conference.

In the analysis of DNA repair, Drosophila provides a logical
bridge between the sophisticated genetic analyses available in
unicellular organisms and extensive biochemical studies being
performed in mammals [2]. Studies of mutagenesis in this organism
have provided extensive evidence for the existence of genetically
controlled repair mechanisms [26]. Primarily as a result of recent
improvements in insect tissue culture, it is now possible to analyze
each of the major forms of DNA repair biochemically by using
procedures developed with mammalian cultures [3]. Application of
this technology to some of the available mutants is reviewed here.
In addition, a new system for analyzing DNA repair in organ culture
is described. This advance places the previously inaccessible
female-sterile mutants within the range of our analysis.

PHOTOREPAIR

Reduction of UV-induced mutagenesis by photoreactivating light
has been documented in Drosophila [12, 21]. An autosomal recessive
factor has also been implicated in photoreversal of UV-induced
lethality [15, 31]. However, it is less certain that this repair

process is acting on DNA damage since repair of uridine dimers has been implicated in photoreactivation in another insect [19].

Subsequent biochemical analyses have documented the capacity of Drosophila cells to abolish pyrimidine dimers from their DNA with the aid of photoreactivating light. Trosko and Wilder [28] directly measured the level of pyrimidine dimers in DNA following UV irradiation of established cell cultures. Of the thymine-containing dimers induced by a fluence of 150 J/m^2, 80% were eliminated after exposure to photoreactivating illumination. Since the level of damage did not change when parallel cultures were incubated in the dark, the loss of lesions is not attributable to dark repair processes. Boyd and Presley [8] have exploited competition between repair pathways to monitor photorepair in whole animals. In that system, photorepair was assayed indirectly as a reduction in excision repair. When larvae were exposed to visible light between UV exposure and excision analysis, the level of excision repair was strongly suppressed. That reduction presumably reflects the light mediated removal of a substrate which is common to both the photo-repair and excision repair pathways.

An enzymatic assay for pyrimidine dimers has recently provided a more sensitive means for the analysis of photorepair [5]. In this system, permeabilized cells are exposed to an endonuclease which nicks DNA in the vicinity of pyrimidine dimers. The frequency of nicking, and thus of dimers, is determined by measuring the molecular weight of the resulting DNA by alkaline sucrose gradient centrifugation. In the experiment described in Fig. 1 the detectable dimers induced by a fluence of 5 J/m^2 were quantitatively removed by subsequent exposure of the cells to visible light. This result suggests, but does not prove, that all dimers are removed by photorepair, since the assay itself detects only 1/5 of the induced lesions. Again, the kinetics of repair are too rapid to be accounted for by dark repair mechanisms. Although the repair capacity of individual mutants has yet to be quantified, a strong photorepair response has been observed in the excision-deficient mutant mei-9[a] [5].

The general agreement of these three biochemical approaches has clearly established the capacity of Drosophila to employ photo-reactivating light to abolish pyrimidine dimers. Although there is no direct evidence that this is accomplished by enzymatic monomerization, analogy with more thoroughly studied systems makes that a highly probable mechanism.

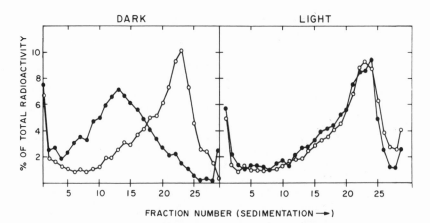

Fig. 1.   Photorepair of pyrimidine dimers. DNA of established
cells (w-1) was uniformly labeled with (● —— ●) ^{3}H or (o —— o)
^{14}C. The ^{3}H-labeled cells received 5 J/m^2 of UV radiation. Cells
labeled with ^{14}C-thymidine were unirradiated. After irradiation
the cells were covered with saline and exposed to light or dark
conditions for 30 min. Permeabilized cells were then incubated
with a UV-specific endonuclease under conditions which nick the
DNA at a frequency equivalent to 20% of the pyrimidine dimers. The
molecular weight of the DNA was monitored with alkaline sucrose
gradient centrifugation. Redrawn from Boyd et al. [5].

NUCLEOTIDE EXCISION

Analysis of Pyrimidine Dimers

Chemical Analysis.   Chromatographic analysis of pyrimidine
dimers permitted the first direct demonstration of excision repair
in Drosophila. Trosko and Wilder [28] found that Drosophila
tissue culture cells can remove 40% of the dimers induced by a UV
fluence of about 35 J/m^2.   Exposure of the cells to caffeine after
UV treatment did not reduce the observed repair. Subsequent studies
conducted in this laboratory [6] have shown that 70% of the induced
thymine dimers are removed from tissue culture cells following a
dose of 15 J/m^2. Cells derived from the recombination-deficient
mutant mei-9^a are devoid of excision repair as measured by this
assay [6].

Enzymatic Analysis.   The chemical assay for pyrimidine dimers
lacks adequate sensitivity to quantify the repair capacity of
certain Drosophila mutants. For example, the extreme radiation
sensitivity of the mei-9 mutants requires the use of UV doses

(15 J/m^2) which are marginally adequate for dimer detection. After
a dose of 25 J/m^2, for which the dimer assay is more reproducible,
the mutant cells detach during postirradiation incubation. To
circumvent this problem we have employed the more sensitive
enzymatic assay which was described under photorepair [5]. After
23 hr of incubation in the dark, 95% of the dimers detected by this
assay have disappeared from the genome of control cells irradiated
with 5 J/m^2. The rate of removal observed in cells of the
established mei-9^{a}-1 culture under these conditions is less than
10% of the control value. Results obtained with the enzymatic
assay, therefore, confirm the conclusions derived from the chemical
assay at a more biologically significant dose.

The use of permeabilized cells to assay pyrimidine dimers still
suffers from two limitations: (1) only about 1/5 of the dimers are
accessible to the exogenous nuclease [5]; and (2) although the
assay is reproducible when applied to established cultures, it is
not reliable with primary cultures. More recently we have employed
a modification of that assay which monitors dimers quantitatively
in primary cells [25]. This procedure differs from the previous
one in that isolated DNA rather than permeabilized cells is exposed
to the UV-specific endonuclease. The two enzymatic assays produced
equivalent results in an analysis of excision kinetics in established
cell cultures. In the experiment depicted in Fig. 2, control cells
assayed by isolating DNA lost 82% of all dimers during a 24 hr
postirradiation incubation.

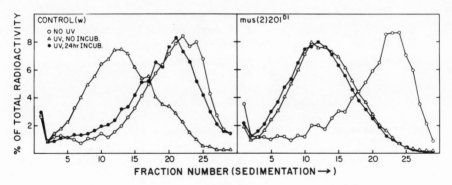

Fig. 2.   Analysis of excision repair in mus(2)201^{D1} cells. DNA of
primary cell cultures was labeled uniformly with ^{3}H or ^{14}C.
Cultures labeled with ^{3}H were irradiated with 5 J/m^2 whereas those
labeled with ^{14}C were untreated. After the indicated incubation
period, DNA was isolated and exposed to a UV-specific-endonuclease.
This treatment produces one break per pyrimidine dimer. The
molecular weight of the DNA was then analyzed by alkaline sucrose
gradient sedimentation. Data from separate gradients are compiled.

The second panel in Fig. 2 reveals a strong excision deficiency in a mutant mapping to the second chromosome. Like the mei-9 mutants, mus(2)201^{D1} is sensitive to such diverse mutagens as MMS, HN2 and AAF. However, it differs from those mutants in that it does not exhibit strong meiotic effects [14]. A total of four loci have been identified which influence excision repair (Table 1). Whereas the mei-9^a and mus(2)201^{D1} mutants are strongly deficient, available mutants at the mus(2)205 and mus(3)308 loci exhibit only a partial reduction in that capacity.

TABLE 1

CAPACITY OF MUTANT CELLS TO EXCISE PYRIMIDINE DIMERS^{a,b}

Strain	% of control (w) repair capacity
w	100%
mei-9^{D2}	0%
mus(2)201^{D1}	0%
mus(2)205^{A1}	40%
mus(3)308^{D2}	59%
mus(3)307^{D1}	109%

^{a}Data of Harris and Boyd [16].

^{b}Excision analysis was performed as described in Fig. 2. The percent of dimers removed by mutant cells during 24 hr postirradiation incubation is divided by the corresponding control value.

Analysis of Base Replacement

Both repair replication and unscheduled DNA synthesis have been employed to study the resynthesis phase of excision repair in Drosophila. The method of Painter and Cleaver [24] for studying repair replication in mammalian cells was originally adapted to study repair in live animals [8]. Replacement of short nucleotide sequences was detected with that procedure after exposure of young larvae to UV. Repair is saturated at doses exceeding 20 J/m^2 and is nearly complete within 5 hr after irradiation with 38 J/m^2. Concentrations of hydroxyurea and caffeine, which strongly reduce semiconservative synthesis, have no detectable effect on repair replication. Application of that technique to two mei-9 mutants has failed to detect repair synthesis after UV treatment [22]. That conclusion applies to established cell cultures of the mutant

as well as to first instar larvae. Lack of repair replication in
these strains is consistent with a block in the early phase of
repair which was suggested by the observations of dimer retention.
Our recent failure to detect unscheduled DNA synthesis in the
$mus(2)201^{D1}$ mutant implicates a related function for these two
loci [10].

Excision-Related DNA Breaks

The nature of the defect in the mei-9 mutants has been
investigated with the highly sensitive alkaline elution procedure
of Kohn et al. [20]. In that study, DNA-synthesis inhibitors were
employed to reduce the resynthesis phase of excision repair. This
inhibition results in the accumulation of UV-stimulated breaks in
DNA of control cells but has little effect on DNA of mei-9 cells
(Fig. 3). A similar observation has been made with cells derived
from the $mus(2)201^{D1}$ mutant. This lack of UV-stimulated breaks in
both strains is most readily explained as a failure of the mutants
to perform the initial endonucleolytic step of excision repair.
Alternative explanations, such as rapid religation of such breaks,
have not been excluded.

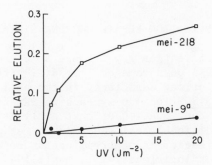

Fig. 3.   Accumulation of single-strand DNA breaks following UV
irradiation. Prior to irradiation established cells were treated
for 20 min with 3 mM hydroxyurea and for an additional 10 min with
a combination of hydroxyurea and 1 mM cytosine-β-D-arabinofuranoside.
After irradiation, incubation was continued for 30 min in the
presence of both inhibitors. Single-strand molecular weight of
the prelabeled DNA was analyzed with the alkaline elution procedure
[20]. Relative elution values are inversely proportional to single-
strand molecular weight.

BASE EXCISION

The base excision form of excision repair is initiated by the sequential action of a glycosylase and an AP-endonuclease rather than by a single damage-specific endonuclease [13]. An extensive search has failed to reveal the presence of a uracil glycosylase in several developmental stages and cell lines of Drosophila [13]. Since this activity is readily detected in a variety of other organisms, Friedberg has speculated that it may be unnecessary in organisms which live primarily below 30°C and thereby experience lower rates of cytosine deamination. A glycosylase which acts on alkylated DNA has recently been isolated from human cells [11]. Such enzymes may be responsible for early observations that MMS and EMS stimulate repair replication in Drosophila larvae [8]. In that study, MMS was found to be 10 times as potent as EMS on a molar basis in stimulating repair synthesis.

An endonuclease activity specific for apurinic sites in DNA is readily demonstrable in crude extracts of Drosophila [23]. Among the sources exhibiting this activity are eggs, embryos, cultured cells, and larval brain ganglia. Optimum assay conditions have been determined for extracts of primary cell cultures. At 25°C the endonuclease activity exhibits a pH optimum of approximately 7.8 and is stimulated by NaCl and divalent cations. The enzyme is inhibited by excess EDTA. Identification of this activity increases the likelihood that a complete base excision process will eventually be documented in Drosophila.

POSTREPLICATION REPAIR AND DNA SYNTHESIS

The term postreplication repair refers to the capacity of a cell to synthesize DNA on a damaged template. Previous studies have demonstrated a strong deficiency in the ability of mutants at the mei-41 and mus(3)302 loci to synthesize DNA following UV irradiation [9]. A continuation of that analysis has uncovered mutants at three additional loci [mus(2)205, mus(3)310, mus(3)311] which express deficiencies in postreplication repair (Table 2). Mutants at four other loci [mus(1)101, mus(1)104, mus(3)307 and mus(3)308] exhibit alterations in DNA metabolism which are less dramatic than the effects observed in the strong postreplication repair deficient mutants [9] (Table 2). Mutants at all four loci exhibit a reduced capacity to synthesize DNA on an undamaged template, and may in addition experience further problems in dealing with a UV-irradiated template [mus(1)101, mus(1)104].

Analysis of postreplication repair to date has been performed with primary cell cultures derived from homozygous embryos. That approach is therefore limited to the analysis of stocks which can be maintained in a homozygous state. In order to analyze stocks

TABLE 2

RELATIVE MOLECULAR WEIGHTS OF PULSE-LABELED DNA[a]

Strain	Relative molecular weight		
	Without prior UV	With prior UV	Difference
mus(3)306^{D1}	1.00	0.99	0.01
mus(3)307^{D1}	0.85[b]	0.84[b]	0.01
mus(3)308^{D2}	0.89[b]	0.84[b]	0.05
mus(3)310^{D1}	1.04	0.58[b]	0.46[c]
mus(3)311^{D3}	0.98	0.86[b]	0.12[d]
mus(2)201^{D1}	1.01	0.93	0.08
mus(2)205^{A1}	0.92[b]	0.63[b]	0.29[c]

[a]Primary cell cultures were exposed to [^{3}H]thymidine for 30 min and incubated in its absence for 3 hr. UV irradiation (10 J/m^2) was administered 30 min prior to labeling. Molecular weights were determined as described in Fig. 4. The average of duplicate values obtained with mutant cells was divided by t e corresponding control value: 165 × 10^6 ± 4.2 [21] without prior UV and 147 ± 4.2 [19] with prior UV. (The standard error is followed by the number of determinations.)

[b]Values are significantly less than 1.00 (control) at the 5% level in a one-sided Student t test.

[c]Influence of UV is significant at the 5% level.

[d]Influence of UV is significant at the 10% level.

in which homozygous females are infertile, a procedure has been developed for assaying postreplication repair in larval brain ganglia. This assay makes it possible to take advantage of genetic procedures for recovering larvae that carry only the mutant allele. The analysis presented in Fig. 4 demonstrates that brain ganglia derived from the mei-41^{D5} mutant exhibit a postreplication repair deficiency after AAAF treatment which is analogous to that expressed in cell cultures following UV treatment [9]. This approach will, therefore, permit a complete survey of the available mutants for alterations in postreplication repair capacity.

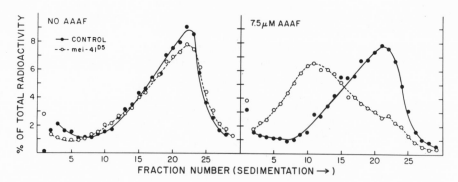

Fig. 4.   Postreplication repair in larval brain ganglia of the
mei-41^{D5} mutant.   Brain ganglia were dissected from late third
instar larvae of the homozygous stocks w and w mei-41^{D5}.   At 10 min
after mutagen treatment the tissue was exposed to [^{3}H]thymidine for
30 min.   The tissue was then incubated for 2 hr in nonradioactive
medium before the labeled DNA was analyzed by sedimentation in
alkaline sucrose gradients.   The mutagen was kindly provided by
Dr. J. A. Miller of the McArdle Laboratory.

RESPONSE TO IONIZING RADIATION

In contrast to the extensive literature available on radiation
genetics in Drosophila [26], relatively little is known at the
biochemical level about the response of Drosophila cells to ionizing
radiation.   Unscheduled DNA synthesis has been observed in polytene
chromosomes following exposure of salivary glands [29] or isolated
polytene nuclei [6] to high doses of x-rays.   Repair replication is
stimulated by x-ray exposure in both first instar larvae [8] and
cultured cells [17] of Drosophila.   Because this response is absent
in tests performed with mei-9 mutants [22], it is likely that these
assays are detecting the repair of x-ray-induced base damage rather
than restitution of strand breaks.   This conclusion derives from
observations that mei-9 cells are deficient in excision repair, yet
possess a normal capacity to repair single-strand breaks induced by
x-rays [5].   An earlier search for mutants with a reduced capacity
to repair single strand breaks was unsuccessful [9].   Current
studies being performed with additional third chromosomal mutants,
however, suggest that this phenotype is represented in the current
mutant collection.

CONCLUSION

A summary of the biochemical analyses is presented in Table 3.
These studies considered in combination with parallel genetic and

cytogenetic investigations are contributing to an increased
understanding of the role of DNA repair mechanisms in mutagenesis
of multicellular eukaryotes.

TABLE 3

GENETIC LOCI KNOWN TO INFLUENCE DNA METABOLISM[a]

	Excision repair	DNA Synthesis	Postreplication repair	Reference
X chromosome				
mei-9	−	+	+	[5]
mei-41	0	+	−	[9]
mus(1)101	0	−	−	[9]
mus(1)104	0	−	−	[9]
2nd chromosome				
mus(2)201	−	+	+	[17]
mus(2)205	−	−	−	[17]
3rd chromosome				
mus(3)302	0	+	−	[9]
mus(3)307	+	−	+	[17]
mus(3)308	−	−	+	[17]
mus(3)310	0	+	−	[17]
mus(3)311	0	+	−	[17]

[a]+, normal phenotype;   −, mutant phenotype;   0, not tested.

ACKNOWLEDGMENTS

We would like to acknowledge the close collaboration with our
previous coauthors which has made this venture so personally
rewarding. Recent work in the Davis laboratory has been supported
by the Department of Energy, Office of Environment under Project
Agreement No. DE-AT03-79EV70210 and National Institutes of Health
Grants GM22221 and GM25562.

REFERENCES

1. Baker, B. S., Effects of repair-deficient loci on mitotic and
     meiotic chromosome behavior, this volume.

2. Baker, B. S., J. B. Boyd, A. T. C. Carpenter, M. M. Green,
    T. D. Nguyen, P. Ripoll, and P. D. Smith, Genetic controls
    of meiotic recombination and somatic DNA metabolism in
    Drosophila melanogaster, Proc. Natl. Acad. Sci. (U.S.A.),
    73 (1976) 4140-4144.
3. Boyd, J. B., DNA repair in Drosophila, In: DNA Repair Mechanisms,
    P. C. Hanawalt, E. C. Friedberg and C. R. Fox (Eds.),
    Academic Press, New York, 1978, pp. 449-452.
4. Boyd, J. B., unpublished observations.
5. Boyd, J. B., M. D. Golino, and R. B. Setlow, The mei-9^a mutant
    of Drosophila melanogaster increases mutagen sensitivity
    and decreases excision repair, Genetics, 84 (1976)
    527-544.
6. Boyd, J. B., and P. V. Harris, Excision repair in Drosophila:
    Analysis of strand breaks appearing in DNA of mei-9 cells
    following exposure to UV and N-acetoxy-N-acetyl-2-amino-
    fluorene, in preparation.
7. Boyd, J. B., and J. M. Presley, Deoxyribonucleic acid synthesis
    in isolated polytene nuclei of Drosophila hydei, Biochem.
    Genetics, 9 (1973) 309-325.
8. Boyd, J. B., and J. M. Presley, Repair replication and photo-
    repair of DNA in larvae of Drosophila melanogaster,
    Genetics, 77 (1974) 687-700.
9. Boyd, J. B., and R. B. Setlow, Characterization of postrepli-
    cation repair in mutagen-sensitive strains of Drosophila
    melanogaster, Genetics, 84 (1976) 507-526.
10. Boyd, S., unpublished observations.
11. Brent, T. P., Partial purification and characterization of a
    human 3-methyladenine-DNA glycosylase, Biochemistry, 18
    (1979) 911-916.
12. Browning, L. S., and E. Alterburg, The proportionality between
    mutation rate and ultraviolet dose after photoreactivation
    in Drosophila, Genetics, 47 (1962) 361-366.
13. Friedberg, E. C., T. Bonura, R. Cone, R. Simmons, and C.
    Anderson, Base excision repair of DNA, In: DNA Repair
    Mechanisms, P. C. Hanawalt, E. C. Friedberg and C. R. Fox
    (Eds.), Academic Press, New York, 1978, pp. 163-173.
14. Green and Smith, unpublished observations.
15. Ghelelovitch, S., La sensibilité des oeufs de la Drosophile
    (Drosophila melanogaster, Meig.) à l'action léthale des
    rayons ultra-violets. I. Évolution de la sensibilité
    avec l'âge de l'embryon, Intern. J. Radiat. Biol., 11
    (1966) 255-271.
16. Harris, P. V., and J. B. Boyd, in preparation.
17. Harris, P. V., K. E. Smith, and J. B. Boyd, in preparation.
18. Hanawalt, P. C., E. C. Friedberg and C. R. Fox, (Eds.),
    DNA Repair, Academic Press, New York, 1978.

19. Kalthoff, K., K. Urban, and J. H. Jäckle, Photoreactivation
       of RNA in UV-irradiated insect eggs (Smittia Sp.,
       Chironomidae, Diptera). II. Evidence for heterogeneous
       light-dependent repair activities, Photochem. Photobiol.,
       27 (1978) 317-322.
20. Kohn, K. W., L. C. Erickson, R. A. G. Ewig, and C. A.
       Friedman, Fractionation of DNA from mammalian cells by
       alkaline elution, Biochemistry, 15 (1976) 4629-4637.
21. Meyer, H. U., Photoreactivation of ultraviolet mutagenesis in
       the polar cap of Drosophila (abstr.), Genetics, 36 (1951)
       565.
22. Nguyen, T. D., and J. B. Boyd, The meiotic-9 (mei-9) mutants
       of Drosophila melanogaster are deficient in repair repli-
       cation of DNA, Molec. Gen. Genet., 158 (1977) 141-147.
23. Osgood, C., unpublished observations.
24. Painter, R. B., and J. E. Cleaver, Repair replication,
       unscheduled DNA synthesis, and the repair of mammalian
       DNA, Radiat. Res., 37 (1969) 451-466.
25. Reynolds, R. J., Removal of pyrimidine dimers from
       Saccharomyces cerevisiae nuclear DNA under nongrowth
       conditions as detected by a sensitive, enzymatic assay,
       Mutat. Res., 50 (1978) 43-56.
26. Sankaranarayanan, K., and F. Sobels, Radiation genetics,
       In: The Genetics and Biology of Drosophila, M. Ashburner
       and E. Novitski (Eds.), Academic Press, New York, 1976,
       Vol. 1c, pp. 1090-1250
27. Smith, P. D., R. D. Snyder, and R. L. Dusenbery, Isolation and
       characterization of repair-deficient mutants of Drosophila
       melanogaster, This volume, p. 175.
28. Trosko, J. E., and K. Wilder, Repair of UV-induced pyrimidine
       dimers in Drosophila melanogaster cells in vitro, Genetics,
       73 (1973) 297-302.
29. Valencia, J. I., and W. Plaut, X-ray-induced DNA synthesis
       in polytene chromosomes (abstr.), J. Cell Biol., 43 (1969)
       151a.
30. Würgler, F. E., and U. Graf, Mutation induction in repair-
       deficient strains of Drosophila, This volume, p. 223.

31. Yegorova, L. A., V. L. Levin and M. A. Kozlova, Heritability
       of UV-sensitivity and photo-reactivation ability in
       Drosophila embryos, Mutat. Res., 49 (1978) 213-218.

CHAPTER 15

MUTATION INDUCTION IN REPAIR-DEFICIENT STRAINS OF DROSOPHILA

F. E. WÜRGLER and U. GRAF

Institute of Toxicology, Swiss Federal Institute of
Technology and University of Zürich,
CH-8603 Schwerzenbach, Switzerland

SUMMARY

Experimental evidence indicates a polygenic control of mutagenesis in <u>Drosophila melanogaster</u>. In oocytes chromosome aberrations detected as half-translocations or dominant lethals depend on
a repair system which in a number of genetically nonrelated strains
shows different repair capacities. Sister chromatid exchanges (SCE)
are easily studied as ring chromosome losses. They develop through
a genotype controlled mechanism from premutational lesions. Stocks
with particular pairs of third chromosomes were discovered in which
increased sensitivity of larvae to the toxic effects of a monofunctional alkylating agent (MMS) correlates with high frequencies
of x-ray induced SCE's.

Sex-linked mutagen-sensitive mutants could be shown to control
mutation fixation: Pronounced maternal effects were found when
sperm carrying particular types of premutational lesions were introduced into different types of mutant oocytes. The mutant $\underline{mus(1)101}^{D1}$
was found to be unable to process lesions induced by the crosslinking
agent **ni**trogen mustard (HN2) into point mutations (measured as sex-
linked recessive lethals). Alkylation damage leads to increased
point mutation frequencies in the excision repair deficient mutant
$\underline{mei-9}^{L1}$, but to reduced frequencies in the post-replication repair
deficient mutant $\underline{mei-41}^{D5}$. It became clear that the study of maternal effects on mutagenized sperm represents an efficient tool to
analyze the genetic control of mutagenesis in the eukaryotic genome
of <u>Drosophila melanogaster</u>.

INTRODUCTION

The study of mutagenesis in repair-deficient mutants is an approach to analysis of the genetic control of mutagenesis in Drosophila. Two principal procedures are possible: that by stock differences and that involving study of maternal effects.

In the stock differences study, differential mutagenesis after treatment of genetically different individuals from repair competent and repair deficient strains is evaluated.

In the maternal effects study, metabolic effects on the processing of premutational lesions are determined in a unique experimental situation. Sperm containing premutational lesions are analyzed for mutation frequencies after introducing them into oocytes with or without repair deficiencies. In this way effects of the maternal repair systems on damaged chromatin can be analyzed. Conceptually the study of such maternal effects is identical with the study of host cell reactivation in microbial systems.

In Drosophila, both types of studies have some advantages and some disadvantages. The main advantage of the analysis of stock differences is the possibility of studying any suitable cell type in any suitable developmental stage. As long as ionizing radiation is used for such studies with the intact animal, one is sure that the mutagenic agent reaches the target cells immediately during exposure. This does not have to be the case if chemical mutagens are studied. As long as genetically different flies or larvae are exposed to chemicals, variations in the mutation frequency may result either from influences of the mutation one is studying or from other genetic variations such as intensity of uptake via different routes, distribution, detoxification, etc. The problems are even more complicated if indirect mutagens are used which need metabolic activation [30]. As no carefully collected data on the dosimetry of the chemical reaching the target cells are available results obtained with mutant flies have to be interpreted very cautiously: In addition to repair deficiencies, the whole pharmacokinetic situation, in particular the balance between activation and detoxification, can profoundly influence the response of a specific strain.

Most of these problems are eliminated if the second procedure is used, the analysis of maternal effects [9, 35]. The basic concept may be described as follows (see Fig. 1).

Premutational lesions in a reproducible amount can be induced in chromosomes of mature sperm by a standard treatment of a standard type of male. There is good evidence that in mature sperm no DNA repair processes are active [21]. Some nonenzymatic changes of primary lesions, such as depurination of alkylated sites, may take place, especially if enough time is provided by storage [11, 31].

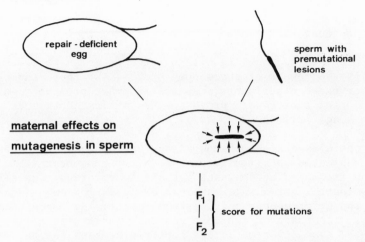

Fig. 1.   Scheme showing the rationale of the experiments for the study of maternal effects on mutagenesis in sperm chromosomes.

        The processing of the lesions by maternal repair systems will take place after the sperm has entered the egg and the sperm chromatin resumes its physiological activity [34].

        Let us now see what the two different approaches can tell us about mutagenesis in Drosophila and how these processes are influenced by repair deficient mutations.   The data will be presented in three sections: First we will see what we know about the genetic control of aberration induction, then we will discuss the induction of sister chromatid exchanges and finally we will turn to point mutations.   The genetic symbols used are those described by Lindsley and Grell [15].

CHROMOSOME ABERRATIONS AND DOMINANT LETHALS

        In crossing tests with Drosophila the consequences of chromosome breaks and their reunion in germ cells can be studied by recording translocations, half translocations (detachments), transvections, etc. [1, 16, 37].   All three tests need suitably marked tester stocks.   The recording of translocations, the "cleanest" test for aberrations, needs two test generations.   On the other hand the recording of half-translocations and transvections are one-generation tests.   Unfortunately at present only a few stocks are available which, in addition to the repair deficiency, contain also the genetic

markers suitable for the scoring of particular chromosome aberrations
in the one-generation tests.

    In one analysis dealing with oocytes we tried to study some
aspects of the repair of chromosome breaks. We chose the class B
oocyte for these experiments, because a number of investigations
have indicated that repair processes are active in this experimentally
suitable stage [21, 25, 26].

    In the classical experimental approach, class B oocytes [12,
19] are subjected to x-radiation, and after the oocytes have matured the frequency of dominant lethals is recorded. Usually only
those dominant lethals which are expressed during embryonic development of the F_1 progeny resulting from fertilizing these oocytes are
analyzed. The shape of the dose response curve with a wide shoulder
permits the assumption of active repair processes in the immature
oocyte. This is further proven by dose fractionation experiments
which demonstrate active repair as soon as the total dose is divided
into at least two fractions separated by 5 to 60 min [22, 26]. An
increasingly larger fraction of damage is repaired if the total dose
is divided into more and more fractions [22]. The recent experiments of Steiner and Würgler [25, 26] show that in class B oocytes
we are dealing with an Elkind-type recovery. The same authors
demonstrated that chromosome aberrations (detachments) show exactly
the same repair kinetics as dominant lethals [25]. This is evident
from the dose response curves for acute and fractionated irradiation
which are indicative of Elkind-type recovery and a very short half-
life of the reparable lesions of only 5-7 min. This time is nearly
as short as the estimated lifetime of lesions in inseminated eggs
which is about 10 min [34]. There is now good evidence that dominant
lethals induced in irradiated oocytes represent one particularly
drastic consequence of chromosome breakage events.

    We tried to take advantage of this situation in the study of
two repair mutants. Before starting with the irradiation experiments, the ovaries of freshly hatched females of mus and mei mutants
were prepared for microscopic analysis. It was found that in all
mutant females oogenesis proceeds with the same kinetics as in wild
type flies [27]. Between 40 and 50 class B oocytes were found in
2.5 hr old females. With acute irradiation it was found that class
B oocytes of repair competent flies (white strain) and those of
mus(1)101^{D1} females have "normal" x-ray sensitivity. In contrast to
this, class B oocytes of mei-41^{D5} females exhibit a clearly increased sensitivity (Fig. 2). Based on the identical kinetics of
oogenesis in all three types of female the increased x-ray sensitivity of mei-41^{D5} oocytes can not be simulated by older oocyte
stages with higher intrinsic sensitivity. The increased x-ray sensitivity of mei-41^{D5} oocytes agrees well with the maternal effects of
this mutant on x-irradiated sperm chromosomes [9] and with the increased gamma-ray sensitivity of mei-41^{D5} larvae [17]. It is

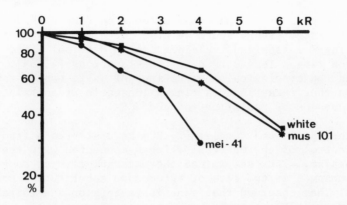

Fig. 2.   X-ray sensitivity of class B oocytes of the strains white,
mus(1)101^{D1}, and mei-41^{D5}.   Females, 0-2 hr old, were irradiated;
24 hr later eggs were collected and tested for survival. Abscissa:
x-ray exposure; ordinate: embryonic survival

interesting to note that mei-41 mutants show strong chromosome instability in somatic cells [5, 23].

    We tested for Elkind-type recovery in the three strains using
fractionated irradiations. We found that the repair competent white
stock shows a comparatively low capacity for Elkind-type recovery
and that both mutants have about the same capacity as the white
stock. Although the mei-41^{D5} exhibits an increased x-ray sensitivity, its capacity to rejoin and rearrange chromosome breaks does
not seem to be strongly reduced. This result is in line with observations of Gatti [6] on somatic cells of mei-41 larvae, indicating
the ability of mei-41 to produce chromosome aberrations.

SISTER CHROMATID EXCHANGE AND RING-CHROMOSOME LOSSES

    Sister chromatid exchanges (SCE) can be demonstrated cytologi-
cally in larval ganglia cells [7]. The study of ring-chromosomes
indicates that SCE's can lead to dicentric ring-X-chromosomes. Such
dicentrics, if present in the paternal pronucleus, can lead either
to loss of the dicentric or act as dominant lethals. In crosses of
ring-X males with suitably marked chromosomes to females with two
free X-chromosomes, ring-X losses can be detected as XO-males.
Therefore, the registration of ring-X losses allows for a quick and
simple test for induced SCE's in Drosophila.

    The study of x-ray-induced ring-X losses has for a long time
given puzzling results which were not easily explained as consequences of the same type of events as those leading to such chromosome aberrations as translocations [13]. In our studies concerned

with the analysis of the maternal effects on ring-X chromosome losses
from x-irradiated mature sperm we also noted a marked difference
between ring-X losses and translocations. Maternal effects were much
stronger on ring-X losses than on translocations [4, 39]. This
result and the cytological observations of Gatti can be taken as an
indication that x-ray induced ring-X losses in Drosophila in fact
are consequences of radiation-induced SCEs.

Racine, Beck, and Würgler [2, 20] have started a study on the
genetic control of the maternal effects connected with the ring-X
loss mechanism. They determined the maternal effects on x-irradiated
ring chromosomes in two sets of chromosome substitution stocks
(Fig. 3). They observed that genetic factors on the third chromosome are responsible for the modification of ring-X loss frequencies.
On the second chromosome at best weak factors could be detected. In
additional studies we tested the chromosome substitution stocks for
methyl methanesulfonate (MMS) sensitivity of larvae (Fig. 4) and
found that increased MMS sensitivity correlated with strong maternal
effects on x-irradiated ring chromosomes. No meiotic effects are
present in the chromosome substitution stocks. Therefore it is
postulated that factors on the third chromosome which belong to the
mus class of mutations possibly influence both MMS sensitivity and
the production of SCEs from x-ray-induced lesions.

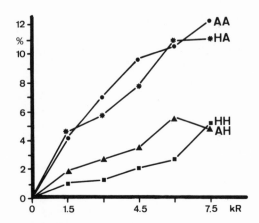

Fig. 3. Maternal effects on x-ray-induced ring-X chromosome losses
with four chromosome substitution stocks. Ring-X males (R(1)2,y
B / B^S Y y$^+$; bw; st p^P) were irradiated and crossed to four
different types of female with substituted second and third chromo-
somes. Genotypes: HH, +/+; +/+ (= Hikone wild type); AH, Cy/Pm;
+/+; HA, +/+; Ubx/Sb; AA, Cy/Pm; Ubx/Sb. Abbreviations: Cy =
In(2LR)SM5,al^{2}Cy lt^{V}cn^{2}sp^2; Pm = In(2LR) bw^{VI}; Ubx = In(2LR)Ubx^{130};
Sb = In(3R) Sb. Abscissa: x-ray exposure to ring-X males;
ordinate: induced ring-X losses scored as XO-males in the progeny.
Details and actual data given elsewhere [20].

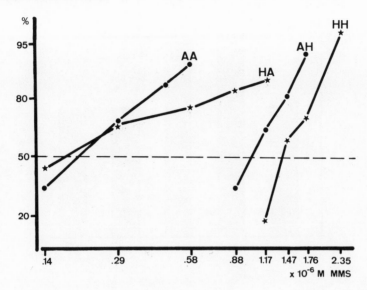

Fig. 4.   MMS sensitivity of first instar larvae of the chromosome
substitution stocks.   Abscissa: Concentration of MMS fed to the
larvae;   ordinate: Induced larva to adult lethality (probit).
Details given elsewhere [2].   Genotypes as in Fig. 3.

     Recently a project to study maternal effects of repair-deficient
mutants on chemically induced SCEs was started.   By testing nitrogen
mustard (HN2)-treated ring-X bearing sperm with different types of
repair deficient oocytes we found that with $\underline{mus(1)101^{D1}}$ and $\underline{mei-41^{D5}}$
increased frequencies of losses and therefore of SCEs are produced
(Fig. 5).   These first results indicate that probing chemically
treated sperm for maternal effects on ring-X losses can be developed
into a powerful tool to study the genetic and metabolic control of
SCE production in Drosophila.

                              POINT MUTATIONS

     In order to study the induction of point mutations in Drosophila
one can score for **sex-linked** recessive lethals.   Cytological and
genetic studies indicate that single gene changes, small deletions,
and certain types of chromosome aberrations can lead to the phenotype of recessive lethality [37].   The relative proportion of the
different types of molecular changes in the chromatin depends on the
mutagen used to induce the mutations.   Among lethals induced by ionizing radiations an appreciable number is connected with structural
changes in the chromosome, including small deletions.   This fact was
demonstrated in complementation tests which indicated that x-ray-
induced mutations often extend over more than one complementation

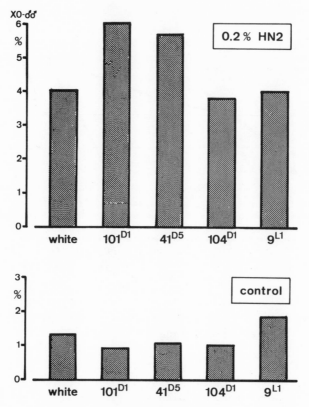

Fig. 5.   Maternal effects on HN2-induced ring-X losses: (top)
Induced ring-X losses;   (bottom) spontaneous ring-X losses.   Ring-X
males $(R(1)2,y B /B^S Y y^+; bw; st p^P)$ were fed with 0.2% HN2 in
5% sucrose for 24 hr and then crossed to females of the strains
white, mus(1)101^{D1}, mei-41^{D5}, mus(1)104^{D1} and mei-9^{L1}.

unit [14].   In contrast to this, mutations induced by monofunctional
alkylating agents in general do not extend over more than one complementation unit [14].   This is true for ethyl methanesulfonate
(EMS) and N-nitrosodiethylamine (DEN), which are unable to break
Drosophila chromosomes; the induction of point mutations of the base
pair substitution type can safely be assumed.

Treatment of Mutant Males

There is only one published experiment in which males carrying a meiotic mutation were exposed to a chemical mutagen and the progeny scored for sex-linked recessive lethals. Vogel reported [30] that 4-dimethylamino-trans-stilbene gives a significantly higher mutation frequency if $mei-9^{L1}$ males are treated instead of males of the standard tester strain Berlin wild K. Vogel [31] has shown that males bearing the $mei-9^a$ $mei-41^{D5}$ mutants, when treated with benzo(a)-pyrene, produced significantly more recessive lethals than did control (yellow) males. Furthermore, experimental work conducted with 2-acetylminofluorene, benzo(a)pyrene, 7,12-dimethylbenzanthracene and 4-dimethylamino-trans-stilbene, revealed a markedly improved detection capacity of strains carrying $mei-9^{L1}$ or $mei-9^a$ $mei-41^{D5}$ relative to the wild type tester strain [31]. All of these carcinogens could be identified as mutagens in repair-deficient stocks following exposure of male larvae or adult males.

Maternal Effects

Since experiments using mutant males pose some problems as discussed in the introduction we chose the study of maternal effects as a mean to analyze the influence of repair defects on mutagenesis. For these studies, which were initiated in collaboration with Mel Green, the following biochemically characterized mutants were used: $mei-9^{L1}$, $mus(1)101^{D1}$, $mus(1)104^{D1}$, $mei-41^{D5}$ and for a comparison the white stock from Davis in which the latter three mutations were induced. The $mei-9^{L1}$ allele used was isolated by Vogel in Leiden [10].

As shown in Fig. 6, larvae of all the mutants used exhibit at least some degree of increased MMS-sensitivity in larval stages. A 30-fold sensitivity difference is found between the white and the $mei-9^{L1}$ as well as the $mei-41^{D5}$ stock [8].

It must be stressed that only a few of the available mutant alleles known at the different loci could be used for the study of maternal effects because the homozygous females have to be fertile. This is, for certain types of studies, a handicap of this experimental approach to study the genetic control of mutagenesis. Fortunately, one of the many $mei-41$ alleles [3], the $mei-41^{D5}$, is female fertile and therefore all the four loci could be included in our study.

In a first experiment x-irradiated sperm were used to study the influence of mutant oocyte cytoplasm on the mutagenesis. Since x-rays induce a wide variety of lesions, some overall picture of the modification by repair defects was expected. As shown in Fig. 7 it was found that with both mutants, $mei-41^{D5}$ and $mei-9^{L1}$ more

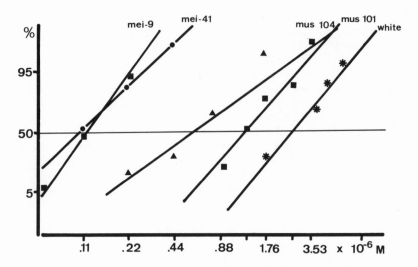

Fig. 6.   MMS-sensitivity of larvae of the five strains white, mus(1)101^{D1}, mus(1)104^{D1}, mei-41^{D5}, and mei-9L1. Details and data given elsewhere [8].

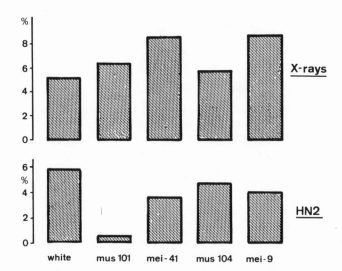

Fig. 7.   Maternal effects on x-radiation-induced and HN2-induced sex-linked recessive lethals. Basc males were x-rayed (2000 R) or fed with HN2 (0.2% for 24 hr) and crossed to females of the strains white, mus(1)101^{D1}, mei-41^{D5}, mus(1)104^{D1}, and mei-9L1. Details given elsewhere [9].

x-ray-induced lesions are processed into recessive lethals than with
the control (white) stock. It might be assumed that in mei-9 oocytes
the reduced excision repair allows more excisable lesions to interfere with the first DNA synthesis than in wild type oocytes. It
might be possible that certain types of lesions which can not be
excised by the mei-9+-dependent pathway normally are eliminated by
the mei-41+-dependent post-replication repair pathway. Therefore,
blocking or reducing the capacity of this pathway in mei-41 mutants
leads to an increased yield of mutations.

Thus the x-ray experiment indicates that mei-9 and mei-41
mutants can modify the mutagenesis initiated by x-ray-induced lesions
and that it may be assumed that the number and the type of lesions
at the time of the beginning of the first DNA replication after
insemination in the S-phase of the pronuclear stage are the most
prominent parameters determining the yield of recessive lethals.

One major problem with the study of x-ray-induced mutations is
the large variety of different lesions present in the chromatin on
which the repair systems act. A somewhat clearer situation may be
expected if chemical mutagens with known mode of action are used.
Studying the influences of repair defects on mutations induced by a
crosslinking agent we found a distinctly different pattern of mutational influences from that in the x-ray experiment.

In a first experiment, standard males were fed with 0.1% nitrogen mustard (HN2) and crossed to four different types of female.
A mutation frequency in the order of the spontaneous one was found
with mus(1)101^{D1} females, whereas a mutation frequency of about 3-4%
was observed with the other types of female. In order to verify this
finding the experiment was repeated with a higher concentration of
HN2. Again practically no HN2-induced mutations were found after
exposing males to 0.2% HN2 and crossing them to mus(1)101^{D1} females.
With the white females nearly 6% mutations were obtained (Fig. 7).

The results of the experiments show that in mus(1)101^{D1} a pathway is missing which in wild type cells generates mutations from
HN2-induced lesions. This may be either the consequence of an
extremely efficient elimination of the premutational lesions or it
may result from the absence of the mutagenic pathway. In view of
the fact that mus(1)101^{D1} larvae are sensitive to the toxic effects
of HN2 [3], the first possibility is unlikely, unless one assumes
that the mutagenic and the toxic lesions are different. On the
other hand, if one assumes crosslinks to be the premutational lesion
and a complete defect in crosslink repair, one would expect that any
crosslink present in any chromosome of the sperm would represent a
dominant lethal event. Such a hypothesis poses some quantitative
problems with respect to the amount of crosslinking in sperm of males
fed with HN2. Any appreciable amount of crosslinking, together with
the mus(1)101^{D1} defect should then lead to sterility.

Unfortunately, due to fluctuations in the spontaneous dominant lethality of progeny from mus(1)101^{D1} females it was not yet possible to determine accurately the frequency of dominant lethals in the progeny from wild type, repair proficient, and from repair deficient mus(1)101^{D1} females after a cross to HN2-treated males. At the moment this problem is still unsolved. We hope to get some additional information from currently running experiments with the half-mustard HN1.

A particularly promising type of DNA lesions to be studied are the alkylations induced by monofunctional alkylating agents. The most attractive reasons [32] are as follows. The reactivity of mono-functional alkylating agents can be described by the Swain-Scott s factor and the dependence of the reaction rate on the nucleophilic strength n of the acceptor atoms [18, 29]. Compounds with high selectivity (high s), such as MMS, alkylate most efficiently the N-7 position of guanine in DNA and various positions in proteins. Conversely, affinity for centers of high nucleophilicity is rela-tively low for compounds with low s, such as ethylnitrosourea (ENU). It has been reported [24, 28] that 80% of the ENU-induced modifica-tions in nucleic acids are on oxygen atoms. Consequently, by using sperm exposed to different types of alkylating agents, it is possible to probe for changes in mutagenesis in repair deficient mutants with different premutational lesions.

A second most interesting point is that Vogel and Natarajan [32, 33] have shown that agents of the ENU type have practically no chromosome-breaking activity in Drosophila. On the other hand, compounds with higher s values such as EMS and MMS, do induce trans-locations, especially if the sperm are stored for several days.

Based on these observations it will be possible not only to study the repair effects on different types of lesions but also to differentiate between the mutants which influence repair pathways related to the production of point mutations and those which affect pathways related to the production of chromosome aberrations.

At the present we can report on the first two series of experi-ments which have been completed within the frame of this project. We have studied the modifications of EMS- and ENU-induced mutagenesis with respect to the appearance of point mutations. The results are shown in Fig. 8. The overall result is that with mei-41^{D5} the mutation frequencies are reduced and with mei-9^{L1} they are increased compared to the standard white stock. With ENU and mei-9^{L1} a most dramatic increase of about 6-fold is found. It seems quite clear that normally the mei-9-dependent repair pathway excises mutagenic O-alkylations (O-6-guanine ?), which in the presence of mei-9 muta-tions remain in the DNA until the pronuclear DNA replication and then lead to mutations.

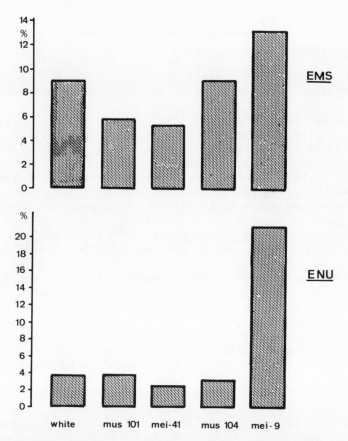

Fig. 8.   Maternal effects on EMS-induced and ENU-induced sex-linked
recessive lethals. Basc males were fed with either EMS (0.024% for
24 hr) or ENU (0.023% for 24 hr) and crossed to females of the
strains white, mus(1)101^{D1}, mei-41^{D5} and mus(1)104^{D1}. In the crosses
with mei-9^{L1} females we used Basc males which were fed the normal
EMS concentration (0.024% for 24 hr) but a ten times lower than
normal concentration of ENU (0.0023% for 24 hr). In order to make
the data comparable, the ENU-induced mutation frequencies obtained
with the higher dose were divided by 10. This calculation assumes
a linear dose response, an assumption which is at present under
experimental test.

On the other hand, if a mei-41 mutation is present, from the
lesions normally persisting until the pronuclear S-phase, less than
normal are translated into mutations. This may mean either, that
mei-41 knocks out or reduces an error-prone pathway, or that in the

presence of the <u>mei-41</u> mutation damage normally acting as premutational lesion now represents lethal damage. Our results do not allow
one to distinguish between these two possibilities at present.

Differentiation between Paternal and Maternal Repair Activities

The observation that <u>mus(1)101</u>^{D1}, in contrast to wild type, is
not able to transform HN2-induced lesions into mutations allows one
to distinguish between paternal and maternal repair activities.
The experimental approach is simply to perform two parallel brood
patterns with HN2-treated males; one by crossing the males to
repair-competent (<u>white</u>) females and the other by crossing identically HN2-treated males to <u>mus(1)101</u>^{D1} females. The results of such
an experiment in which males fed 0.1% HN2 were crossed in five
successive broods to <u>white</u> and <u>mus(1)101</u>^{D1} are shown in Fig. 9. In
the first three broods, which correspond to HN2-treated mature sperm
and middle to late spermatids, no HN2-induced lethals are found with
<u>mus(1)101</u>^{D1} females. In the later broods, in which early spermatids,
spermatocytes, and spermatogonia were tested, the mutation frequencies are identical in both series. These results indicate that in
spermatogonia and meiotic cells the paternal DNA metabolism, including replication and repair, processes the induced lesions. After
meiosis, probably in early spermatids, these processes are turned
off as the postmeiotic cells go into spermiohistogenesis.

Lesions induced in spermatids and sperm chromatin remain, depending on their physicochemical stability, for a long time in the chromatin and most of them are still present when the mature sperm
inseminates an oocyte. Only when the sperm chromatin decondensates
and has changed its structure so that the DNA becomes accessible for
maternal enzyme systems, the enzymatic repair of lesions can start.

The observations are important with respect to the biological
implications, but they have practical consequences as well. If
adult mutant males are treated with a mutagen, repair activities in
male germ cells can only be studied in later broods and not with
mature sperm and spermatids.

CONCLUSIONS

The experimental data available on maternal effects from repair
deficient mutants lead to the following conclusions.

(1) Polygenic genetic controls of mutagenesis exist in Drosophila for all three genetic endpoints studied (chromosome aberrations, SCE and point mutations).

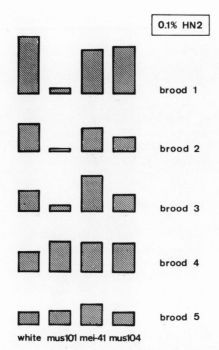

Fig. 9.   Brood-pattern analysis of the maternal effects on HN2-
induced sex-linked recessive lethals. Basc males were fed with 0.1%
HN2 (24 hr) and crossed to females of the strains white, mus(1)101^{D1},
mei-41^{D5}, mus(1)104^{D1}, and mei-9^{L1}. Every two or three days the
males were crossed to fresh females. Details given elsewhere [9].

        (2) Individual loci connected with repair pathways acting on
specific types of premutational lesions can be identified: e.g.
mus(1)101^{+} acts on lesions induced by crosslinking agents and mei-9^{+}
acts on particular alkylation products preferentially induced by
monofunctional alkylating agents with a low Swain-Scott constant.

        (3) The degree of overlap between the different pathways with
respect to mutagenesis can only be determined after more loci have
been studied.

        (4) Mutants which lead to increased mutation frequencies are
interpreted to be deficient in the removal of premutational lesions.

        (5) The mechanisms of action of mutants leading to reduced muta-
tion frequencies remain to be determined. In particular the extent
of delayed mutation fixation which leads to mosaics has to be determined for these mutants.

(6) Our experiments indicate that the study of maternal effects on mutagenized sperm represents an efficient tool for the analysis of radiation and chemically induced mutagenesis in Drosophila.

ACKNOWLEDGEMENTS

We thank Dr. E. Vogel (Leiden) and Dr. P. Schweizer (Zürich) for permission to quote unpublished data from work in progress. Original work included in this paper was supported by the Swiss National Science Foundation, project Nos. 3.3620.74 and 3.156-0.77.

REFERENCES

1. Abrahamson, S., I. H. Herskowitz, and H. J. Muller, Identification of half-translocations produced by x-rays in detaching attached-X chromosomes of Drosophila melanogaster, Genetics, 41 (1956) 410-419.
2. Beck, A., R. R. Racine, and F. E. Würgler, Genes controlling sensitivity to alkylation and x-ray damage on chromosome 3 of Drosophila melanogaster, In preparation.
3. Boyd, J. B., M. D. Golino, T. D. Nguyen, and M. M. Green, Isolation and characterization of X-linked mutants of Drosophila melanogaster which are sensitive to mutagens, Genetics, 84 (1976) 485-506.
4. Bürki, K., Röntgenbestrahlung reifer Drosophila-Spermien: Mutationsraten nach Besamung gealterter und frisch gebildeter Eier, Arch. Genet., 47 (1974) 105-126.
5. Gatti, M., Genetic control of chromosome breakage and rejoining in Drosophila melanogaster: Spontaneous chromosome aberrations in X-linked mutants defective in DNA metabolism, Proc. Natl. Acad. Sci. (U.S.), 76 (1979) 1377-1381.
6. Gatti, M., Unpublished data.
7. Gatti, M., G. Santini, S. Pimpinelli, and G. Olivieri, Lack of spontaneous sister chromatid exchanges in somatic cells of Drosophila melanogaster, Genetics, 91 (1979) 255-274.
8. Graf, U., and F. E. Würgler, Mutagen-sensitive mutants in Drosophila: relative MMS-sensitivity and maternal effects, Mutat. Res., 52 (1978) 381-394.
9. Graf, U., M. M. Green, and F. E. Würgler, Mutagen-sensitive mutants in Drosophila melanogaster. Effects on premutational damage, Mutat. Res., 63 (1979) 101-112.
10. Graf, U., E. Vogel, U. P. Biber, and F. E. Würgler, Genetic control of mutagen sensitivity in Drosophila melanogaster. A new allele at the mei-9 locus on the X-chromosome. Mutat. Res., 59 (1979) 129-133.

11. Janca, F. C., W. R. Lee, and C. S. Aaron, Stability of induced
     DNA alkylations in sperm and embryos of Drosophila melano-
     gaster (Abstract), Ann. Meeting American Environmental
     Mutagen Soc., San Francisco, 1978.
12. Koch, E. A., P. A. Smith, and R. C. King, Variations in the
     radiosensitivity of oocyte chromosomes during meiosis in
     Drosophila melanogaster. Chromosoma, 30 (1970) 98-108.
13. Leigh, B., Ring chromosomes and radiation induced chromosome
     loss, In: The Genetics and Biology of Drosophila, Vol. 1b,
     M. Ashburner and E. Novitski, Eds., Academic Press, New
     York, 1976, pp. 505-528.
14. Lifschytz, E., and R. Falk, Fine structure analysis of a
     chromosome segment in Drosophila melanogaster: Analysis of
     ethyl-methanesulfonate-induced lethals, Mutat. Res., 8
     (1969) 147-155.
15. Lindsley, D., and E. H. Grell, Genetic Variations of Drosophila
     melanogaster, Publ. 627, Carnegie Institution, Washington,
     D.C., 1968.
16. Mendelson, D., The improved "bithorax method" for the detection
     of rearrangements in Drosophila melanogaster, Mutat. Res.,
     41 (1976) 269-276.
17. Nguyen, T. D., M. M. Green, and J. B. Boyd, Isolation of two
     X-linked mutants in Drosophila melanogaster which are sensi-
     tive to gamma-rays. Mutat. Res., 49 (1978) 139-143
18. Osterman-Golkar, S., L. Ehrenberg, and C. A. Wachtmeister,
     Reaction kinetics and biological action in barley of mono-
     functional methanesulfonic esters, Rad. Bot., 10 (1970)
     303-327.
19. Parker, D. R., Dominant lethal mutations in irradiated oocytes.
     Biological Contributions, The University of Texas,
     Publication No. 5914 (1959) 113-127.
20. Racine, R. R., A. Beck, and F. E. Würgler, The genetic control
     of maternal effects on mutations recovered from x-rayed
     mature Drosophila-sperm, Mutat. Res., 63 (1979) 87-100.
21. Sankaranarayanan, K., and F. H. Sobels, Radiation genetics,
     In: The Genetics and Biology of Drosophila, Vol. 1c,
     M. Ashburner and E. Novitski, Eds., Academic Press, New
     York, 1976, pp. 1089-1250.
22. Sankaranarayanan, K., and W. S. Volkers, Exposure fractionation
     effects for x-ray-induced dominant lethals in immature
     (Stage 7) oocytes of Drosophila melanogaster: A re-analysis,
     Mutat. Res., in press.
23. Schweizer, P., Unpublished data.
24. Singer, B., All oxygens in nucleic acids react with carcinogenic
     ethylating agents, Nature, 264 (1976) 333-339.
25. Steiner, T., and F. E. Würgler, Repair of x-ray-induced sub-
     lethal damage in class B oocytes of Drosophila melanogaster,
     Int. J. Radiat. Biol., 36 (1979) 201-216.

26. Steiner, T., and F. E. Würgler, Time dependence of Elkind-type
     recovery in class B oocytes of <u>Drosophila melanogaster</u>,
     Int. J. Radiat. Biol., 36 (1979) 201–216.
27. Steiner, T., and F. E. Würgler, Oocyte stages in newly hatched
     females of some <u>mus</u> and <u>mei</u> mutants, Drosophila Inform.
     Serv., 55 (1980) in press.
28. Sun, L., and B. Singer, The specificity of different classes of
     ethylating agents toward various sites of HeLa cell DNA
     in vitro and in vivo, Biochemistry, 14 (1975) 1795–1802.
29. Swain, C. G., and C. B. Scott, Quantitative correlation of
     relative rates: Comparison of hydroxide ion with other
     nucleophilic reagents toward alkyl halides, esters, epoxides
     and acyl halides, J. Am. Chem. Soc., 75 (1953) 141–147.
30. Vogel, E., Mutagenicity of carcinogens in Drosophila as function
     of genotype-controlled metabolism, In: In Vitro Metabolic
     Activation in Mutagenicity Testing, F. J. de Serres, J. R.
     Fouts, J. R. Bend, and R. M. Philpot, Elsevier/North
     Holland, 1976, pp. 63–79.
31. Vogel, E., Unpublished data.
32. Vogel, E., and A. T. Natarajan, The relation between reaction
     kinetics and mutagenic action of monofunctional alkylating
     agents in higher eukaryotic systems. I. Recessive lethal
     mutations and translocations in Drosophila, Mutat. Res.,
     62 (1979) 51–100.
33. Vogel, E., and A. T. Natarajan, The relation between reaction
     kinetics and mutagenic action of monofunctional alkylating
     agents in higher eukaryotic systems. II. Total and partial
     sex-chromosome loss in Drosophila, Mutat. Res., 62 (1979).
34. Würgler, F. E., Radiation-induced translocations in inseminated
     eggs of <u>Drosophila melanogaster</u>, Mutat. Res., 13 (1971)
     353–359.
35. Würgler, F. E., and P. Maier, Genetic control of mutation
     induction in <u>Drosophila melanogaster</u>. I. Sex-chromosome
     loss in x-rayed mature sperm, Mutat. Res., 15 (1972) 41–53.
36. Würgler, F. E., U. Graf and W. Berchtold, Statistical problems
     connected with the sex-linked recessive lethal test in
     <u>Drosophila melanogaster</u>. I. The use of the Kastenbaum-
     Bowman test, Arch. Genet., 48 (1975) 158–178.
37. Würgler, F. E., F. H. Sobels, and E. Vogel, Drosophila as an
     assay system for detecting genetic changes, In: Handbook
     of Mutagenicity Test Procedures, B. J. Kilbey, M. Legator,
     W. Nichols, and C. Ramel, Eds., Elsevier, Amsterdam, 1977,
     pp. 335–373.
38. Würgler, F. E., T. Steiner, and U. Graf, Strain differences in
     repair capacity of class B oocytes of <u>Drosophila melano-
     gaster</u>, Arch. Genet., 51 (1978) 99–105.
39. Würgler, F. E., U. Graf, P. Ruch, A. Beck, and T. Steiner,
     Mutagen sensitivity of wild type and recombination deficient
     c(3)G strains of <u>Drosophila melanogaster</u>, Arch. Genet., 51
     (1978) 217–242.

CHAPTER 16

REPAIR AND MUTAGENESIS IN DROSOPHILA: A SUMMARY AND PERSPECTIVE

M. M. GREEN

Department of Genetics, University of California
Davis, California 95616 (U.S.A.)

The contributions of genetic experiments with Drosophila melanogaster to the relationship between chromosome breakage and mutagenesis antedate the demonstration of DNA as the genetic material. One of the earliest observations was that the spontaneous rate of mutations in females is no greater than that of males. The fact that meiotic crossing over, a chromosome breakage and rejoining process, occurs in females and not in males implied that the "repair" of the broken chromatids involved in crossing over must occur with such precision as to preclude the generation of new mutations. Subsequently, the genetic versatility of D. melanogaster was exploited to demonstrate first that x-rays and later that mustard gas and other chemicals can be powerful mutagenic agents. The post Watson-Crick era and the dominance of microorganisms in genetic research deferred, for obvious reasons, research on DNA repair and mutagenesis in eukaryotes. From the series of reports that are included here, it is eminently clear that much progress has been made in our understanding the process of repair in eukaryote DNA and its relationship to mutagenesis. It is also evident from the research results presented that experimentation with D. melanogaster will further our understanding on DNA repair and mutagenesis.

Why use D. melanogaster as an experimental organism? Clearly, a number of advantages accrue when the vast cytogenetic knowledge of this organism is exploited. These advantages include genetic methods which permit one to measure spontaneous or induced mutation rates with comparative ease either, for example, as X-linked recessive lethals, or at specific loci. Polytene chromosome cytology allows one to define in detail the nature of chromosome aberrations, if any, associated with specific mutational events. An array of balancer chromosomes and genetic markers permits one to measure quantitatively disturbances in regular meiotic chromosome disjunction or alterations

241

in the frequency of meiotic crossing over. To the germinal cytogenetic tools can be added somatic cytogenetic methods which permit
one to assay both genetically and cytologically disturbances to
somatic cells. These are but a sample of the available genetic tools
which may be employed in the characterization mutants which affect
DNA repair and mutagenesis.

Finally, primary somatic cell culture of Drosophila cells is
feasible and thereby opens the road to the biochemical description
of Drosophila DNA replication and repair by methods identical to or
derived from methods which have been instructive in studying microbial DNA repair and replication.

What has been achieved to date? In a relatively short period
of time, it has been possible to induce and isolate a class of
conditional lethal mutants which are presumably defective in DNA
repair or replication. The rationale of the mutant search is
simple: flies bearing a mutant defective in DNA repair or replication will die if their chromosomes are broken but survive when their
chromosomes are unaltered. To overcome the technical difficulties
of breaking chromosomes with x-ray or other high-energy radiation,
quasi-radiomimetic compounds, such as methyl methanesulfonate (MMS),
have been successfully employed in the mutant search. Appropriate
genetic selection systems combined with feeding of MMS to developing
larvae have led to the isolation of an array of conditional lethal
mutants which die in the presence of MMS and survive in its absence.
Presumably, the mutants die because they cannot repair DNA damaged
by MMS and thus are inferred to be repair defective.

To date more than 100 MMS-sensitive mutants have been isolated.
These mutants fall into a minimum of 12 complementation groups on
the X chromosome, 7 complementation groups on the second chromosome
and 12 on the third chromosome.

The characterization of some of these mutants, reported in
extenso in the contributions, can be summarized as follows.

1. Some MMS-sensitive mutants are also sensitive to x-rays,
UV, and nitrogen mustard, others to UV and nitrogen mustard, others
to x-rays, others to UV, and one to nitrogen mustard.

2. Some MMS-sensitive mutants exhibit both somatic and germinal
defects, the latter as increased chromosome nondisjunction and
decreased meiotic crossing.

3. Some MMS-sensitive mutants bring about a significant
increase in somatic chromosome aberrations, both euchromatic and/or
heterochromatic, implying their normal alleles function to maintain
chromosome integrity.

4. Some MMS-sensitive mutants are responsible for increased mutation frequencies, spontaneous or mutagen-induced, presumably because they cannot properly repair premutationally altered DNA.

Combined together this array of phenotypic effects associated with one or another MMS-sensitive mutant leads to the conclusion that each is in some way defective in DNA repair and/or replication. That this conclusion has merit is supported by the biochemical investigation of a sample of MMS sensitive mutants. At least four mutants are excision repair-defective, seven mutants are post-replication repair-defective, and five mutants are defective in DNA synthesis.

What are the needs and prospects for the future? There can be little doubt that only the surface has been scratched in the analysis and characterization of DNA repair deficient mutants in Drosophila. The phenotypic effects of most MMS sensitive mutants are incomplete. The relationship between DNA repair and/or synthesis and mutator (or antimutator) effects has hardly been explored. A good start on the biochemical characterization of the mutants has been made but more detailed information is needed. The biochemistry will be enormously facilitated when established Drosophila cell lines can be routinely made.

Finally, by analogy with other organisms there is an entire class of repair-defective mutants, the UV-sensitive, yet to be isolated and characterized.

Much research work has been done but much remains to be done. However, the progress made to date generates a note of optimism that in the forseeable future experiments with Drosophila will significantly advance our knowledge and understanding of eukaryote DNA repair and mutagenesis.

CHAPTER 17

RELATIONSHIP OF DNA LESIONS AND THEIR REPAIR TO CHROMOSOMAL

ABERRATION PRODUCTION

MICHAEL A BENDER

Medical Department, Brookhaven National Laboratory
Upton, NY 11973 (U.S.A.)

SUMMARY

Though the roles of some specific DNA lesions in the production
of chromosomal aberrations is clearly established, those of others
remain unclear. While the study of aberration production in human
genetic DNA repair deficiency diseases has been extremely rewarding
already, eukaryotic repair systems are obviously complex, and one
is tempted to feel that such studies may have raised as many
questions as they have provided answers. For example, the "standard"
sort of xeroderma pigmentosum is chromosomally sensitive to ultraviolet light and to those chemical agents inducing ultraviolet-type
DNA repair. But both it and the variant form have been reported to
also be sensitive to the crosslinking agent mitomycin C in one study
[18], implying a common step or steps in the repair of pyrimidine
cyclobutane dimers and DNA crosslinks. However, just to complicate
matters, another study of chromosomal aberration production in
xeroderma pigmentosum cells had found them no more sensitive to
mitomycin C than normal cells [50]. Similarly, Fanconi's anemia
cells, which are chromosomally sensitive to crosslinking agents,
and appear to be defective in the "unhooking" of linked polynucleotide strands [15, 16, 49, 51], are reported to be chromosomally
sensitive to ethyl methanesulfonate as well [29], and to be sensitive to ionizing radiation [7, 19,]0], again implying overlapping
repair systems. It seems certain that further study of chromosomal
aberration production in repair deficient cells by agents inducing
various DNA lesions will reveal even greater complexity in eukaryotic
DNA repair systems and their role in chromosomal aberration production. Nevertheless, there seems hope, at least, that such studies
may also ultimately lead to a complete understanding of the molecular
mechanisms involved.

INTRODUCTION

Perhaps one of the most notable developments in cytogenetics
of the past decade is the integration of the ideas and techniques
of molecular biology and genetics that has occurred over the past
few years. Though the production of chromosomal aberrations by
radiation has of course been studied intensively from the biophysical
point of view for over four decades [30], and by chemicals from the
biochemical for over three [26], and despite occasional perceptions
of the implications of DNA synthesis and repair biochemistry [12, 60],
I think it fair to state that recent work on the roles of specific
DNA lesions and their repair has led to a real breakthrough in our
understanding of the molecular mechanisms involved in what has come
to be called clastogenesis. Reviewing such a rapidly developing
field is always difficult and the result never completely up to
date, so what follows is necessarily selective rather than comprehensive, and certainly presents a personal and not necessarily
generally accepted view of the topic.

A striking consequence of recent cytogenetic developments is
that it is now possible to interpret chromosomal aberration
production in terms of general molecular models in much the same
manner as it earlier became possible to interpret gene mutation in
molecular terms. Any specific model may always, of course, prove
inadequate in the light of new data, or even totally wrong.
Nevertheless, the testing of such models is productive, and it has
been the study of the cytogenetic results of the introduction of
specific lesions into DNA at specific points in the cell cycle and
the study of the influence of specific DNA repair systems using
genetic repair deficiencies, repair poisons such as caffeine, or
other manipulations of repair capacities such as "liquid holding
recovery" that has led to our recent rapid progress. The parallel
with molecular genetics is striking.

A MODEL

While other models are possible, and many features have not as
yet been rigorously proven, I believe that the very simple one we
formalized some years ago [3] still constitutes, with a few
additions, an acceptable framework within which to understand the
molecular mechanisms involved in chromosomal aberration production
and the roles of specific DNA lesions and their enzymatic repair
systems. Briefly, it contains the following elements.

First, the eukaryote chromosome is considered to be mononeme,
each prereplication (G_1) chromosome or post-replication (G_2)
chromatid containing a single DNA double helix. The double helices
of each G_2 chromatid are, of course, comprised of one "old" polynucleotide strand from the G_1 molecule and one new one synthesized

by using the old one as a template [62]. Whether there is just one DNA molecule or a series joined by "linkers," with respect to aberration production, the chromosome or chromatid behaves empirically as though the DNA runs continuously from one end to the other.

Second, whatever intermediates there might be, the ultimate target for aberration production is the DNA. Changes in other chromosomal constituents will result in aberrations only if they lead in turn to alterations in DNA.

Third, aberrations consist of polynucleotide chain breaks and of recombinations between their broken ends. Almost by definition, a chromosome or chromatid break involves a DNA double-strand break. Aberrations of the chromosome type, with both daughter metaphase chromatids affected at the same distance from their ends or centromere, result from replication of double-strand breaks or of "illegitimate" products of rejoining between their broken ends. Aberrations of the chromatid type, affecting (with one exception) only one of the two daughter metaphase chromatids, arise from double-strand breaks in already replicated (S and G_2 phase) DNA. Achromatic lesions (or "gaps"), whether considered true aberrations or not, are manifestations of breaks and possibly other DNA alterations involving only one polynucleotide strand, and thus constitute "half chromatid aberrations." Again by definition, half chromatid exchanges are between single polynucleotide strands, though it seems likely that the rejoining involved is actually between double strand breaks occurring in palindromic or reverse tandem complementary repeat base sequence regions of single polynucleotide strands while paired in the "hairpin" configuration. Figures 1 and 2 illustrate these ideas schematically.

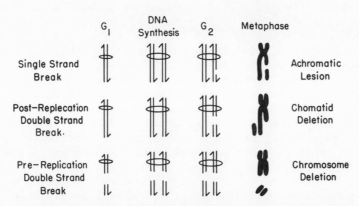

Fig. 1. Schematic representation of the roles of single and double polynucleotide strand breaks in the production of achromatic lesions and chromatid and chromosome type breaks.

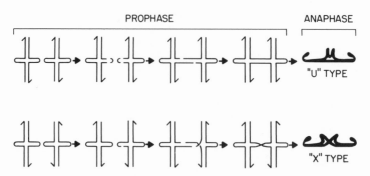

Fig. 2.   A possible mechanism for the origin of half-chromatid
exchanges from the recombination of "double strand" breaks occurring
within palindromic base sequence regions of single polynucleotide
strands while paired in the "hairpin" configuration.

Fourth, double polynucleotide strand breaks may arise directly,
but are frequently generated secondarily as a consequence of normal
DNA synthesis, of enzymatic DNA repair processes, or through the
action of specific nucleases not necessarily related to DNA repair.
Single polynucleotide strand breaks present in template strands
during local DNA synthesis are duplicated in the nascent strand,
thus yielding double strand breaks in the daughter molecule; other
lesions can also interfere with the template function and result in
the "synthesis" of single strand breaks in the nascent strand.
Single-strand breaks can further be converted to double-strand
breaks by either specific repair endonucleases or endonucleases
specific for single-stranded DNA. Some of the possibilities are
illustrated schematically in Fig. 3.

Fifth, the process of rejoining of double strand breaks
probably arises through precisely the same mechanisms as are now
so widely employed in the deliberate construction of recombinant
DNA molecules for cloning, namely, the creation of single stranded
"sticky" ends by specific exonuclease activity like that of lambda
exonuclease or DNA polymerase I, the annealing of sticky ends
posessing sufficient complementarity, trimming or filling out of
the free ends by exonuclease and/or polymerase activity, and final
closing of the chains by ligase activity. This is shown in Fig. 4.
Essentially this mechanism was proposed by J. H. Taylor many years
ago [60]; some of the evidence supporting it, particularly that
relating to repetitive DNA base sequences, was recently summarized
by Chadwick and Leenhouts [9].

It seems quite possible that the temporal decrease in the
capacity of "old" chromosome breaks to rejoin with "new" ones induced
later on in the cell cycle, which gives rise to the well-known
fractionation effect for exchange aberrations, as well as the

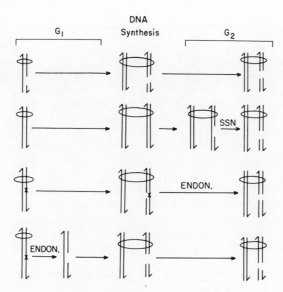

Fig. 3.   Diagramatic illustration of the possible conributions of
single polynucleotide strand breaks and of "base damage" to
chromatid breaks through single strand nuclease (SSN) attack,
normal DNA synthesis and/or endonucleolytic base damage excision
(ENDON).

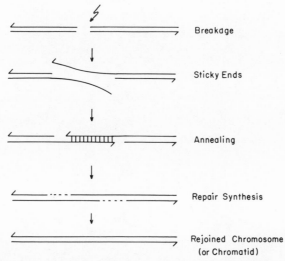

Fig. 4.   Diagram showing steps in proposed mechanism by which
broken chromosome ends may rejoin. Ends of broken DNA double
helices are rejoined through exonuclease activity, annealing of
sticky ends, and repair of the remaining single polynucleotide
strand breaks, just as is deliberately done in the construction of
recombinant DNAs.

intriguing ability of chromatid breaks occurring in sister chromatids
(isochromatid deletions) to rejoin with each other in sister union
configurations may also arise through a similar mechanism involving
the production and then annealing of sticky ends. Cavalier-Smith
[8] some time ago proposed that chromosome ends or telomeres might
consist of palindromic base sequences as an explanation of how the
synthesis of the 5' ends of linear DNA molecules might be accomplished. The terminal hairpin configuration is ligated in this
model so that there are literally no free polynucleotide strand
ends except while synthesis is actually in progress. A similar
annealing of sticky ends of chromosome breaks containing palindromic
base sequences would lead to the creation of the telomeric
configuration as shown in Fig. 5, with the consequence that the
breaks would no longer be available for interactions with other
breaks. A similar process, also illustrated in Fig. 5, and akin
to that proposed by Chadwick and Leenhouts [9], would also result
in isochromatid sister unions.

Simple as is this model of chromosomal aberration production,
it appears adequate at least for the present. While the idea that
established molecular mechanisms can satisfactorily explain cytogenetic phenomena is a relatively new one to many cytogeneticists,
current information on the effects of both specific DNA lesions and
their enzymatic repair mechanisms appears to support it, as I shall
attempt to show.

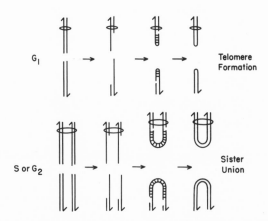

Fig. 5.   Illustration of the way that breaks in palindromic base
sequence regions of DNA could anneal to form "unavailable" break
ends (telomeres?), or, in S or G_2 cells, sister unions.

STRATEGIES

Several approaches to the elucidation of the roles of various DNA lesions and their repair mechanisms have been employed, including the introduction of specific lesions into cells' DNA at specific points in their cell cycle, the comparison of responses of cells differing genetically in DNA repair capacities, selective removal of specific DNA lesions after treatment with agents inducing more than one type of DNA lesion, and the use of agents or conditions that increase or decrease the effectiveness of various DNA repair processes. These are powerful strategies, as a few examples will show.

Introduction of Specific Lesions

The simplest way to relate aberration production to specific kinds of DNA lesions is to induce them in a cell at a specific point in its cell cycle and then to examine the consequence at the next mitosis. The requirement that the lesions be introduced at a known time stems partly from the fact that some DNA lesions produce aberrations only when the lesion-bearing DNA is used as template for the synthesis of new DNA. In addition, some lesions result in one kind of aberration at one point in the cell cycle and quite another, or even none at all, when introduced at a different point. Ionizing radiation, for example, produces chromosome type aberrations in G_1, chromatid types in S and G_2, and subchromatid exchanges in prophase, while UV light probably usually produces only chromatid types and these only (or mainly) if the cells synthesize new DNA.

Unfortunately, most agents produce DNA lesions of more than one type. Again, ionizing radiation is a good example, for it produces both single and double polynucleotide breaks as well as various kinds of base damage, all of which, it appears, can give rise to aberrations. However, a few systems do appear to produce only one, or at least mainly one type of lesion, and their study has proven profitable. An example is the induction of single polynucleotide strand breaks by photolysis of DNA in which 5-bromodeoxyuridine has been substituted for thymidine [2].

Lesion Removal

It is sometimes possible to selectively remove one specific type of DNA lesion from among a variety that may have been induced by treatment with a given agent, and thus to elucidate its role in aberration production by observing what cytogenetic effects no longer result following its removal. For example, cells from some (but not all) eukaryotes possess a photoreactivating enzyme which

in the presence of visible light of the right wavelength efficiently
monomerizes pyrimidine cyclobutane dimers. By such selective
elimination of this lesion from the DNA of cells treated with UV
light we were able to demonstrate the role of such dimers in the
production of chromosomal aberrations [17]. Comparisons of the
effects of related agents differing in their ability to induce one
specific class of lesion from among a spectrum of lesions also
constitutes a valuable "subtraction" approach, as was shown for
example by Sasaki in his study of the sensitivity of Fanconi's
anemia cells to crosslinking agents and to a monofunctional
derivative [49, 51].

Genetic Repair Defects

A classical stratagem in microbial mutation research has been
the identification of specific genetic DNA repair deficiencies and
the study of their influence on the induction of mutation. The
specificities of repair systems for particular lesions or families
of lesions has allowed important insights into the nature of
mutagenesis itself and the molecular mechanisms involved in the
production of mutations by particular DNA lesions. Several genetic
repair defects have now been identified in humans, and study of
their influence on chromosomal aberration production by various
clastogens has begun. Perhaps the best known is xeroderma pigmentosum (XP), a defect in the excision repair of pyrimidine cyclobutane
dimers and certain other DNA lesions. A number of studies have
shown that UV light induces more chromosomal aberrations in XP than
in normal human cells in tissue culture [38]. XP cells are also
more sensitive to some chemical mutagens, for example, as Sasaki
[48] has shown for aberration production by 4-nitroquinoline 1-oxide.

Two other human genetic disorders, ataxia telangiectasia (AT)
and Fanconi's anemia (FA), appear to involve specific DNA repair
deficiencies, and are being used currently in chromosome aberration
studies, as I will describe presently.

Because species also differ in DNA repair capacities, similar
comparisons are possible between the cytogenetic responses of cells
of these species. For example, cells from murine rodents excise
UV-induced dimers from their DNA only poorly, while those from
normal humans excise them rapidly. As would be expected, treatment
with UV light in G_0 or G_1 induces aberrations much more efficiently
in Chinese hamster tissue culture cells than in human lymphocytes
[4, 34, 38].

Repair Modification

Modification of the abilities of cells to repair DNA damage
is a classical method of demonstrating the existence of systems
capable of repairing the damage and their influence on mutation
induction, as exemplified by "liquid holding recovery," or the use
of caffeine as a repair "poison" in bacteria. The same strategies
have been employed in the study of chromosomal aberration production,
as for example in recent experiments on the influence of holding
cells in the confluent state on aberration yields [14] or in
numerous studies of the influence of caffeine on yields of chromosomal aberrations induced by a variety of mutagens [27].

SPECIFIC LESIONS

Though there remain gaping holes in the picture, there is
already enough evidence to allow us to be fairly certain regarding
the roles of certain DNA lesions or classes of lesion in aberration
production, and to begin, at least, to catalog them and the
influences of their specific repair systems.

Single Polynucleotide Strand Breaks

The role of single-strand breaks in aberration production is
clearly complex. Such breaks are, of course, one of the consequences
of exposure to ionizing radiation, and apparently of treatment with
certain chemicals such as the chemotherapeutic agents bleomycin and
neocarzinostatin as well [35, 40]. From their study of the cytogenetic effects of treatment with the base analog 5-fluorodeoxy-
uridine, Taylor, Haut, and Tung [61] deduced that S-phase cells so
treated arrived at metaphase with gaps left in the nascent polynucleotide strands, and that these gaps could appear as achromatic
lesions. Precocious condensation of S-phase chromosomes in which
the nascent strand is still incomplete also yields metaphase
chromosomes with achromatic lesions [24]. Our own study of the
effect of photolysis of 5-bromodeoxyuridine incorporated into only
one of the polynucleotide strands of each DNA double helix yielded
similar results, and further led us to conclude that single-strand
breakage could also result in chromatid and isochromatid aberration
production, processes we postulated to arise from single strand
nuclease activity, normal DNA synthesis, and the operation of a
recombinational DNA repair mechanism [2], all of which would, as
already noted, result in the conversion of single-strand breaks
into double ones. Interestingly enough, Natarajan and Obe [36]
have recently reported an increase in induced chromatid aberration
yields in cells treated with exogenous single-strand nuclease in
the presence of inactivated Sendai virus. Single polynucleotide
strand breaks are quite rapidly repaired by most cells [55], so one

might expect that achromatic lesion yields would be greatest for cells irradiated in late G_2 and that they would decrease quite rapidly for progressively earlier irradiations as more time was allowed for repair prior to their becoming "caught" by chromatin condensation in preparation for cell division. This is, of course, precisely what happens.

From the classical observation that treatment with ionizing radiation during the G_1 phase of the cell cycle normally does not result in the production of chromatid type aberrations, I conclude that single-strand breakage is not normally an important contributor to chromosomal aberration production during this phase of the cell cycle [3]. However, Wolff [64] and others have shown that if G_1 cells are irradiated very close to the G_1-S border, some chromatid type aberrations can result. It seems likely that the reason chromatid aberrations are not usually observed following G_1 irradiation is because the repair of single strand breaks is usually very rapid, so that none are left as such by the time the S phase commences, though some may, of course, be converted to double-strand breaks by single-strand endonuclease activity, and thus contribute to chromosome type aberration production. However, if the lesions are induced very shortly before the beginning of S, such repair would still be incomplete and would produce chromatid aberrations in the same manner as if they were induced by S phase irradiation.

Two rare human recessive genetic disorders, ataxia telangiectasia and Fanconi's anemia, previously reported to be characterized by an abnormal chromosomal sensitivity to ionizing radiation of their peripheral lymphocytes when irradiated in G_0 [19, 20], have both been found to be radiosensitive when irradiated in G_2, exhibiting increased yields of both achromatic lesions and chromatid deletions [7, 41, 57]. Such a finding suggests the possibility of a strand break repair deficiency. Several investigations, however, have failed to demonstrate any such deficiency on the biochemical-biophysical level, at least in AT [58, 63].

Double Polynucleotide Strand Breakage

As noted earlier, given a mononeme model for the eukaryote chromosome and the overwhelming evidence that DNA is at least the principal target in clastogenesis, direct induction of double-strand breaks must, almost by definition, constitute chromosome or chromatid breakage. Furthermore, those agents known to induce double-strand breaks directly, or at least promptly, produce chromosome type aberrations; those that do not do not appear to produce prompt double-strand breakage either. Though this is true for most biological effects of ionizing radiation, it is perhaps worth noting that the well known observation that chromosomal aberrations are produced with greater efficiency per unit dose with increasing linear energy transfer is paralleled by an increasing DNA double-strand breakage efficiency [10, 25], a finding at least consistent with their postulated role in aberration production.

Though there has been some confusion on the point, it now seems clear that there is repair of radiation-induced double-strand breaks in eukaryotes [11, 21, 46]. Resnick [45] has proposed a recombinational model of double-strand break repair through the formation of heteroduplexes with intact homologous molecules, and he and Martin [46] have verified some of the predictions of the model in yeast, as have Krasin and Hutchinson [28] in E. coli. However, it remains to be seen whether this is the only, or even a predominant, mode of repair in the cells of higher eukaryotes.

Chadwick and Leenhouts [9] have recently proposed the recombinational double strand break repair model of Resnick as an explanation of certain features of chromosomal aberration production by ionizing radiation. Though their theory that chromosomal exchange aberrations must arise from single double-strand breaks, rather than from two independently induced breaks seems to me unnecessary for reasons some of which have been discussed by Savage [52], the proposal remains an interesting possibility. We proposed a recombinational repair process as an explanation for the ability of lesions in one polynucleotide strand to "spread" and result in the formation of isochromatid deletions [4] Chadwick and Leenhouts have shown that not only could the Resnick mechanisms account for "spreading", but that it could also, if occurring in the region of a palindromic base sequence, account for the sister union phenomenon.

Among the human genetic diseases conferring sensitivity to mutagens, ataxia telangiectasia has been investigated to determine whether cells from these patients might be deficient in their ability to repair DNA double-strand breaks. Taylor et al., [58] and Lehman and Stevens [31] both report, however, a normal double-strand break repair capacity for such cells.

The earlier-reported G_1 chromosomal radiosensitivity of lymphocytes from AT patients [20] has also been reported by Taylor [57], though the increased yield he reported in G_0-irradiated AT lymphocytes was, unlike that seen by Higurachi and Conen [20], largely in the fragment (i.e., deletion) class rather than in rings and dicentrics. Though Taylor argues that the techniques used to measure double-strand break repair might not be sensitive enough to detect a deficiency sufficient to account for it, the G_0 chromosomal radiosensitivity in AT lymphocytes nevertheless seems to be in conflict with the apparently normal double strand break repair in AT cells, and the idea that double strand DNA break production is the basic mechanism by which aberrations are formed, unless possibly, the DNA of AT cells is simply more easily broken by ionizing radiation. The available data, however, do not suggest an increased double strand break yield [31, 58]. We have therefore reinvestigated the reported AT G_0 lymphocyte sensitivity [6], employing a 5-bromodeoxyuridine substitution-differential staining technique [65] to allow both the scoring of only cells unequivocally in their first post-irradiation mitosis and also the determination of whether there are differences in cell proliferation dynamics [53] between AT lymphocytes and control lymphocytes from normal individuals. Preliminary experiments showed that the addition of 5-bromodeoxy-uridine to lymphocyte cultures to a level of 25 μM following irradiation neither increases aberration yields nor produces appreciable changes in proliferation dynamics.

The preliminary results from two such experiments involving four different AT patients and three normal controls are summarized in Table 1. Neither the two experiments nor the results from fixations at either 72 or 96 hr appears to differ appreciably, so they are pooled in the Table for the purpose of illustration. Two features of the chromosome type aberration yields are immediately apparent: first, the yields of rings and dicentrics are no higher in the AT cells than the controls, and second, there is a large excess of deletions in the AT cells. Though I shall return to this point in my discussion of DNA base damage, it is necessary to note here that AT cells display the peculiarity of being susceptible to the induction of chromatid type aberrations by G_0 or G_1 irradiation; this is seen in Table 1. Because isochromatid deletions and chromosome type deletions are indistinguishable except when sister union occurs (an event that appears to be relatively rare in human cells) the aberrations scored as chromosome deletions actually include an unknown number of isochromatid deletions as well. If their frequency is increased in G_0-irradiated AT cells as is the frequency of other chromatid types, as seems reasonable, then much if not all of the apparent increase in chromosome deletions might disappear were we but able to distinguish between them.

When examined in this light, the reports of G_0 AT lymphocyte radiosensitivity of Taylor et al. [57, 59] also suggests that in fact the difference from normal cells may be accounted for entirely by the chromatid aberration increase. As noted already, the ring and dicentric yields he observed were not much, probably not statistically, greater. Furthermore, Taylor [57] reports that many of the exchange aberrations seen in both normal control and AT lymphocytes lacked the expected acentric fragments, and the controls more often than the AT cells, particularly at the higher doses. This suggests to me that second post-irradiation mitoses were included in his sample, and with higher frequency in the normal than in the AT cultures, though Taylor argues otherwise.

TABLE 1

FREQUENCIES OF CHROMOSOMAL ABERRATIONS IN UNIRRADIATED
AND G_0-IRRADIATED PERIPHERAL LYMPHOCYTE CULTURES
FROM PATIENTS WITH ATAXIA TELANGIECTASIA AND NORMAL CONTROLS[a]

Dose (R)	Subjects	Cells	Chromatid type (%)			Chromosome type (%)		
			Al	Cd	Ex	Del	Ring	Dic
0	3 Controls	461	18	6	1	0.2	0	0.2
	4 AT	289	5	8	1	5	1	4
200	3 Controls	544	10	4	0.2	31	7	39
	4 AT	504	23	33	6	70	7	42

[a]Only first post-irradiation mitoses were scored. Irradiations were 200 R of 250 kVp x-rays or 200 R of ^{60}Co gamma-rays in two separate experiments, the results of which were not significantly different.

We therefore conclude that the reported G_0 sensitivity of AT lymphocytes is not in fact a sensitivity to the induction of chromosome type aberrations. In the earlier experiments no means of excluding second or later post-irradiation mitoses from the sample scored was available, and it seems likely that the difference can in part be attributed to the inclusion of such cells, which would have a lower aberration frequency because of losses at the first mitosis. Not only do the data of Taylor on exchanges lacking fragments suggest this, but our data on the relative frequencies of first, second and third or later metaphases in the experiments of Table 1 also strongly support this view; the frequencies of first metaphases in the AT cultures, which are always higher even in the unirradiated samples, are notably elevated in the irradiated ones as compared to the irradiated control cultures. Thus it does not appear that the case of AT offers any real argument against the proposed central role of DNA double strand breakage in aberration formation.

Base Damage

This category of DNA lesions includes a variety of alterations frequently defined in terms of their recognition by specific endo-nucleases. It appears that most chemical mutagens produce lesions

of this general class. Those that produce chromosomal aberrations
seem to do so through local interference with the lesion-bearing
polynucleotide strand's ability to serve as template for nascent
strand synthesis; aberration induction is "S-dependent." Only
chromatid aberrations are produced, and often, at least, only if the
treated cells pass through at least part of an S phase. Chemically
produced alkylations, apurinic and apyrimidinic sites, and lesions
of the 5,6-dihydroxydihydrothymine type fall in this class, though
little is as yet known of the specific roles played by them in
chromosome aberration production.

It appears that cells from some, but not all, cases of the
human recessive genetic disease Fanconi's anemia are deficient in
their ability to excise lesions of the 5,6-dihydroxydihydrothymine
type from their DNA [43]. As already noted, FA lymphocytes have
been reported to be chromosomally sensitive to ionizing radiation
administered in G_0 [19, 20], though Sasaki and Tonomura [51] were
unable to confirm this. Nevertheless, we have found both lymphocytes and fibroblasts from FA patients to be abnormally sensitive
to irradiation in G_2 [7]. However, FA cells have also been reported
to be sensitive to aberration induction by alkylating agents,
including tetramethansulfonil-d-manitol [54], nitrogen mustard and
mitomycin C [51], ethyl methanesulfonate [29] and diepoxybutane [1].
As will be discussed later, FA appears to be defective in DNA
crosslink repair, but since some of the agents to which FA cells
are reported to be sensitive are nonfunctional, FA must also be
deficient in the removal of at least some simple alkylations,
perhaps in an enzyme common to several DNA repair systems.

Though perhaps most often thought of as being deficient in
repair of pyrimidine cyclobutane dimers, cells from patients
afflicted with the excision repair forms of xeroderma pigmentosum
are also sensitive to aberration production by some, but not all,
alkylating agents. Those to which XP cells are sensitive are those
inducing DNA repair of the "long patch" type induced by UV light
[42], including N-acetoxy-2-acetylaminofluorene, polycyclic hydrocarbons and 4-nitroquinoline 1-oxide [33, 48, 56]. Those to which
they are not abnormally sensitive induce ionizing-radiation-type
("short patch") DNA repair [42], and include methyl methanesulfonate
and N-methyl-N-nitronitrosoguanidine [48, 56]. Sensitivity of XP
cells to mitomycin C has also been reported [18], and since repair
of DNA crosslinks appears to be normal in XP cells [50], it seems
probable that the monoadducts produced by this agent produce the
excess aberrations.

Ataxia telangiectasia clearly confers abnormal sensitivity to
ionizing radiation, and like FA cells, AT cells are reported to be
deficient in the ability to remove a form of base damage, the gamma
endonuclease sensitive site, from their DNA [39]. The deficiencies
involved in the two diseases are different, however, since AT cells

have a normal capacity to remove the lesions of the 5,6-dihydroxy-dihydrothymine type [44] the repair of which is deficient in FA.

If this is the only repair deficiency in AT, the abnormal chromosomal sensitivity of G_2 AT lymphocytes to ionizing radiation implicates this form of base damage in the production of chromatid aberrations and also achromatic lesions, since the yields of both are abnormally elevated [6, 41, 57]. However, AT cells are not totally unable, but rather just slow to remove gamma-endonuclease-sensitive base damage, and this could arise if the defect affected an intermediate step in excision. Thus it is possible that the additional aberrations are actually the consequence of repair-induced strand breaks.

A most notable cytogenetic consequence of the repair defect characterizing AT cells was discovered by Taylor et al. [59] and is illustrated by the data in Table 1. In sharp contrast to the classical observation that irradiation of G_0 or G_1 cells (except very close to the onset of the S phase) produces only aberrations of the chromosome type, G_0 irradiation of AT lymphocytes produces chromatid aberrations as well. Though Taylor [57] has argued that an undetected strand break repair deficiency might be involved, the implication seems clear to me that the gamma endonuclease sensitive lesions, though normally repaired rapidly enough so that few if any are left when DNA synthesis begins, are capable, if present during S, of producing aberrations by precisely the same route as other forms of base damage caused by chemical mutagens.

DNA Crosslinks

Bifunctional alkylating agents are capable of crosslinking a polynucleotide strand to either protein or another polynucleotide strand. Unfortunately, it is difficult to distinguish between the two, or to sort out effects caused by crosslinks from those caused by the monoadducts these agents also produce. However, Sasaki and Tonomura have quite clearly demonstrated that FA cells are particularly sensitive to those mutagens capable of crosslinking, including mitomycin C, nitrogen mustard and treatment with 8-methoxypsoralen plus 355 nm ultraviolet light, but not notably so to the monofunctional derivative decarbamoyl mitomycin C or other monofunctional agents [49-51], thus implicating a defect in the repair of crosslinks in this disease. This has been confirmed by direct biophysical measurements on DNA from treated FA cells [15, 16]. Thus it seems certain that crosslinks do in fact give rise to chromosomal aberrations. Just how a DNA interstrand crosslink might do so is still unclear, however, since one might expect both chromatids to be affected, but some, at least, of the excess aberrations induced by crosslinking agents in FA cells appear to be types involving only one [51].

Pyrimidine Cyclobutane Dimers

These lesions are the predominant form of DNA damage induced by irradiation with ultraviolet light. As already mentioned, the existence of the photoreactivation phenomenon, which appears to be specific for removal of lesions of this type only, made it possible to be certain that virtually all of the cytogenetic consequences of ultraviolet irradiation (if not all) are produced by dimers [17]. Aberration production appeared to be entirely S-dependent; in Chinese hamster and amphibian cells in culture, it was found that only chromatid aberrations resulted, and only in cells that had passed through at least part of an S phase [4, 23]. However, this may not be an entirely universal phenomenon.

Several authors have studied aberration production by ultraviolet light in normal human cells and reported that though the efficiency with which aberrations of any kind are produced appears much lower than in rodent or amphibian cells, presumably because of the much higher efficiency of the excision repair system in human cells, a few chromosome type aberrations appear in apparent first post-irradiation mitoses [22, 34]. Furthermore, Orr and Griggs [37] have also found a few chromosome type aberrations in apparent first metaphases of synchronized Chinese hamster and amphibian cell cultures given doses in excess of 20 J/m^2.

Such an exception to strict S-dependence could arise if the prereplication excision repair of dimers occasionally resulted in creation of a double polynucleotide strand break through either coincidence of dimers close enough to each other in the two strands of a double helix to result in such a break if simultaneously excised (i.e., within an average long patch length of each other), or through occasional nuclease attack on the temporarily single stranded region of the other polynucleotide strand. With the intent of investigating this possibility, we have recently done experiments in which we irradiated separated normal human G_0 peripheral lymphocytes with 254 nm ultraviolet light and scored unequivocal first post-irradiation mitoses in cultures made with 25 μM 5-bromodeoxyuridine and differentially stained after fixation [5]. However, after scoring almost a thousand cells given doses of up to 10 J/m^2 and fixed at intervals of up to 128 culture hours (when only about 10% of the metaphases seen in 5 J/m^2 cultures were still first divisions), we have yet to find an unequivocal chromosome type aberration in a first metaphase at any dose or time. Clearly, though the role of the pyrimidine cyclobutane dimer in S-dependent aberration production seems unequivocal, the mechanisms involved in chromosomal aberration production by ultraviolet light need further study.

The common forms of XP are deficient in pre-replication excision of ultraviolet-induced dimers, and XP cells, as already

noted, are also more sensitive than cells from normal humans to
chromosomal aberration induction by ultraviolet irradiation [34,
38]. The so-called "variant" form of XP, on the other hand, appears
to have normal excision repair but to be defective in a post-
replication repair system for ultraviolet-induced DNA damage
[13, 32, 47]. However, the induction of chromosomal aberrations by
ultraviolet light in XP variant cells has not yet been investigated,
so the role in aberration production of whatever the lesions are for
which repair is deficient in such cells remains unknown. They
could, since their repair is post-replicational, simply by the gaps
left in nascent strands because of dimers remaining unremoved in the
template strands, and the repair system itself the recombinational
one we postulated to account for the production of isochromatid
deletions [4].

ACKNOWLEDGEMENT

    This work was supported by the U.S. Department of Energy under
Contract EY-76-C-02-0016 and the U.S. Environmental Protection
Agency under Contract 79-D-X-0533.

REFERENCES

1. Auerbach, A. D., and S. R. Wolman, Susceptibility of Fanconi's
        anemia fibroblasts to chromosome damage by carcinogens,
        Nature, 261 (1976) 494-496.
2. Bender, M. A, J. S. Bedford, and J. B. Mitchell, Mechanisms of
        chromosomal aberration production. II. Aberrations
        induced by 5-bromodeoxyuridine and visible light, Mutat.
        Res., 20 (1973) 403-416.
3. Bender, M. A, H. G. Griggs, and J. S. Bedford, Mechanisms of
        chromosomal aberration production. III. Chemicals and
        ionizing radiation, Mutat. Res., 23 (1974) 197-212.
4. Bender, M. A, H. G. Griggs, and P. L. Walker, Mechanisms of
        chromosomal aberration production. I. Aberration induction
        by ultraviolet light, Mutat. Res., 20 (1973) 387-402.
5. Bender, M. A, J. L. Ivett, and S. M. Jacobs, Chromosomal
        aberrations induced by ultraviolet light, in preparation.
6. Bender, M. A, J. M. Rary, and R. P. Kale, Mechanisms of
        chromosomal aberration production. IV. Chromosomal
        radiosensitivity in ataxia telangiectasia, in preparation.
7. Bigelow, S. B., J. M. Rary, and M. A Bender, G_2 chromosomal
        radiosensitivity in Fanconi's anemia, Mutat. Res., 63
        (1979) 189-199.
8. Cavalier-Smith, T., Palindromic base sequences and replication
        of eukaryote chromosome ends, Nature, 250 (1974) 467-470.

9. Chadwick, K. H., and H. P. Leenhouts, The rejoining of DNA
    double-strand breaks and a model for the formation of
    chromosomal rearrangements, Intern. J. Radiat. Biol., 33
    (1978) 517-529.

10. Christensen, R. C., C. A. Tobias, and W. D. Taylor, Heavy-ion-
    induced single- and double-strand breaks in ϕX174 repli-
    cative form DNA, Intern. J. Radiat. Biol., 22 (1972)
    457-477.

11. Cory, P. M., and A. Cole, Double strand rejoining in mammalian
    DNA, Nature, 245 (1973) 100-101.

12. Dubinin, N. P., and U. N. Soyfer, Chromosome breakage and
    complete genic mutation production in molecular terms,
    Mutat. Res., 8 (1969) 353-365.

13. Fornace, A. J., K. W. Kohn, and H. E. Kann, DNA single strand
    breaks during repair of UV damage in human fibroblasts
    and abnormalities of repair in xeroderma pigmentosum,
    Proc. Natl. Acad. Sci. (U.S.), 73 (1976) 39-43.

14. Fornace, A. J., H. Nagasawa, and J. B. Little, Relationship of
    DNA repair and chromosome aberrations to potentially lethal
    damage repair in X-irradiated mammalian cells, This volume,
    p. 267.

15. Fujiwara, Y., and M. Tatsumi, Repair of mitomycin C damage to
    DNA in mammalian cells in Fanconi's anemia cells, Biochem.
    Biophys. Res. Comm., 66 (1975) 592-598.

16. Fujiwara, Y., M. Tatsumi, and M. S. Sasaki, Cross-link repair
    in human cells and its possible defect in Fanconi's
    anemia cells, J. Mol. Biol., 113 (1977) 635-649.

17. Griggs, H. G., and M. A Bender, Photoreactivation of ultra-
    violet-induced chromosomal aberrations, Science, 179
    (1973) 86-88.

18. Hartley-Asp, B., The influence of caffeine on the mitomycin C-
    induced chromosome aberration frequency in normal human
    and xeroderma pigmentosum cells, Mutat. Res., 49 (1978)
    117-126.

19. Higurachi, M., and P. E. Conen, In vitro chromosomal radio-
    sensitivity in Fanconi's anemia, Blood, 38 (1971) 336-342.

20. Higurachi, M., and P. E. Conen, In vitro chromosomal radio-
    sensitivity in "chromosomal breakage syndromes," Cancer,
    32 (1973) 380-383.

21. Ho, K. S. Y., Induction of DNA double-strand breaks by X-rays
    in a radiosensitive strain of the yeast Saccharomyces
    cerevisiae, Mutat. Res., 30 (1975) 327-334.

22. Holmberg, M., Lack of synergistic effect between X-ray and
    UV irradiation on the frequency of chromosome aberrations
    in PHA-stimulated human lymphocytes in the G_1 stage,
    Mutat. Res., 34 (1976) 141-148.

23. Ikushima, T., and S. Wolff, UV-induced chromatid aberrations
    in cultured Chinese hamster cells after one, two or three
    rounds of DNA replication, Mutat. Res., 22 (1974) 193-201.

24. Johnson, R. T., and P. N. Rao, Mammalian cell fusion: induction of premature chromosome consensation in inter-phase nuclei, Nature, 226 (1970) 717-722.

25. Kelley, J. E. T., and M. A Bender, On the relationship between polynucleotide strand breakage and chromosome aberration production as a function of LET: I. Single strand/double strand break ratios; in preparation (1979).

26. Kihlman, B.A., Actions of Chemicals on Dividing Cells, Prentice-Hall, Englewood Cliffs, 1966.

27. Kihlman, B. A., Caffeine and Chromosomes, Elsevier, Amsterdam, 1977.

28. Krasin, F., and F. Hutchinson, Repair of DNA double-strand breaks in E. coli by recombination, Radiat. Res., 67 (1976) 534.

29. Latt, S. A., G. Stetten, L. A. Juergens, G. R. Buchanan, and P. S. Gerald, Induction by alkylating agents of sister chromatid exchanges and chromatid breaks in Fanconi's anemia, Proc. Natl. Acad. Sci. (U.S.), 72 (1975) 4066-4070.

30. Lea, D. E., Actions of Radiations on Living Cells, 2nd ed., Cambridge, 1955.

31. Lehman, A. R., and S. Stevens, The production and repair of double strand breaks in cells from normal humans and from patients with ataxia telangiectasia, Biochem. Biophys. Acta, 474 (1977) 49-60.

32. Lehman, A. R., S. Kirk-Bell, C. F. Arlett, M. C. Paterson, P. M. H. Lohman, E. A. DeWeerd-Kastelein and D. Bootsma, Xeroderma pigmentosum cells with normal levels of excision repair have a defect in DNA synthesis after UV-irradiation, Proc. Natl. Acad. Sci. (U.S.), 72 (1975) 219-233.

33. Maher, V. M., J. J. McCormick, P. L. Grover, and P. Sims, Effect of DNA repair on the cytotoxicity and mutagenicity of polycyclic hydrocarbon derivatives in normal and xeroderma pigmentosum human fibroblasts, Mutat. Res., 43 (1977) 117-138.

34. Marshall, R. R., and D. Scott, The relationship between chromosome damage and cell killing in UV-irradiated normal and xeroderma pigmentosum cells, Mutat. Res., 36 (1976) 397-400.

35. Muller, W. E. G., and R. K. Zahn, Bleomycin, an antibiotic that removes thymine from double-stranded DNA, Progr. Nucleic Acid Res. Mol. Biol. 20 (1977) 21-57.

36. Natarajan, A. T., and G. Obe, Molecular mechanisms involved in the production of chromosomal aberrations. I. Utilization of Neurospora endonuclease for the study of aberration production in G_2 stage of the cell cycle, Mutat. Res., 52 (1978) 137-149.

37. Orr, T. V., and H. G. Griggs, Chromosomal aberrations resulting from UV exposures to G_1 Xenopus cells, Photochem. Photobiol., 30 (1979) 363-368.

38. Parrington, J. M., J. D. A. Delhanty, and H. P. Baden,
    Unscheduled DNA synthesis, UV-induced chromosome aberrations
    and SV40 transformation in cultured cells from <u>xeroderma
    pigmentosum</u>, Ann. Human Genet., 35 (1971) 149-160.
39. Paterson, M. C., B. P. Smith, P. M. H. Lohman, A. K. Anderson,
    and L. Fishman, Defective excision repair of x-ray-damaged
    DNA in human (ataxia telangiectasia) fibroblasts, Nature,
    260 (1976) 444-447.
40. Poon, R., T. A. Beerman, and I. H. Goldberg, Characterization
    of DNA strand breakage in vitro by the antitumor protein
    neocarzinostatin, Biochemistry, 16 (1977) 486-493.
41. Rary, J. M., M. A Bender, and T. E. Kelly, Cytogenetic studies
    of ataxia telangiectasia, Am. J. Human Genet., 26 (1974)
    70a.
42. Regan, J. D., and R. B. Setlow, Two forms of repair in the
    DNA of human cells damaged by chemical carcinogens and
    mutagens, Cancer Res., 34 (1974) 3318-3325.
43. Remsen, J. F., and P. A. Cerutti, Deficiency of gamma-ray
    excision repair in skin fibroblasts from patients with
    Fanconi's anemia, Proc. Natl. Acad. Sci. (U.S.), 73 (1976)
    2419-2423.
44. Remsen, J. F., and P. A. Cerutti, Excision of gamma-ray induced
    thymine lesions by preparations from ataxia telangiectasia
    fibroblasts, Mutat. Res., 43 (1977) 139-146.
45. Resnick, M. A., The repair of double-strand breaks in DNA:
    a model involving recombination, J. Theor. Biol., 59 (1976)
    97-106.
46. Resnick, M. A., and P. Martin, The repair of double-strand
    breaks in the nuclear DNA of Saccharomyces cerevisiae and
    its genetic control, Mol. Gen. Genet., 143 (1976) 110-129.
47. Robbins, J. H., W. R. Lewis, and A. E. Miller, Xeroderma
    pigmentosum epidermal cells with normal UV-induced
    thymidine incorporation, J. Invest. Dermatol., 59 (1972)
    5402-5408.
48. Sasaki, M. S., DNA repair capacity and susceptibility to
    chromosome breakage in Xeroderma pigmentosum cells,
    Mutat. Res., 20 (1973) 291-293.
49. Sasaki, M. S., Is Fanconi's anemia defective in a process
    essential to the repair of DNA cross links? Nature, 257
    (1975) 501-503.
50. Sasaki, M. S., Cytogenetic evidence for the repair of DNA
    cross-links: its normal functioning in Xeroderma
    pigmentosum and its impairment in Fanconi's anemia, Mutat.
    Res., 46 (1977) 152-153.
51. Sasaki, M. S., and A. Tonomura, A high susceptibility of
    Fanconi's anemia to chromosome breakage by DNA cross-
    linking agents, Cancer Res., 33 (1973) 1829-1836.
52. Savage, J. R. K., Radiation-induced chromosomal aberrations
    in the plant Tradescantia: Dose-response curves. I. Pre-
    liminary considerations, Radiat. Bot., 15 (1975) 87-140.

53. Schneider, E. L., R. R. Tice, and D. Kram, Bromodeoxyuridine-
     differential staining technique: a new approach to
     examining sister chromatid exchange and cell replication
     kinetics, In: Methods in Cell Biology, Vol. 20, D. M.
     Prescott (Ed.), Academic Press, New York, 1978, pp. 379-
     409.
54. Schuler, D., A. Kiss, and F. Fabian, Chromosomal pecularities
     and "in vitro" examinations in Fanconi's anemia,
     Humangenetik, 7 (1969) 314-422.
55. Setlow, R. B., and J. K. Setlow, Effects of radiation on
     polynucleotides, In: Annual Review of Biophysics and
     Bioengineering, M. F. Morales, W. A. Hagins, L. Stryer,
     and W. S. Yamamoto (Eds.), Vol. 1, Annual Reviews Inc.,
     Palo Alto, Calif., 1972, pp. 293-346.
56. Stich, H. F., W. Stich, and R. H. C. San, Chromosome aberrations
     in xeroderma pigmentosum cells exposed to the carcinogens
     4-nitroquinoline-1-oxide and N-methyl-N'-nitro-nitroso-
     guanidine, Proc. Soc. Exp. Biol. Med., 142 (1973) 1141-
     1144
57. Taylor, A. M. R., Unrepaired DNA strand breaks in irradiated
     ataxia telangiectasia lymphocytes suggested from cyto-
     genetic observations, Mutat. Res., 50 (1978) 407-418.
58. Taylor, A. M. R., D. G. Harnden, C. F. Arlett, S. A. Harcourt,
     S. Stevens, and B. A. Bridges, Ataxia telangiectasia: a
     human mutation with abnormal radiation sensitivity, Nature,
     258 (1975) 427-429.
59. Taylor, A. M. R., J. A. Metcalfe, J. M. Oxford, and D. G.
     Harnden, Is chromatid type damage in ataxia telangiectasia
     after irradiation at G_0 a consequence of defective repair?
     Nature, 260 (1976) 441-443.
60. Taylor, J. H., Radioisotope studies on the structure of the
     chromosome, In: Radiation-Induced Chromosome Aberrations,
     S. Wolff (Ed.), Columbia University Press, New York, 1963.
61. Taylor, J. H., W. F. Haut, and J. Tung, Effects of fluoro-
     deoxyuridine on DNA replication, chromosome breakage and
     reunion, Proc. Natl. Acad. Sci. (U.S.), 48 (1962) 190-198.
62. Taylor, H. J., P. S. Woods, and W. L. Hughes, The organization
     and duplication of chromosomes as revealed by autoradio-
     graphic studies using tritium-labeled thymidine, Proc.
     Natl. Acad. Sci. (U.S.), 43 (1957) 122-128.
63. Vincent, R. A., R. B. Sheridan, and P. C. Huang, DNA strand
     breakage repair in ataxia telangiectasia fibroblast-like
     cells, Mutat. Res., 33 (1975) 357-366.
64. Wolff, S., The doubleness of the chromosome before DNA
     synthesis as revealed by combined x-ray and tritiated
     thymidine treatments, Radiat. Res., 14 (1961) 517-518.
65. Wolff, S., and P. Perry, Differential Giemsa staining of
     sister chromatids and the study of sister chromatid
     exchanges without autoradiography, Chromosoma, 48 (1974)
     341-353.

CHAPTER 18

RELATIONSHIP OF DNA REPAIR AND CHROMOSOME ABERRATIONS TO

POTENTIALLY LETHAL DAMAGE REPAIR IN X-IRRADIATED MAMMALIAN CELLS

A. J. FORNACE, JR., H. NAGASAWA, AND J. B. LITTLE

Department of Physiology, Laboratory of Radiobiology
Harvard School of Public Health, Boston, MA   02115
(U.S.A.)

SUMMARY

By the alkaline elution technique, the repair of x-ray-induced DNA single strand breaks and DNA-protein cross-links was investigated in stationary phase, contact-inhibited mouse cells. During the first hour of repair, approximately 90% of x-ray induced single strand breaks were rejoined whereas most of the remaining breaks were rejoined more slowly during the next 5 hr. The number of residual non-rejoined single strand breaks was approximately proportional to the x-ray dose at early repair times. DNA-protein cross-links were removed at a slower rate – $T_{\frac{1}{2}}$ approximately 10-12 hr. Cells were subcultured at low density at various times after irradiation and scored for colony survival (potentially lethal damage repair), and chromosome aberrations in the first mitosis after sub-culture. Both cell lethality and the frequency of chromosome aberrations decreased during the first several hours of repair, reaching a minimum level by 6 hr; this decrease correlated temporally with the repair of the slowly rejoining DNA strand breaks. The possible relationship of DNA repair to changes in survival and chromosome aberrations is discussed.

INTRODUCTION

Many lesions have been identified in the DNA of mammalian cells exposed to x-rays, but the relation of these particular types of damage to biologic parameters such as cell killing, chromosome aberrations, mutation, and malignant transformation remains far from resolved. DNA single-strand breaks (SSB) can be readily detected after x-ray, but most are rapidly rejoined in mammalian

267

cells even after supralethal doses [21]. It has been proposed that approximately 1 DNA double-strand break induced by x-irradiation per cell is a lethal event [5], and that these lesions are not re-paired [5, 19]. However, there has been wide variability in the reported efficiency of double-strand break induction by x-ray [2, 5, 10, 19, 24, 33], and in at least one report repair of most double-strand breaks was observed [24]. DNA alkaline labile sites have also been implicated as possible lethal events since these lesions are more persistent with incubation after x-ray than are SSB [24]. With moderate to long incubation times after x-ray, a very small fraction of the DNA SSB are not rejoined [5, 30]; interest in the biologic significance of these residual breaks was raised when the fraction of nonrejoined SSB in cells exposed to ionizing radiation of varying linear energy transfer (LET) was found to correspond to the relative biological effectiveness of the particular radiation for cell killing [30]. Several investigations have revealed the presence of x-ray-induced lesions in mammalian DNA which appear to be enzymatically excised [20, 25, 26, 28]. The possible biologic importance of enzymatic excision was raised when radiosensitive cells from some, but not all, ataxia telangiectasia patients were found to remove these lesions at a much slower rate than normal cells [26].

All of the studies cited above were performed with very high doses of x-irradiation, usually in excess of 10,000 rad. At lower doses, few molecular lesions can be identified with conventional techniques. Yet, cellular effects such as cell lethality and the induction of chromosome aberrations occur following much lower radiation doses. There is a strong correlation between cell killing by x-rays and the frequency of chromosome aberrations [1]. In split dose recovery experiments, and in experiments in which DNA repli-cation was delayed by holding at 22°C (potentially lethal damage repair), the decreases in cell killing observed corresponded to the decreases in the aberration frequency [4]. These decreases were not observed when the cells were incubated at 0°C or with inhibitors of protein synthesis, suggesting that inhibition of repair mechanisms prevented the restitution of chromosome aberrations.

The repair of potentially lethal damage (PLDR) has been studied primarily by irradiating contact-inhibited confluent (stationary phase) cultures and then comparing the clonogenic survival of cells immediately replated at a lower density versus cells held for several hours in the confluent phase [22]. This phenomenon is somewhat analogous to liquid holding recovery in bacterial cells. A maximum enhancement in survival is seen by holding in confluency for 2-4 hr [32]. The possible relationship of PLDR to molecular DNA repair processes was strengthened when pyrimidine dimer excision-deficient xeroderma pigmentosum fibroblasts were also found to be deficient in their PLDR capacity after UV radiation [34].

PLDR also appears to influence the frequency of x-ray-induced malignant transformation in vitro [32].

The alkaline elution technique has been shown to be a sensitive assay for detecting DNA SSB produced directly by x-rays [7, 17] and various chemical agents [16], as well as excision breaks which occur during repair of UV-radiation damage [8]. By an adaptation of this technique, low levels of both DNA-DNA and DNA-protein crosslinks can also be detected [7, 16]. Recently, DNA-protein crosslinks were detected after irradiation of mammalian cells with moderate and high doses of x-rays [9]. This has enabled us to assess quantitatively both DNA crosslinking and, with removal of the crosslinking by proteinase, DNA SSB after moderate and low doses of x-rays.

In the present investigation, we have employed the alkaline elution technique with the mouse C3H/10T½ system [32] to measure the rates of repair of DNA SSB and DNA-protein crosslinks at varying times during the repair of potentially lethal x-ray damage in stationary cells and to correlate these with the frequency of chromosome aberrations. Our aim has been to determine the extent to which repair of these molecular DNA lesions may correlate with cell survival and cytogenetic changes.

MATERIALS AND METHODS

Cells and Cell Labeling

Mouse C3H 10T½ clone 8 embryo-derived fibroblasts were grown as previously described [29,32]. For experiments, cells at passage 8 to 13 were grown until confluent; they were held in the confluent state for 2 days prior to the experiments with medium changes every 24 hr. At this time, the cultures were in nearly complete stationary growth; less than 2% of the cells were in the S phase, and only an additional 1% entered S every 24 hr as determined by autoradiographic techniques, whereas over 90% of the cells were in G_1 as determined by flow microfluorimetry (H. Nagasawa, unpublished data). After subculture, the labeling index reaches 70-75% by 24 hr, indicating a high degree of synchrony. For alkaline elution experiments, [2-^{14}C]thymidine (0.02 µCi/ml, 57 mCi/mM, New England Nuclear) was added to the growing cells for 2 days before they reached confluency. The cells were then returned to a nonradioactive medium; otherwise the labeled cells were handled identically to the other samples. Exponentially growing L1210 mouse leukemia cells were prepared as previously described [7].

Irradiation

Confluent cultures were aerobically x-irradiated at 37°C at a dose rate of 80 rad/min with a G.E. Maximar x-ray generator operated at 220 kV and 15' mA. Following irradiation, the medium was replaced with fresh warm medium, the cultures incubated at 37°C for the indicated times, trypsinized, and either analyzed by alkaline elution or replated as described below. For alkaline elution experiments, the cells were treated as previously described [9]; the cells were irradiated while suspended in cold medium when no repair incubation followed x-ray exposure.

Cell Survival

Cell survival was measured by the colony formation assay [27]. The cells in confluent cultures were trypsinized at appropriate times after x-ray and seeded at low density in 100 mm plastic Falcon Petri dishes. Cell numbers were adjusted to yield 40-80 viable colony-forming cells per dish; six replicate dishes were seeded per point. Colonies were scored after 10-15 days as described previously [32], and the results expressed as the fraction surviving as compared with non-irradiated controls.

Chromosome Aberrations

The cells were subcultured from plateau phase cultures, resuspended in fresh medium and seeded at a density of 3×10^5 per T-30 Falcon flask. Colchicine (final concentration 2×10^{-6}M) was added to the flasks for a 4-hr interval prior to fixation to arrest the cells in metaphase. To ensure that only first-division cells were scored for aberrations, cultures were fixed at 4-hr intervals from 20 to 32 hr after subculture. Aberrations were scored in the first-division cells that were harvested at the interval when the mitotic index was highest; the types and distribution of aberrations were similar in all first-division cells. These results as well as the determination of optimal times to harvest first mitosis cells will be reported in detail elsehwere.

The cells were fixed by the hypotonic method, prepared for chromosomal scoring by the air drying technique, and stained with 2% aceto-orcein [13]. About 50 cells from each sample from one experiment were analyzed for chromosome aberrations as described by Dewey et al. [3]. The total number of aberrations was defined as the number of chromatid deletions, chromatid exchanges, isolocus deletions, dicentrics, and ring chromosomes per cell. About 70-80% of the aberrations scored were chromosomal type aberrations.

Alkaline Elution

The procedure used [7-9] is a modification of that described by Kohn et al. [18]. Briefly, the cells were filtered into a polyvinylchloride filter, lysed with 2 M NaCl/0.02 M Na_3 EDTA/ 0.2% Sarkosyl (pH 10.2), washed with 0.02 M Na_3 EDTA (pH 10.3), and then eluted at 0.04 ml/min with a solution consisting of 0.02 M EDTA (Acid Form) plus tetrapropylammonium hydroxide added in the amount required to give a pH of 12.2. Eluted fractions were collected and assayed for radioactivity as previously described [7]. In some experiments, the cell lysates were digested with proteinase prior to elution [6]. Proteinase-K, dissolved in the lysing solution described above to a concentration of 0.5 mg/ml, was added to the cells on the filter instead of the regular lysing solution. They were allowed to incubate at room temperature for 1 hr following which alkaline elution was carried out as described previously. In order to provide for an internal standard, ^{3}H-labeled L1210 cells which had received 150 rad at 0°C were included in each assay. To improve quantification, the elution of sample DNA was normalized against the elution of the internal reference DNA [9], and plotted on a corrected time scale.

Extensive evidence has been presented that the alkaline elution technique can quantitatively measure DNA single strand breaks (SSB) produced by low doses of x-ray [7, 8, 17]. The retention of DNA on the filter, as measured by the relative retention (fraction of DNA retained on the filter after 12 hr), has been seen to decrease according to a first-order relation of the x-ray dose. Treatment of the cells with a crosslinking agent, however, diminishes the effect of subsequent x-irradiation on alkaline elution [9, 17]. This crosslinking effect, seen with alkaline elution as measured by the crosslink factor, has been quantified by comparing the increase in elution produced by a small test dose of x-rays in treated cells to the increase produced by the same test dose of x-rays in untreated cells. This value, the crosslink factor, was shown to be approximately directly proportional to the dose of crosslinking agent used with various DNA crosslinking agents [9].

RESULTS

All experiments were performed with density-inhibited, confluent (stationary phase) cultures of mouse C3H 10T½ cells. The effect of x-ray on the alkaline elution of cellular DNA is demonstrated in Fig. 1. With control cells, most of the DNA was retained on the filter, while after exposing the cells to 300 rads at 0°C, there was a marked near-linear decrease in the retention of DNA on the filter. When the cells were exposed to 5 krad and incubated in confluency for an additional 2 hr, most of the DNA SSB were rejoined [9, 17], yielding the elution profiles seen in

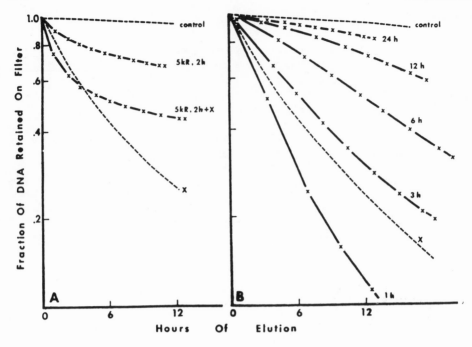

Fig. 1.   Effect of x-ray on alkaline elution. Cells were x-
irradiated with 5 krad at 37°C, incubated for the indicated times
and analyzed by alkaline elution. In A, cells which had been
previously irradiated and incubated for 2 hr were suspended in
medium and irradiated at 0°C with 300 rad where indicated (+X);
control cells were also included with (X) and without (control)
a similar 300 rad dose. In B, conditions were the same as in A
except cell lysates were digested with proteinase-K prior to
alkaline elution.

Fig. 1A. At later elution times, however, the elution rate
decreased in this sample with a resultant nonlinear profile
characteristic of crosslinked DNA [9]. This observation was
confirmed by exposing cells treated in the same manner to a test
dose of 300 rad at 0°C; the increase in elution was markedly less
than when the same test dose was given to control (nonirradiated)
cells. This crosslink effect has not been seen in cells treated
with agents which induced SSB only [9]; in this case, the test
dose of x-rays was additive with the effect induced by these
agents.

     Proteinase digestion of the cell lysates has been shown to
remove the DNA crosslinking effect induced by high dose x-ray,
allowing an accurate determination of the SSB frequency to be made
[9]. This phenomenon is demonstrated in Fig. 1B. The effect of

proteinase is slight in control cells or cells treated with the
small test dose of x-rays at 0°C, but there is a significant increase
in elution of the samples exposed to 5 krad when the DNA-protein
crosslinking effect has been removed by incubation with proteinase-K.
With the sensitivity of alkaline elution, the level of SSB present
3 hr or more after 5 krad exposure is measurable even when the effect
is less than that induced by the 300 rad test dose at 0°C.

The effect of repair incubation in confluent cells after
various doses of x-ray is demonstrated in Fig. 2. Since the elution
profiles are approximately linear when the crosslink effect has been
removed by proteinase, the value "the relative retention" is representative of the slope of the elution profiles in a logarithmic plot,
which has been shown to reflect the DNA SSB frequency [7, 9, 16, 17].
These values can thus be directly compared to various test doses of
x-ray as shown on the right ordinate. When this comparison is made,

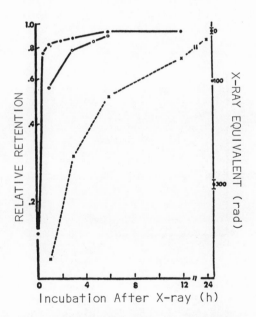

Fig. 2.   Effect of repair incubation on x-irradiated cells with
proteinase digestion of the cell lysates. Cells were exposed to
(●) 0.4, (○) 1.2, and (X) 5.0 krad as in Fig. 1 and incubated at
37°C. Relative retention is defined as the fraction of DNA
retained on the filter after 12 hr of alkaline elution. On the
right ordinate, the effect of x-ray alone at 0°C is included for
comparative purposes and is expressed with S.E.M.

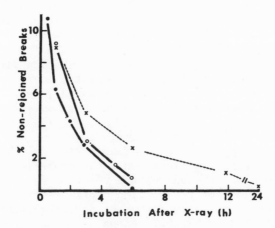

Fig. 3.   Fraction of nonrejoined single-strand breaks (SSB) after
various doses of x-ray and repair incubation.   These data are taken
from Fig. 2.   The fraction of nonrejoined SSB was determined by
comparing the relative retention of these samples to that of x-ray
alone, which induced the same relative retention;   this value was
then divided by the original x-ray dose.   Symbols are taken from
Fig. 2 after the same x-ray exposures.

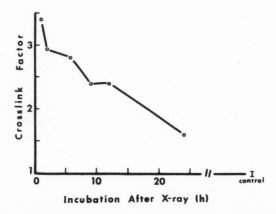

Fig. 4.   Repair of DNA-protein crosslinks induced by 5 krad of
x-ray.   Cells were handled as in Fig. 1A and the crosslink factor
was determined at various incubation times.   The crosslink factor
(see text) is defined [9] as
        [mean (log relative retention of control - log relative
        retention of cells exposed to 300 R at 0°)] ÷
        [log relative retention of cells preirradiated with 5kR -
        log relative retention of cells preirradiated with 5kR, and
        exposed to 300 R at 0° at the end of incubation).

the rad equivalent at various repair incubation times can be divided
by the original X-ray dose to derive the fraction of nonrejoined
SSB at these various repair times. As seen in Fig. 3, greater than
90% of the SSB are rejoined in the first hour after doses of 0.4
to 5 krad. By 6 hr of repair, the 0.4 and 1.2 krad dose groups are
within 1 S.D. of the control, while less than 3% of the DNA SSB
induced by the 5 krad dose remain. At longer repair times, most of
the SSB induced by 5 krad are rejoined, such that by 24 hr less than
1% (0.3%) remain.

An estimate of the level of DNA-protein crosslinking present
after high doses of x-ray can be made by comparing the effect of a
second small test dose of x-rays on these cells, as illustrated in
Fig. 1A, with the effect on controls [9]. By use of such a
comparison, a crosslink factor may be obtained which reflects the
magnitude of the crosslinking effect. In Fig. 4, the crosslink
factor is plotted as a function of repair time for cells irradiated
with 5 krad; this factor decreased slowly over 24 hr with less
than 25% of the crosslinks remaining at this time.

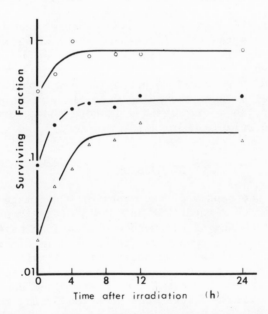

Fig. 5.   Change in survival of mouse 10T½ cells during the repair
of potentially lethal x-ray damage (PLD): (◯) 200 rad; (●)
400 rad; (△) 800 rad.   Cells were x-irradiated while in the
density-inhibited phase of growth, and were subcultured at low
density 0-24 hr later to assay for colony forming ability. Results
of one representative experiment with 6 replicate dishes per point
containing 40-80 macroscopic colonies. Cloning efficiency was 26%.

The results of PLDR experiments after various doses of x-ray are presented in Fig. 5. A marked enhancement in clonogenic survival was observed when the cells were held in confluence for 2-4 hr after irradiation before replating; survival remained approximately constant with repair intervals of 6 hr or more. As the enhancement of survival reflects a change in the slope of the survival curve [23], the relative increase in survival is greater with higher x-ray doses.

A similar protocol was used for the experiments shown in Fig. 6, but the cells were arrested in the first mitosis after replating and the total number of chromosome aberrations were scored in 50 cells, and the results expressed as the mean number of aberrations per mitotic cell (see Methods). After both a 200 or a 400 rad dose, there was a significant decrease in the number of chromosome aberrations during the first 6 hr of PLDR. With longer incubation in confluence, no further decline in the frequency of chromosome aberrations occurred. The types of aberrations seen were similar in all experimental groups; 70-80% were chromosome type aberrations, primarily isochromatid breaks. The precise distribution of aberrations will be described in detail elsehwere.

In Fig. 7, the number of chromosome aberrations induced per cell is plotted as a function of cell survival after x-irradiation; as can be seen there is a near linear relation on a first order plot. As reported previously [4], 37% survival was sustained at the x-ray dose which resulted in approximately 1 chromosome aberration per cell. When the cells were allowed to undergo PLDR, there was recovery such that changes in both these parameters still indicate the same relationship.

DISCUSSION

In summary, the repair of two types of DNA damage induced in confluent cultures by x-rays (SSB and DNA-protein crosslinks), and changes in the frequency of chromosome aberrations have been compared under identical conditions to changes in clonogenic survival which occurred when the cells were maintained under conditions which favored the repair of potentially lethal damage. A rapid decrease in the frequencies of nonrejoined DNA strand breaks and of chromosome aberrations occurred during the first several hours of PLDR: these coincided in time with the enhancement in survival seen after irradiation with similar doses of x-rays. After 6 hr of PLDR, no further decrease in the frequency of chromosome aberrations occurred after 200 or 400 rad; by this time essentially all the DNA SSB had been rejoined after 400 or 1200 rad as measured by alkaline elution. After 5 krad of x-ray, the level of DNA-protein crosslinks slowly decreased with a half-removal time of approximately 10-12 hr.

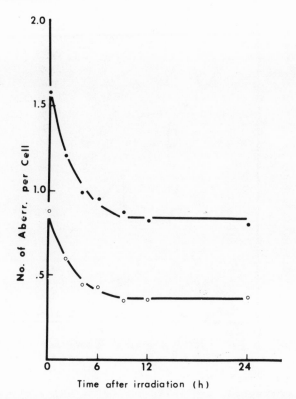

Fig. 6.   Effect of potentially lethal damage repair on the
frequency of chromosome aberrations after x-irradiation: (○)
200 rads;   (●) 400 rads.   The cells were treated as in Fig. 5.
Chromosome aberrations were scored in 50 cells for each experimental
point as described in Materials and Methods.   The aberration
frequency in nonirradiated cells was 0.047 ± 0.009 (data pooled
from several experiments).

        The number of nonrejoined DNA SSB at early repair times after
x-ray was approximately directly proportional to dose, implying a
1-hit type of production.   After 1 hr of repair, for example,
6.3 to 9.2% of the original breaks remained at 400, 1200, and 5000
rad;   after 3 hr, 2.5 to 4.8% remained with the same doses.   These
results are in general agreement with those reported by Ritter
et al. [30], who used the alkaline gradient sedimentation technique
with higher doses of x-rays;   they found that the number of
nonrejoined SSB was proportional to dose.   These results are in
contrast however, to those reported by Dugle et al. [5], who found
that the number of nonrejoined SSB after 210 min repair was
proportional to the square of the original dose at doses greater

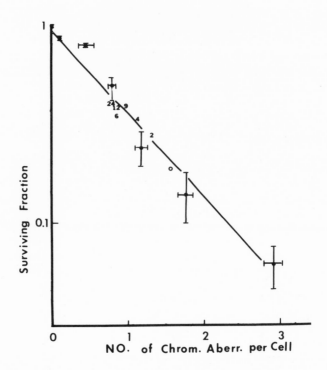

Fig. 7.   Relationship of cell lethality to the frequency of
chromosome aberrations. Density inhibited cells were irradiated
with 50 to 600 rads and subcultured immediately (●), as well as
with cultures irradiated with 400 rads and subcultured 0 to 24 hr
after irradiation (PLDR). Data points designated by numbers
indicate these repair times.

than 20 krad. This latter relationship would be expected with a
2-hit type event, but, at the relatively low doses used in our
investigation, these events should be rare for the target size of
mammalian DNA.

Most previous investigations have found approximately one
double-strand break per 10 SSB. This would correspond approximately
to the fraction of nonrejoined SSB seen 1 hr after irradiation. It
should be noted that all these SSB are rejoined by 6 hr after 400
or 1200 rad (within 1 S.D. of control) as are most (0.3% remaining)
by 24 hr with the superlethal dose of 5000 rad. It is clear from
the data in Fig. 3, however, that there are two components to the
rejoining curve for SSB. This fact suggests the existence of two
types of lesions: breaks which are rapidly rejoined (within 1 hr)
and a second class of more slowly rejoining breaks.

During the excision of UV-photoproducts, a low level of
enzymatically induced excision breaks has been detected by alkaline
elution; with higher doses of UV these breaks persisted longer [8].
The possibility exists that some of the SSB seen after x-ray may
reflect similar DNA lesions which are also being enzymatically
excised. This hypothesis is supported by the fact that a low level
of SSB are persistent longer after 5 krad than after lower doses.
After 50 krad, however, most of the x-ray-induced base products
sensitive to gamma endonuclease are reportedly removed by 3 hr [26];
this contrasts with the presence of significant levels of DNA SSB
at longer repair times after 5 krad in our study.

DNA-protein crosslinks appeared to be slowly repaired after
5 krad with a half-removal time ($T\frac{1}{2}$) of 10-12 hr. Various investigators have reported that DNA-DNA crosslinks are removed faster in
mammalian cells with a $T\frac{1}{2}$ of 2-8 hr [6, 11, 14, 31, 35]. In the
same cell line used in the present study, DNA-protein crosslinks
were also slowly removed after UV irradiation, $T\frac{1}{2}$ approximately
24 hr after 10 J/M^2 (unpublished results). Therefore, these lesions
appear to be relatively persistent after high doses of x-ray, but
their relation to lethality, mutation, and other cellular parameters
remains to be determined.

As stated earlier, evidence has been presented that the
enhancement in survival after radiation damage seen by holding cells
in stationary growth for several hours before seeding at a lower
density (PLDR) is related to DNA repair. This enhanced survival
appears to parallel the slowly rejoining component of DNA SSB during
the first several hours of repair after x-irradiation. As discussed
earlier, there is some evidence that the presence of nonrejoined SSB
is related to lethality in mammalian cells [30]. Also, 1, 3 - bis
(cyclohexyl)-1-nitrosourea has been recently shown to inhibit strand
rejoining after x-ray at relatively non-toxic doses of the drug;
the same dose of this agent was found to markedly enhance cell
killing when given to the cells at the time of x-irradiation [15].
If the fraction of nonrejoined DNA SSB at the time of replating to
lower density does indeed determine cell lethality (or a portion of
it), then this damage must be "fixed" in the cell at the time of
replating, since the cells do not enter S phase for an additional
18-20 hr (Nagasawa, unpublished results). We have found that the
rejoining of SSB proceeds at an approximately equivalent rate during
this period (G_1) after trypsinization and replating, before the onset
of the S phase (data not shown). By premature chromosome condensation, however, a significant qualitative difference can be seen
between cells in G_1 and G_0 [12]. It would not be unreasonable to
speculate that, once cells have been committed to divide by release
from confluent conditions, changes in the chromatin occur which
determine cell lethality regardless of further SSB repair before
the initiation of DNA synthesis.

The above speculation is supported by the observation that the frequency of chromosome aberrations is approximately directly proportional to the fraction of nonrejoined SSB from 1 to 6 hr of PLDR after 400 rad. By 6 hr, when essentially all the SSB have been rejoined after 400 or 1200 rad, no further change in the frequency of chromosome aberrations occurs. Chromosome aberrations have been considered to represent a lethal event after x-ray [4] With radiation of higher LET, an enhancement of both chromosome aberrations [1], double-strand breaks [1], nonrejoined SSB [30], and cell killing [30] have been reported. It is tempting to speculate that when the cells enter a G_1-type phase after release from stationary growth, changes in the chromatin occur which fix the damage of a nonrejoined DNA SSB (which may represent double strand breaks) such that a chromosome aberration is produced which is a lethal event. With PLDR, this damage is repaired before this critical time such that the chromosome aberration frequency is reduced.

ACKNOWLEDGEMENTS

      This study was supported by Research Grants CA-11751 and ES-00002 and Training Grant CA-09078 from the National Institutes of Health.

REFERENCES

1. Altman, K. I., G. B. Gerber, and S. Okada, Radiation Biochemistry, Vol. I, Academic Press, New York, 1970, pp. 308-326.
2. Corry, P. M., and A. Cole, Radiation-induced double-strand scission of the DNA of mammalian metaphase chromosomes, Radiat. Res., 36 (1968) 528-543.
3. Dewey, W. C., and H. M. Miller, X-ray induction of chromatid exchanges in mitotic and G1 Chinese hamster cells pretreated with colcemid, Exptl..Cell Res., 57 (1969) 63-70.
4. Dewey, W. C., H. H. Miller, and D. B. Leeper, Chromosomal aberrations and mortality of x-irradiated mammalian cells: emphasis on repair, Proc. Natl. Acad. Sci. (U.S.), 68 (1971) 667-671.
5. Dugle, D. L., C. J. Gillespie, and J. D. Chapman, DNA strand breaks, repair, and survival in x-irradiated mammalian cells, Proc. Natl. Acad. Sci. (U.S.), 73 (1976) 809-812.
6. Ewig, R. A. G., and K. W. Kohn, DNA damage and repair in mouse leukemia L1210 cells treated with nitrogen mustard, 1,3-bis(2-chloroethyl)-1-nitrosourea, and other nitroso-ureas, Cancer Res., 37 (1977) 2114-2122.

7. Fornace, Jr., A. J., and K. W. Kohn, DNA-protein cross-
    linking by ultraviolet radiation in normal human and
    xeroderma pigmentosum fibroblasts, Biochim. Biophys. Acta,
    435 (976) 95-103.
8. Fornace, Jr., A. J., K. W. Kohn, and H. E. Kann, Jr., DNA-
    single-strand breaks during repair of UV damage in human
    fibroblasts and abnormalities of repair in xeroderma
    pigmentosum, Proc. Natl. Acad. Sci. (U.S.), 73 (1976)
    39-43.
9. Fornace, Jr., A. J., and J. B. Little, DNA crosslinking induced
    by x-rays and chemical agents, Biochim. Biophys. Acta,
    477 (1977) 343-355.
10. Freifelder, D., Lethal changes in bacteriophage DNA produced
    by x-rays, Radiat. Res. Suppl., 6 (1966) 80-96.
11. Fujiwara, Y., and M. Tatsumi, Cross-link repair in human cells
    and its possible defect in Fanconi's anemia cells, J.
    Mol. Biol., 113 (1977) 635-649.
12. Hittelman, W. N., and P. N. Rao, Predicting response or
    progression of human leukemia by premature chromosome
    condensation of bone marrow cells, Cancer Res., 38 (1978)
    416-423.
13. Hsu, T. C., and O. Klatt, Mammalian chromosomes in vitro, on
    genetic polymorphism in cell population, J. Natl. Cancer
    Inst., 21 (1958) 437-473.
14. Jolley, G. M., and M. G. Ormerod, An improved method for
    measuring crosslinks in the DNA of mammalian cells: the
    effect of nitrogen mustard, Biochim. Biophys. Acta, 308
    (1973) 242-251.
15. Kann, Jr., H. E., A. Petkas, and M. A. Schott, Cytotoxic
    synergism between radiation and various nitrosoureas,
    Proc. Amer. Assoc. Cancer Res., 19 (1978) 214.
16. Kohn, K. W., DNA as target in cancer chemotherapy: Measure-
    ment of macromolecular DNA damage produced in mammalian
    cells by anti-cancer agents and carcinogens, In: Methods
    in Cancer Research, (1978) in press.
17. Kohn, K. W., L. C. Erickson, R. A. G. Ewig, and C. A.
    Friedman, Fractionation of DNA from mammalian cells by
    alkaline elution, Biochemistry, 15 (1976) 4628-4637.
18. Kohn, K. W., C. A. Friedman, R. A. G. Ewig, and Z. M. Iqbal,
    DNA chain growth during replication of asynchronous L1210
    cells. Alkaline elution of large DNA segments from cells
    lysed on filters, Biochemistry, 13 (1974) 4134-4139.
19. Lehmann, A. R., and M. G. Ormerod, Double-strand breaks in
    the DNA of a mammalian cell after x-irradiation, Biochim.
    Biophys. Acta. 217 (1970) 268-277.
20. Lennartz, M., T. Coquerelle, and U. Hagen, Modification of
    end-groups in DNA strand breaks of irradiated thymocytes
    during early repair, Int. J. Radiat. Biol., 28 (1975)
    181-185.

21. Lett, J. T., I. Caldwell, C. J. Dean, and P. Alexander,
    Rejoining of x-ray induced breaks in the DNA of leukaemia
    cells, Nature 214 (1967) 790-792.
22. Little, J. B., Repair of sub-lethal and potentially lethal
    radiation damage in plateau phase cultures of human cells,
    Nature, 224 (1969) 804-806.
23. Little, J. B., Repair of potentially-lethal radiation ramage
    in mammalian cells: Enhancement by conditioned medium
    from stationary cultures, Int. J. Radiat. Biol., 20 (1971)
    87-92.
24. Matsudaira, H., I. Furuno, A. Ueno, K. Shinohara, and K.
    Yoshizawa, Induction and repair of strand breaks and 3'-
    hydroxy terminals in the DNA of mammalian cells in culture
    following γ-ray irradiation, Biochim. Biophys. Acta, 476
    (1977) 97-107.
25. Mattern, M. R., P. V. Hariharan, B. E. Dunlap, and P. A.
    Cerutti, DNA degradation and excision repair in γ-irradiated
    Chinese hamster ovary cells, Nature New Biol., 245 (1973)
    230-232.
26. Paterson, M. C., B. P. Smith, P. H. M. Lohman, A. K. Anderson,
    and L. Fishman, Defective excision repair of γ-ray-damaged
    DNA in human (ataxia telangiectasia) fibroblasts, Nature
    260 (1976) 444-446.
27. Puck, T. T., and P. I. Marcus, Action of x-ray in mammalian
    cells, J. Exp. Med., 103 (1956) 653-666.
28. Remsen, J. F., and P. A. Cerutti, Deficiency of gamma-ray
    excision repair in skin fibroblasts from patients with
    Fanconi's anemia, Proc. Natl. Acad. Sci. (U.S.), 73 (1976)
    2419-2423.
29. Reznikoff, C. A., D. W. Brankow, and C. Heidelberger,
    Establishment and characterization of a cloned line of
    C3H mouse embryo cells sensitive to postconfluence
    inhibition of division, Cancer Res., 33 (1973) 3231-3238.
30. Ritter, M. A., J. E. Cleaver, and C. A. Tobias, High-LET
    radiations induce a large proportion of non-rejoining
    DNA breaks, Nature, 266 (1977) 654-655.
31. Ross, W. E., R. A. G. Ewig, and K. W. Kohn, Differences between
    melphalan and nitrogen mustard in the formation and removal
    of DNA cross-links, Cancer Res., 38 (1978) 1502-1506.
32. Terzaghi, M., and J. B. Little, Repair of potentially lethal
    radiation damage in mammalian cells is associated with
    enhancement of malignant transformation, Nature, 253 (1975)
    548-549.
33. Veatch, W., and S. Okada, Radiation-induced breaks in DNA in
    cultured mammalian cells, Biophys. J., 9 (1969) 330-346.
34. Weichselbaum, R., J. Nove, and J. B. Little, Deficient recovery
    from potentially lethal radiation damage in ataxia
    telangiectasia and xeroderma pigmentosum, Nature, 271
    (1978) 261-262.

35. Yin, L., E. H. I. Chun, and R. J. Ruiman, A comparison of the
         effects of alkylation on the DNA of sensitive and resistant
         lettre-ehrlich cells following in vivo exposure to nitrogen
         mustard, Biochim. Biophys. Acta, 324 (1974) 472-481.

CHAPTER 19

CHROMOSOME ABERRATION FORMATION AND SISTER CHROMATID EXCHANGE IN

RELATION TO DNA REPAIR IN HUMAN CELLS[*]

MASAO S. SASAKI

Radiation Biology Center, Kyoto University
Sakyo-Ku, Kyoto 606, Japan

SUMMARY

Apparent association between the ability to induce chromosome
aberrations and sister chromatid exchanges and mutagenic-carcino-
genic potential found in a variety of physical and chemical agents
has led us to speculate that these cytogenetic changes might be
reflection of DNA damage and repair and might provide indices
of mutagenic changes. However, the mechanisms of their formation
and their relation to DNA repair as well as the mechanism of their
linking to mutation are by no means well understood. Studies in
some human genetic mutant cells defective in their ability to repair
DNA damage indicate, as a testable proposition, that sister
chromatid exchanges and chromsome aberrations are cytological manifestations of replication-mediated dual-step repair pathways that
are in operation to tolerate DNA damage when damage-bearing DNA
enters and passes through semiconservative replication. The observations are also in line with idea that the majority of sister
chromatid exchanges can arise when damage DNA attempts replication
possibly by a process relating with the replicative bypass repair
mechanisms such as those proposed by Fujiwara and Tatsumi [34] and
Higgins et al. [54], while chromosome aberration formation and some
fraction of sister chromatid exchanges are related with the post-
replication repair processes which attempt to rescue damaged
template post-replicationally by de novo synthesis or recombination
type repair systems. The former sister chromatid exchange-relating
process seems to link mutation to less extent, if any, than the
latter process, which is caffeine sensitive and likely to be error-
prone.

INTRODUCTION

Chromosome aberrations and sister chromatid exchanges (SCEs) are two types of cytological changes which can arise in response to a wide variety of agents, including x-ray and UV-irradiation, chemicals, and viruses. Their response to DNA damaging agents suggests that they are reflections of the basic DNA repair processes, and their genesis has been suggested to be intimately related with DNA metabolism, and explained in terms of the operation of repair, replication and recombination systems in lesions induced in chromosomal DNA [3-5, 22, 26, 69, 73, 74]. Recently, evidence has been accumulated in favor of the idea that a mammalian chromosome in the prereplication phase of the cell cycle contains a single array of DNA double helix [72, 77, 133]. This mononeme model applies especially to the study of the molecular mechanism underlying chromosome breakage and rejoining, and the mechanism of chromosome mutation and its relationship to DNA metabolism are subjects that have received wide attention in recent years. However, molecular mechanisms of these chromosomal changes and their relevance to DNA metabolism are poorly understood. One approach to insight into these mechanisms might be an analysis using mutants affecting different aspects of DNA metabolism, such as those relating to chromosome instability, DNA repair processes, hypersensitivity to mutagens, or disturbances in DNA replication and recombination. By this approach, considerable progress has been achieved with several rare human genetic diseases that exhibit defects in DNA repair or chromosome instability or both and cause a predisposition to cancer. Insight into the mechanisms linking chromosome aberration formation, SCE, DNA metabolism, and such pro-cancer class of genes is particularly interesting in elucidating the involvement of these biological processes in other deleterious consequences such as mutation and mutation toward cancer.

CHROMOSOME INSTABILITY IN HUMAN GENETIC DISEASES

Some human genetic diseases have been demonstrated to show an increased level of spontaneous chromosome breakage and/or enhanced susceptibility to chromosome breakage by some mutagens. Among these, several are known to be defective in the repair of damaged DNA. To investigate the interrelation between chromosome aberrations, SCE, and DNA repair, it is of interest to study the situation in these genetic diseases. Table 1 summarizes observations carried out along this line. Genetic diseases categorized into chromosome breakage syndrome [45], such as Bloom syndrome (BS), Fanconi's anemia (FA), ataxia telangiectasia (AT), and incontinentia pigmenti (IP) show abnormally high rate of spontaneous chromosome aberrations [24, 44, 46, 50, 52, 122]. However, only BS cells show an abnormally high level of spontaneous SCEs [10], and the rate of SCEs in FA, AT, and IP is within normal, despite a large number of

TABLE 1

CHROMOSOME INSTABILITY OF PERIPHERAL BLOOD LYMPHOCYTES FROM VARIOUS HUMAN DISEASES[a]

Diseases	Spontaneous		Relative susceptibility to chromosome breakage by:						
	Chromosome aberrations	SCE	γ-Ray	UV	4NQO	DCMMC	MMC	MMS	MNNG
Xeroderma pigmentosum[b]									
Excision defective	0.17 (5)	10.92 (8)	0.9 (1)	16.6 (2)	8.7 (4)	15.6 (2)	0.9 (4)	1 (3)	1.2 (2)
Variant[c]	0.07 (2)	10.50 (2)	1.0 (1)	1.1 (2)	1 (2)	1.2 (2)	1.0 (2)	1.1 (2)	----
XP25JTO	0.12 (1)	12.24 (1)	----	1.2 (1)	1 (1)	1.7 (1)	1 (1)	1 (1)	----
Fanconi's anemia	1.10 (14)	8.24 (4)	1.1 (3)	2.8 (5)	1.1 (4)	2.9 (4)	32.3 (12)	1.1 (7)	1 (2)
Ataxia telangiectasia	0.30 (2)	11.59 (2)	2.2 (2)	----	1.1 (2)	----	1 (2)	1 (2)	----
Werner's syndrome	0.10 (1)	----	0.8 (1)	1 (1)	1.0 (1)	----	0.9 (1)	0.8 (1)	----
Progeria	0.10 (1)	----	1.1 (1)	----	1.1 (1)	----	1.3 (1)	0.9 (1)	----
Incontinentia pigmenti	0.26 (3)	7.88 (1)	----	----	3.2 (2)	----	0.7 (2)	3.7 (2)	----
Dyskeratosis congenita	0.10 (1)	7.60 (1)	1.1 (1)	1 (1)	1 (1)	----	1 (1)	1 (1)	----
Achiasmatic men	0.08 (3)	8.24 (3)	1.1 (3)	0.9 (3)	0.9 (3)	1 (2)	0.8 (3)	1.2 (3)	0.8 (1)
Control	0.06 (8)	8.24 (6)	1	1	1	1	1	1	1

[a]To study the susceptibility to chromosome aberration formation by mutagens, lymphocyte cultures were treated with chemicals for the last 24 hrs. UV irradiation was performed 18 hrs prior to harvest. For γ-ray sensitivity, whole blood was exposed to ^{60}Co γ-rays and chromosome aberrations were scored at 50 hr of total incubation time with the last 20–24 hr treatment with colcemid. Doses used in these experiments were 160, 200, or 300 rad of γ-rays, 75 or 100 ergs/mm^2 of UV, 10^{-6} M 4-nitroquinoline 1-oxide (4NQO), 1 μg/ml decarbamoyl mitomycin C (DCMMC), 0.01 μg/ml mitomycin C (MMC), 1 μg/ml methylmethanesulfonate (MMS), and 1 μg/ml N-methyl-N'-nitro-N-nitrosoguanidine (MNNG). The relative susceptibility was obtained by the ratio of net induced aberrations in patient's cells to the net induced aberrations in normal cells at a given dose of mutagen. Values underlined are significantly abnormal compared with the values in normal cells. Numbers in parentheses are numbers of patients studied.

[b]Patients belonging to complementation group A or those showing unscheduled DNA synthesis less than 5% of normal.

[c]XP4JTO and XP27JTO. Spontaneous chromosome aberrations and SCEs are shown on a per cell basis.

spontaneous chromosome aberrations [10, 38, 126]. Such apparent
dissociation of chromosome aberrations and SCEs readily leads us to
a perennial notion that chromosome aberration formation and SCE are
not simply related. This notion will receive further support from
the observations that x-ray is rather inefficient in inducing SCEs
while it produced a large number of chromosome aberrations [40, 88,
97, 125]; on the contrary UV and chemical mutagens induce a significant amount of SCEs even at doses that induce only a negligible or
low aberration frequency [64, 66, 70, 80, 97, 127].

    Spontaneous chromosome aberrations and SCEs can not be
simply explained by any known DNA repair mechanisms, since spontaneous levels of chromosome aberrations and SCEs are within a normal
range in xeroderma pigmentosum (XP) cells that are known to be
defective in excision repair and XP variant cells that are thought
to be defective in their ability to carry out post-replication
repair [71, 110, 145]. This may be interpreted as an indication
that neither of these repair systems are themselves directly
involved in the formation of spontaneous chromosome aberrations
or SCEs. However, DNA excision repair capacity plays an important
role in the induction of chromosome aberrations when DNA damage is
introduced exogeniously. This is clearly seen in Table 1. XP cells
with defective excision repair capacity show high susceptibility to
chromosome aberration formation only when they are treated with
mutagens that produce DNA damage unexcisable in XP cells. XP cells
have little capacity to repair damage induced by UV [12], 4-nitro-
quinoline 1-oxide (4NQO) [62, 128], and decarbamoyl mitomycin C
(DCMMC) [33, 115] and hence show high susceptibility to chromosome
aberration formation by these agents, but respond normally to x-
or γ-ray, mitomycin C (MMC), methyl methanesulfonate (MMS), and
N-methyl-N'-nitro-N-nitrosoguanidine (MNNG), major damage induced
by these agents being excised even in XP cells [13, 15, 17, 33].

    Cells from patients with FA are highly sensitive to chromosome
aberration formation by MMC and other DNA crosslinking agents [116].
A defect in repair of DNA interstrand crosslinks has been suggested
by a lack of apparent recovery from chromosome aberrations in MMC-
treated FA cells [111, 113] and more directly by an absence of the
operation of the initial half-excision step in the removal of DNA
interstrand crosslinks in FA cells after treatment with MMC [33,
35]. AT cells have been demonstrated to be abnormally sensitive to
chromosome aberration formation and cell killing by x- or γ-rays
[55, 130, 131]. A defect in the repair of x- or γ-ray-induced DNA
damage has been implicated in the AT cells [60, 95, 129, 132]. The
XP variants have clinical XP but normal excision repair capacity
[16, 106]. They have been found to be defective in their ability to
carry out post-replication repair of DNA and hence sensitive to the
caffeine post-treatment potentiation of cell killing by UV [1, 28,
86]. In contrast to the excision-defective XP, the variants are
not abnormally sensitive to the induction of chromosome aberrations

by UV, 4NQO, and DCMMC (Table 1), but recently Hartley-Asp [53]
reported that the XP variant cells were slightly more sensitive to
chromosome breakage by MMC and had higher sensitivity to
caffeine potentiation of MMC-induced chromosome aberrations than
normal cells. These lines of experimental evidence strongly
point to the possibility that the unexcised DNA damage is
responsible for the induction of chromosome aberrations and that
such DNA damage is translated into chromosome structural change as
a result of errors in the DNA replication-mediated, possibly post-
replicational, repair process(es).

The involvement of unexcised .DNA damage in the formation of
chromosome aberrations is more clearly seen in the results shown in
Figs. 1 and 2. In these experiments, lymphocyte cultures were
treated with chemicals for a short period, allowed to grow, and the
frequencies of chromosome aberrations in the subsequent mitoses
were studied as a function of cell cycle position at the time of
treatment [110, 113]. It is evident that, when XP cells were
treated with 4NQO and DCMMC, and FA cells with MMC, reduction of the
chromosome breaking activity was minimal during G_1 phase even
damages were introduced at the cell cycle position away from the
DNA synthesis (S) stage. The results indicate that DNA damages are
translated into chromosome aberrations when they pass through the S
phase and the aberration frequency is related with the amount of
DNA damage that has not been repaired before the damage-bearing
DNA enters semiconservative DNA synthesis.

There is some suggestive evidence for the association between
DNA repair capacity and meiotic recombination in higher eukaryotes.
The altered sensitivity to radiation and chemicals or defective
DNA repair has been associated with the defective meiotic recombination in Drosophila [6, 7, 39, 41, 139], barley [105], and in the human
male [96]. During the course of study on meiotic chromosomes in
subfertile men, we found three patients with azoospermia who had a
gross reduction of chiasma counts in their spermatocyte metaphase I
cells. In the somatic cells from these achiasmatic men, however,
no abnormality was found in the spontaneous level of chromosome
aberrations and SCEs, and susceptibility to chromosome aberration
formation by several mutagens (Table 1) as well as in their excision
repair capacity as measured by unscheduled DNA synthesis after UV
irradiation [117]. These observations may be in accord with the
idea that the genetic control mechanism of the meiotic process is
complex, and some mutations affect both meiotic and somatic cells
while the others are restricted to the meiotic cells [7].

DNA REPAIR AND SCE RESPONSE TO MUTAGENS

The induction of SCEs by UV and chemical mutagens resembles
that of chromosome aberrations in many respects. The induction of

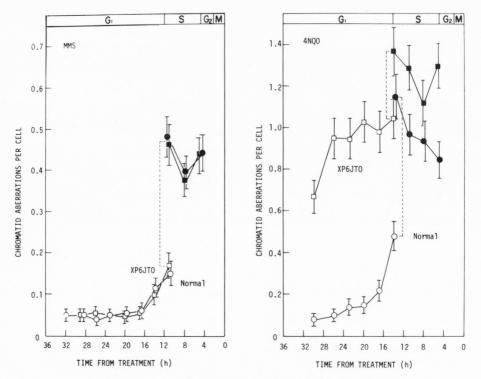

Fig. 1.   Induction of chromosome aberrations in (O, ●) normal
and (□, ■) XP cells by MMS and 4NQO as a function of cell cycle
position at the time of treatment; (●, ■) cells in S phase at
the time of treatment; (O, □) cells in G$_1$ phase at the time of
treatment. Lymphocytes in PHA cultures were treated with chemicals
together with ^{3}H-thymidine for 30 mins at indicated time before
fixation, and chromosome aberrations were scored in labeled (S) and
unlabeled (G$_1$) cells.

SCEs also requires a coincident occurrence of DNA damage and DNA
replication [65, 91, 143], and more precisely, for the SCE to be
formed it is necessary for the damage-bearing DNA to pass through
semiconservative DNA replication before the damage is repaired
[143]. As is the case for chromosome aberration formation, excision-
defective XP cells have been demonstrated to be highly sensitive to
the induction of SCEs by UV [2, 11, 25, 120].

However, when studied in XP cells with different excision
repair capacity, the amount of UV-induced SCEs has not been simply
related with excision repair capacity as measured by UV-stimulated
unscheduled DNA synthesis [11, 25]. For instance, XP complementation group B cells differ in their susceptibility to SCE formation

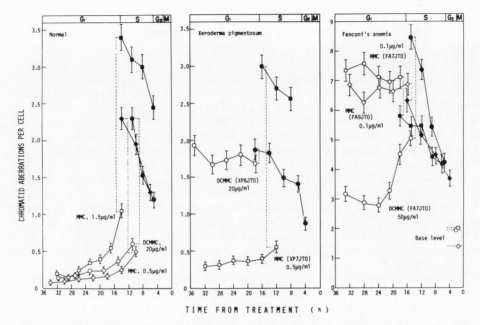

Fig. 2. Changes in the frequency of chromosome aberrations in
normal, XP and FA cells as a function of cell cycle position at the
time of treatment with MMC and DCMMC. Experimental procedures are
the same as those in Fig. 1. XP6JTO and XP7JTO belong to complementation group A. FA7JTO and FA9JTO are characterized by high
susceptibility to chromosome breakage by MMC.

by UV only slightly from that in normal cells in spite of their
very limited rate (3-7% of normal) of unscheduled DNA synthesis,
and furthermore they are less sensitive to the induction of SCE by
UV than XP group C and group D cells which have higher residual
repair activity. The situation in XP cell lines belonging to
group C is paradoxical. Some XP group C cell lines show as high an
SCE rate as repair-defective group A cells in response to UV, while
others are insensitive to the induction of SCE by UV, although they
all have 10-20% of the normal rate of unscheduled DNA synthesis
[11, 25]. Thus, there is considerable complexity in attempting in
a meaningful way to correlate UV-induced SCE with DNA repair
capacity as expressed by unscheduled DNA synthesis.

Recently, Wolff et al. [145] compared the frequencies of SCEs
in normal and XP group A cells after treatment with various chemicals
including 4NQO, MMS, ethyl methanesulfonate (EMS), MNNG, MMC, ethyl
nitrosourea (ENU), and dimethyl sulfate (DMS), and found that, in

contrast to chromosome aberration formation and cell killing, the XP cells were uniformly sensitive to the induction of SCEs by these chemicals whether they were chemicals that could not induce unscheduled DNA synthesis in XP cells (UV-like chemicals), or they were chemicals that induced the normal rate of unscheduled DNA synthesis (x-ray-like chemicals). These observations led the authors to conclude that lesions that gave rise to chromosome aberrations might be different from those leading to SCEs. They postulated that the SCEs were reflecting the unexcised minor fraction of DNA damage, the repair of which was usually unresolvable by unscheduled DNA synthesis, possibly O^6 alkylation of guanine, which was DNA damage unexcisable in XP cells [49]. Since these experiments were based on SV40-transformed cells, the influence of the induction of viruses by mutagens and its consequences in the formation of SCEs [63, 92] cannot be fully excluded. However, more recently, Perry et al. [98] also found a higher incidence of SCEs in XP than normal cells in blood lymphocyte cultures after in vitro exposure to nitrogen mustard (HN2), 4NQO, and even after exposure to the x-ray like-chemical, EMS. In both of these experiments, chemicals were present during a period long enough to cover two cell cycles. We repeated similar experiments using peripheral blood lymphocytes in PHA culture. The cells were grown for 72 hr in the presence of bromodeoxyuridine (BrdU), but in this experiment test chemicals were present only for the last 24 hr, which covered the 2nd S phase in two replication cycles. The frequencies of SCEs are shown in Fig. 3. As seen in this figure, the spectrum of sensitivity to SCE of XP cells differs from those reported by Wolff et al. [145] and Perry et al. [98], but is apparently in parallel with that for the induction of chromosome aberrations; the XP cells responding normally to MMS, EMS, MNNG and MMC while they are highly sensitive to 4NQO and DCMMC in terms of the induction of SCEs. Does this mean that the lesions leading to SCEs are the same as those leading to chromosome aberrations?

Since for the SCE to be formed it is necessary for the DNA damage to pass through DNA replication, and also the efficiency of damage to link to SCE formation may depend on types of damage, the difference between XP and normal cells in the induction of SCE by a given chemical must be closely related with the types and relative amount of each damage as well as their repair types. The excision of DNA damage is a rate-limitimg process. Therefore, the amount of DNA damage yet unrepaired and then linking to SCEs is also dependent on time left for the damage to be repaired before the damage-bearing DNA enters the replication phase. The reaction of chemical to DNA is diverse and various types of DNA damage are produced even with a single chemical, and moreover, the rate of repair differs among different types of damage [20]. XP cells might differ from normal cells in their capacity to repair certain types of DNA damage. If such damage is the fast-repair type and constitutes a major fraction, the difference in the cellular repair capacity can be manifested by

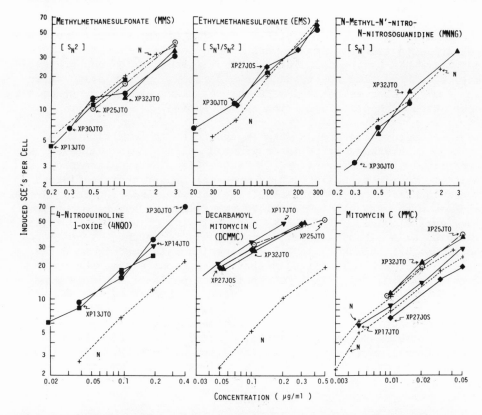

Fig. 3.   Induction of SCEs by chemicals in blood lymphocyte cultures from normal and XP patients.   Peripheral blood lymphocytes in PHA culture were grown for 72 hr in the presence of 40 μM BrdU. The cultures were treated with chemicals for the last 24 hr.   SCEs were scored in chromosome slides prepared according to the FPG method of Perry and Wolff [99].   N: normal cells.   All XP patients except XP25JTO show UDS of less than 5% of normal.   For XP25JTO, see text.

the difference in the number of SCEs even if a limited time is allowed to excise the damage before entering S, as is the case for the treatment for only 24 hr before harvest.   However, if such damage is the slow-repair type and constitutes a minor fraction, the difference in the cellular repair capacity can be reflected by differing SCE rate only when enough time is left before the damage bearing DNA enters S, as is the case for long term treatment. Therefore, these observations might not necessarily dissociate the damage leading to SCE from those leading to chromosome aberrations but rather points to the possibility that the SCEs and chromosome aberrations are the cytological manifestations of the multiple (at least dual) pathways for replication-mediated repair that are operating to tolerate damage when damage-bearing DNA enters semiconservative DNA synthesis. The relative dependency to each process may be related with the types of DNA damage. Such relative dependency might also be related with the cellular regulatory mechanisms associated with differentiation and evolution.

Although there are no data on the relative sensitivity to chromosome breakage by UV in XP group C cells showing different UV sensitivity to SCE formation, it is tempting to correlate such multiple repair pathways with the unusual repair characteristics found in one of our XP patients. The patient, XP25JTO, is a 59-year-old man with very mild clinical XP symptoms. He has no cancer. The level of unscheduled DNA synthesis is 10% of normal, but his cultured skin fibroblasts are considerably resistant to the lethal action of UV. As shown in Table 1, peripheral blood lymphocytes of this patient are only slightly sensitive to chromosome aberration formation by UV and DCMMC. However, this patient is highly sensitive to the induction of SCE by in vitro treatment with a UV-like chemical, DCMMC (Fig. 3). These data may be interpreted as reflecting the genetically determined modification of repair pathways to tolerate unexcised damage. The mild clinical symptoms and high level of cell survival after UV irradiation characteristic of this patient suggest that the SCE pathway links to less extent to the detrimental outcome afforded by exposure to UV than that relating with chromosome aberration formation.

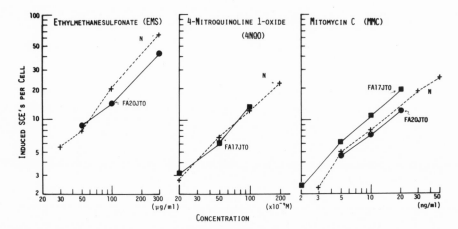

Fig. 4.   Induction of SCEs by chemicals in blood lymphocyte cultures by normal and FA patients. Experimental procedures are the same as in Fig. 3.

Figure 4 shows the induction of SCEs by chemicals in cultured peripheral blood lymphocytes obtained from FA patients. The SCE responses of the FA cells to EMS, 4NQO, and MMC are close to normal. These results are in contrast to those reported by Latt et al. [82], who found a reduced increment of SCE induction by MMC and EMS in FA cells compared with normal cells. They tested the SCE responses in the presence of deoxycytidine, which also augmented the SCE levels in normal cells but only slightly in the FA cells. In another experiment, deoxycytidine was found rather to depress SCE frequency in another genetic mutant, AT cells, as compared with normal cells [37]. However, these observations clearly show that the situation in FA differs from that in XP cells. In FA cells, defective removal of DNA crosslinks induced by MMC does not result in the production of SCE, suggesting that the interstrand DNA crosslink is a type of damage that can not be bypassed or tolerated by the SCE mechanism but can readily link to the formation of chromosome aberrations when crosslink-bearing DNA enters the S phase [113].

AT is another class of genetic disease which has been implicated to be defective in the repair of diverse classes of radiation products [94, 95]. The incidence of SCEs was reported to be normal in AT lymphocytes after treatment with x-rays or chemicals such as MMC, EMS and adriamycin [37]. However, in another AT patient, although based on a single experiment, AT lymphocytes showed a high sensitivity to the induction of SCEs by γ-ray irradiation (Fig. 5). Paterson et al. [94, 95] reported that different AT patients have different rates of loss of endonuclease-sensitive sites in their γ-irradiated DNA. The difference in the SCE response to radiation may be a reflection of such genetic heterogeniety in terms of the ability to carry out excision repair of radiation products.

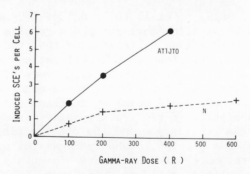

Fig. 5.   Frequencies of γ-ray-induced SCEs in AT and normal lymphocytes. Whole blood was exposed to ^{60}Co γ-rays, and then cultured for 72 hr in the presence of 40 μM BrdU and 3% PHA.

Recent development of new techniques to differentiate sister
chromatids and to detect their exchanges at high resolution [67,
79, 99] greatly stimulated the studies on the mechanisms of SCE and
its relevance to DNA damage with its repair in relation to their
biological consequences [18, 19, 27, 36, 68, 69, 141], and in recent
years, a considerable number of papers has been published on the SCE
responses of mammalian cells to a variety of physical and chemical
agents under a variety of conditions. However, clearly there remain
many unanswered questions about the mechanism and molecular basis
of SCE. Obviously, we are not yet in a position to draw conclusions
on the relationship between SCE, chromosome aberration formation
and any known DNA repair mechanism, yet information available at
present in studies with human genetic mutant cells defective in DNA
repair processes is in line with the idea that the SCEs and
chromosome aberrations reflect the presence of at least two types
of damage-tolerating mechanisms which are in operation when damage-
bearing DNA enters the semiconservative DNA synthesis, both
reflecting the unexcised DNA damage. However, the relative burden
to each process may depend on types of damage and also may be
modified by the cellular regulatory mechanisms to tolerate damage.

SCE AND CHROMOSOME ABERRATIONS AS CYTOLOGICAL MANIFESTATIONS OF DUAL-STEP REPAIR PATHWAY

The basic separateness of induction of SCEs and chromosome
aberrations found spontaneously or in response to mutagens in
human genetic diseases leads to the idea that there might be more
than one major pathway for tolerating unexcised DNA damage. Using the
strand breaks introduced by photolysis of a BrdU-substituted DNA
strand, Kato [68, 69] studied the path of involvement of damage in
SCE formation in relation to DNA replication. In two types
of condition, one in which unifilarly substituted DNA replicates in
the absence of BrdU, to yield one out of four strands BrdU-substituted, and another in which unifilarly substituted DNA replicates
in the presence of BrdU, to yield three out of four strands BrdU-
substituted, the illumination during S phase results in very little
difference in the SCE frequency, indicating that the SCE is
generated at a place very close to the replication fork, However,
when caffeine is present after illumination, more SCEs are formed
in trifilarly substituted chromosomes. These observations led him
to a hypothesis that SCE could arise by at least two different
mechanisms, one operating at replicating points probably utilizing
the machinary of DNA replication and the other acting only in the
post-replicational DNA portion, probably in a similar fashion as
assumed in a general model of crossingover in eukaryotes such as
those proposed by Holliday [56] and Whitehouse [140].

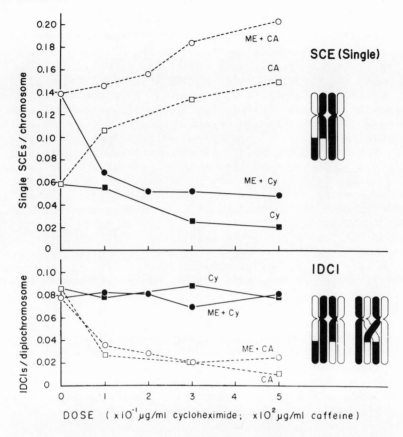

Fig. 6. Effects of caffeine (CA) and cycloheximide (Cy) on the frequencies of SCE and chromatid interchange (IDCI) in diplo-chromosomes. Caffeine and cycloheximide were present for the last 24 hr which covered the second S phase. The experiment was done in the presence or absence of 0.005% β-mercaptoethanol (ME).

Recently, I compared the response of SCEs and chromatid exchanges to caffeine and cycloheximide in diplochromosomes in human cells. Diplochromosomes result from two successive DNA replications without intervening cytokinesis. I found an indication that the process leading to SCE differed from that leading to chromatid exchange aberrations [112]. Cyclo-heximide suppressed SCEs but had no effect on chroma-tid exchange aberrations, whereas caffeine reduced exchange aberrations but rather increased SCE (Fig. 6). The observation strongly points to the possibility that the induction of chromosome aberrations is related with the caffeine sensitive pathways and can be distinguished from the SCE formation. As is generally the case for chromosome aberrations, chromatid exchange aberrations in diplochromosomes, here referred to as IDCIs, seem to reflect unexcised DNA damage, since XP cells are highly sensitive to the induction of such aberrations by treatments with UV, 4NQO and DCMMS, and FA cells are super sensitive to MMC (Fig. 7). However, it should be noted that such exchanges when they occur between sister chromatids in ordinary diploid mitosis, would be manifested as SCEs, but these SCEs constitute the caffeine-sensitive fraction and can be distinguished from cycloheximide-sensitive SCEs. This also suggests the dual nature of the SCE formation. Again assuming that the relative burden to each process is dependent on types of damage and also on the cellular regulatory mechanism to tolerate unexcised damage, such a dual nature of SCE formation provides a reason for the difference in the effect of caffeine on SCEs among mutagens as well as among species [75, 101, 102, 138]. In eukaryotes, caffeine effects on DNA repair processes seem to be complicated [74]. In addition to the pronounced effects on post-replication repair in mammalian [21, 29, 32, 84, 85, 93, 107, 135, 136] and some human cells [86], there are some indications that caffeine also interferes with pre-replicational, possibly excision type, repair in mammalian cells [61, 68, 69], though there are also counterindications [14, 104]. Caffeine inhibits post-replication repair [21, 29, 32, 84-86, 107, 135, 136], which is thought to involve the formation of gaps in the daughter strand during replication on a damaged DNA template and the filling in of these gaps by de novo synthesis [83]. Similar types of lesions are likely to be responsible for chromatid exchange formation and the induction of a caffeine sensitive fraction of SCEs. possibly through a recombinational process.

The mechanism of the effect of cycloheximide on SCEs is not clear, but it is tempting to correlate the reduction of SCEs with the action of cycloheximide with the modification of DNA replication process. Although the action of cycloheximide may be diverse, it has been demonstrated to have an effect on DNA replication [30, 42, 58]. In this regard, it is interesting to find that the SCEs in Bloom syndrome cells can be suppressed by cycloheximide and also by spermidine [114]. The cationic nature of polyamines suggests that they may directly interact with DNA and modify DNA replication [43, 89]. A depressed rate of DNA chain elongation has been demonstrated in Bloom syndrome cells [48, 51] and implicated for the high spontaneous SCE rate in these cells. The retarded rate of DNA chain elongation might expose unwinded DNA for a longer time to increased opportunities for exchange. However, during in vitro senescence of cultured cells [100] and in Werner's syndrome fibroblasts in culture [31], retarded DNA chain elongation has been also found in spite of the absence of an abnormally elevated rate of SCEs [2, 71, 118, 119]. Moreover, treatment with cycloheximide, which reduces SCE, inhibits DNA chain elongation [58]. These observations suggest a strong linking of SCE formation to a process associated

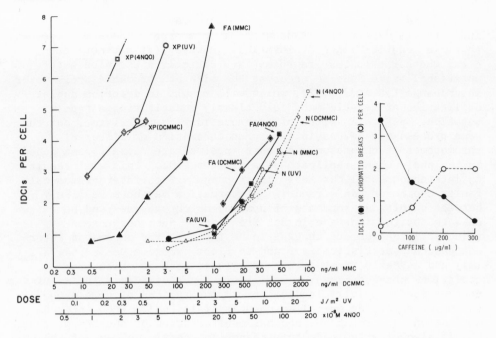

Fig. 7.   Chromatid interchanges in diplochromosomes (IDCIs) in cultured skin fibroblasts.   Cultures were exposed to UV or treated for 30 min with chemicals and allowed to grow for 60-70 hr in the presence of 0.005% β-mercaptoethanol.   Chromatid interchanges were scored in the endoreduplicated mitoses.   The interposed figure shows the effect of caffeine on the MMC-induced chromatid interchanges.   Caffeine was present for the last 24 hr in cultures which were treated and processed otherwise in the same way. Caffeine reduced chromatid interchanges, but instead, increased the chromatid breaks.

with replication itself rather than post-replicational processes. DNA replication involves a multienzyme system, and little is known about its mechanism particularly in eukaryotes;   therefore, we cannot pinpoint the location of the process involved, but it is probable that the cell has an excellent system for bypassing damage when damage-bearing DNA enters replication, and SCE is likely to be a reflection of an error in such a process.

MECHANISMS OF SCE AND CHROMOSOME ABERRATION FORMATION IN RELATION TO MUTATION

The relationship between SCE and mutation has been a subject of repeated discussion.   Since many of the mutagen-carcinogens

induce SCEs at subtoxic doses, SCE might provide a sensitive
indicator in detecting DNA damaging agents or provide a measure of
possible genetic damage or mutation. However, it has not been
clear whether the SCEs are themselves directly associated with
mutations. Some SCEs do occur at the site of chromatid breakage or
interchange [59, 137, 142], which will result in deletion and/or
duplication of genetic material, clearly constituting a type of
mutation. SCE is a switch of a chromatid with its sister, but the
same process may be possible between chromatids of different
chromosomes if chromosome segments involved are closely positioned
in the nucleus and replicate at a similar time. This will result
in interchromosomal chromatid interchange. Such interchromosomal
faulty choice of DNA strand in SCE formation may be more likely
between homologous segments of homologous chromosomes and be
enhanced by the increase in SCE frequency. Such chromosome
structural changes are thought to be the case for chromatid interchanges characteristically found in Bloom syndrome cells [44, 47,
121] and in cells treated with MMC [123], both of which are
conditions characterized by a high frequency of SCEs. These interchanges preferentially involve homologous regions of homologous
chromosomes forming so-called quadriradials [44]. Such interchange
aberration is nothing but another manifestation of the SCE process,
but it also clearly leads to a change in genetic make-up of the cell
through recombination if it involves homologous chromosomes, or
duplication and deletion of genetic material if it involves nonhomo-
logous chromosomes. The induction of SCEs by the tumor promoter,
12-o-tetradecanoylphorbol 13-acetate (TPA), has been implicated for
its tumor promotion by such SCE-related somatic recombination [76].

In these cases at least, the SCEs themselves associate with
mutation, more particularly with chromosome mutation. However, we
have no experimental evidence to show the involvement of any
mutagenic changes in the SCE process itself. But instead, there
are some indications that SCEs might not be directly related with
mutation. In spite of its ability to induce SCE [76, 91], TPA is
not mutagenic in mammalian cells [78, 134]. In XP, susceptibility
of the cells to the induction of SCE by UV is not simply related
with the degree of clinical symptoms. Moreover, XP variant cells
show a high mutation level in response to UV irradiation [87]
while they show normal response to UV in terms of the induction of
SCE [25]. Recently, Carrano et al. [9] compared the SCE rate and
mutation to 8-azaguanine resistance in Chinese hamster ovary
(CHO) cells after treatment with various mutagens, and failed to
correlate the potency of chemicals to induce SCE with their
efficiency to induce mutation in general, although for each chemical
there was an internal linear relationship between SCE and mutation
rate.

At the present state of our knowledge, it is obviously premature
to integrate all available cytogenetic data into a single model to

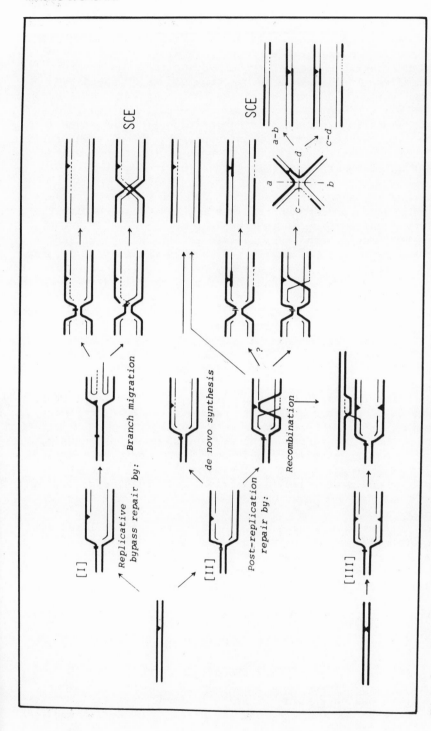

Fig. 8.   Diagram illustrating principal features of the processes possibly leading to SCE and
chromosome aberration when damaged DNA attempts to pass through S phase: (I) replicative bypass
repair and its possible consequence leading to SCE: (II) post-replication repair pathways and
their possible role in the formation of SCE and chromosome changes;   (III) If both strands are
damaged, neither can be used to guide repair replication.   They readily develop into chromatid
aberrations, or repaired or misrepaired if appropriate templates can be found in other chromosomes.

explain SCE and chromosome aberration formation by any known mechanisms of DNA repair and replication. However, assuming rather an error-free nature of the SCE process, it is tempting to correlate the SCE with a faulty choice of strand during ligation after replicative bypass repair through branch migration, as proposed by Fujiwara and Tatsumi [34] and Higgins et al. [54] (Fig. 8). Such replicative bypass repair seems to be error-free, and its process is shown to be caffeine-insensitive in untransformed human cells [34]. Initiation of the exchange may be influenced by the altered stability of a replicating portion of the DNA as well as functional states of replication machenaries such as gyrase, unwinding protein, etc.

As we see it, a possible candidate for the process involved in the formation of chromosome aberrations might be related with the post-replicational portion of the repair pathways. It is known that gaps are formed in the daughter strand during replication on a damaged DNA template [83, 108]. They can be the initial lesions leading to aberrations. These gaps may be either left unrepaired to be transformed into chromatid gaps or breaks, or filled in by de novo synthesis [8, 29, 32, 83] to restore original integrity, or repaired by recombinational processes[108, 109]. The strand exchange between sister chromatids, possibly through a process similar to those proposed for genetic recombination [57,90,103, 124] will also result in SCE (caffeine-sensitive fraction of SCEs), and chromosome aberrations may also arise as a result of incomplete exchange or exchange occurring between chromatids belonging to different chromosomes. Post-replication repair of this kind is thought to be error-prone and the gap filling process has been demonstrated to be caffeine sensitive [84, 85, 107]. Many of the clastogens, particularly those which can induce exchange-type aberrations, have been recognized as mutagens and/or carcinogens. How does the mutation relate with the chromosome aberration formation? The recent finding of Cox and Masson [23] is intriguing in this respect. They found that a significant fraction of radiation-induced mutations to 6-thioguanine resistance in cultured human cells were associated with gross chromosomal changes. This indicates that at least some of the mutational changes reside in chromosome aberration formation itself. As depicted in Fig. 8, a continuing strand transfer during the maturation of Holliday structure can account for the development of regions of heterozygous DNA during recombination [56], which will result in duplication and deletion of the genetic region in the subsequent mitoses when the process involves two chromosomes.

ACKNOWLEDGEMENT

*This work was supported by grants from the Ministry of Education, Science and Culture, and the Ministry of Health and Welfare.

REFERENCES

1. Arlett, C. F., S. A. Harcourt, and B. C. Broughton, The influence of caffeine on cell survival in excision proficient and excision-deficient xeroderma pigmentosum and normal human cell strains following ultraviolet light-irradiation, Mutat. Res., 33 (1975) 341-346.

2. Bartram, C. R., T. Koske-Westphal, and E. Passarge, Chromatid exchange in ataxia telangiectasia, Bloom syndrome, Werner syndrome, and xeroderma pigmentosum, Ann. Hum. Genet., 40 (1976) 79-86.

3. Bender, M. A, J. S. Bedford, and J. B. Mitchell, Mechanisms of chromosomal aberration production. II. Aberrations induced by 5-bromodeoxyuridine and visible light, Mutat. Res., 20 (1973) 403-416.

4. Bender, M. A, H. G. Griggs, and J. S. Bedford, Mechanisms of chromosomal aberration production. III. Chemicals and ionizing radiation, Mutat. Res., 23 (1974) 197-212.

5. Bender, M. A, H. G. Griggs, and P. L. Walker, Mechanisms of chromosomal aberration production. I. Aberration induction by ultraviolet light, Mutat. Res., 20 (1973) 387-402.

6. Boyd, J. B., and R. B. Setlow, Characterization of postreplication repair in mutagen-sensitive strains of Drosophila melanogaster, Genetics, 84 (1976) 507-526.

7. Boyd, J. B., M. D. Golino, and R. B. Setlow, The mei-9[a] mutant of Drosophila melanogaster increases mutagen sensitivity and decreases excision repair, Genetics, 84 (1976) 527-544.

8. Buhl, S. N., R. B. Setlow, and J. D. Regan, Steps in DNA chain elongation and joining after ultra-violet irradiation of human cells, Int. J. Radiat. Biol., 22 (1972) 417-424.

9. Carrano, A. V., L. H. Thompson, P. A. Lindl, and J. L. Minkler, Sister chromatid exchange as an indicator of mutagenesis, Nature, 271 (1978) 551-553.

10. Chaganti, R. S. K., S. Schonberg, and J. German, A manifold increase in sister chromatid exchange in Bloom's syndrome lymphocytes, Proc. Natl. Acad. Sci. (U.S.), 71 (1974) 4508-4512.

11. Cheng, W.-S., R. E. Tarone, A. D. Andrews, J. S. Whang-Peng, and J. H. Robbins, Ultraviolet light-induced sister chromatid exchanges in xeroderma pigmentosum and Cockayne's syndrome lymphocyte cell lines, Cancer Res., 38 (1978) 1601-1609.

12. Cleaver, J. E., Defective repair replication of DNA in xeroderma pigmentosum, Nature, 218 (1968) 652-656.

13. Cleaver, J. E., Xeroderma pigmentosum: A human disease in which an initial stage of DNA repair is defective, Proc. Natl. Acad. Sci. (U.S.), 63 (1969) 428-435.

14. Cleaver, J. E., Repair replication of mammalian cell DNA:
     Effects of compounds that inhibit DNA synthesis or dark
     repair, Radiation Res., 37 (1969) 334-348.
15. Cleaver, J. E., Repair of alkylation damage in ultraviolet-
     sensitive (xeroderma pigmentosum) human cells, Mutat. Res.,
     12 (1971) 53-462.
16. Cleaver, J. E., Xeroderma pigmentosum: Variants with normal
     DNA repair and normal sensitivity to ultraviolet light,
     J. Invest. Dermatol., 58 (1972) 124-128.
17. Cleaver, J. E., DNA repair with purines and pyrimidines in
     radiation- and carcinogen-damaged normal and xeroderma
     pigmentosum human cells, Cancer Res., 33 (1973) 362-369.
18. Cleaver, J. E., DNA repair mechanisms and the generation of
     sister chromatid exchanges in human cell lines from
     xeroderma pigmentosum patients, In: Molecular Human
     Cytogenetics, R. S. Sperkes, D. E. Comings and C. F. Fox
     (Eds.), Academic Press, New York, 1977, pp. 341-354.
19. Cleaver, J. E., Repair replication and sister chromatid
     exchanges as indicators of excisable and nonexcisable
     damage in human (xeroderma pigmentosum) cells, J. Toxicol.
     Environ. Health, 2 (1977) 1377-1394.
20. Cleaver, J. E., DNA repair and its coupling to DNA replication
     in eukaryotic cells, Biochim. Biophys. Acta, 516 (1978)
     489-516.
21. Cleaver, J. E., and G. H. Thomas, Single strand interruptions
     in DNA and the effects of caffeine in Chinese hamster cells
     irradiated with ultraviolet light, Biochem. Biophys. Res.
     Comm., 36 (1969) 203-208.
22. Comings, D. E., What is a chromosome break? In: Chromosomes
     and Cancer, J. German (Ed.), John Wiley & Sons, New York,
     1974, pp. 95-133.
23. Cox, R., and W. K. Masson, Do radiation-induced thioguanine-
     resistant mutants of cultured mammalian cells arise by
     HGPRT gene mutation or X-chromosome rearrangements?
     Nature, 276 (1978) 629-630.
24. De Grouchy, J., J. Bonnette, J. Brussieux, M. Roidot, and
     P. Begin, Cassures chromosomiques dans l'incontinentia
     pigmenti. Etude d'une famille, Ann. Génet., 15 (1972)
     61-65.
25. De Weerd-Kastelein, E. A., W. Keijzer, G. Rainaldi, and
     D. Bootsma, Induction of sister chromatid exchanges in
     xeroderma pigmentosum cells after exposure to ultraviolet
     light, Mutat. Res., 45 (1977) 253-261.
26. Evans, H. J., Effect of ionizing radiation on mammalian
     chromosomes, In: Chromosomes and Cancer, J. German (Ed.),
     John Wiley & Sons, New York, 1974, pp. 191-237.
27. Evans, H. J., Molecular mechanisms in the induction of chromo-
     some aberrations, In: Progress in Genetic Toxicology,
     D. Scott, B. A. Bridges, and F. H. Sobels (Eds.), Elsevier/
     North-Holland Biomedical Press, Amsterdam, 1977, pp. 57-74.

28. Fornace, A. J., Jr., K. W. Kohn, and H. E. Kann, Jr., DNA
    single-strand breaks during repair of UV damage in human
    fibroblasts and abnormalities of repair in xeroderma
    pigmentosum, Proc. Natl. Acad. Sci. (U.S.), 73 (1969)
    39-43.
29. Fujiwara, Y., Characteristics of DNA synthesis following
    ultraviolet light irradiation in mouse L cells: postrepli-
    cation repair, Exptl. Cell Res., 75 (1972) 483-489.
30. Fujiwara, Y., Effects of cycloheximide on regulatory protein
    for initiating mammalian DNA replication at the nuclear
    membrane, Cancer Res., 32 (1972) 2089-2095.
31. Fujiwara, Y., T. Higashikawa, and M. Tatsumi, A retarded rate
    of DNA replication and normal level of DNA repair in
    Werner's syndrome fibroblasts in culture, J. Cell. Physiol.,
    92 (1977) 365-374.
32. Fujiwara, Y., and T. Kondo, Caffeine-sensitive repair of ultra-
    violet light-damaged DNA of mouse L-cells, Biochem. Biophys.
    Res. Comm., 47 (1972) 557-564.
33. Fujiwara, Y., and M. Tatsumi, Repair of mitomycin C damage to
    DNA in mammalian cells and its impairment in Fanconi's
    anemia cells, Biochem. Biophys. Res. Comm., 66 (1975)
    592-598.
34. Fujiwara, Y., and M. Tatsumi, Replicative bypass repair of
    ultraviolet damage to DNA of mammalian cells: Caffeine
    sensitive and caffeine resistant mechanisms, Mutat. Res.,
    37 (1976) 91-110.
35. Fujiwara, Y., M. Tatsumi, and M. S. Sasaki, Crosslink repair
    in human cells and its possible defect in Fanconi's
    anemia cells, J. Mol. Biol., 113 (1977) 635-649.
36. Galloway, S. M., What are sister chromatid exchanges? In: DNA
    Repair Processes, W. W. Nichols and D. G. Murphy (Eds.),
    Stralton Intern. Med. Book Coop., New York, 1977, pp. 191-
    201.
37. Galloway, S. M., Ataxia telangiectasia: the effect of chemical
    mutagens and x-rays on sister chromatid exchanges in blood
    lymphocytes, Mutat. Res., 45 (1977) 343-349.
38. Galloway, S. M., and H. J. Evans, Sister chromatid exchanges
    in human chromosomes from normal individuals and patients
    with ataxia telangiectasia, Cytogenet. Cell Genet., 15
    (1975) 17-29.
39. Gatti, M., Genetic control of chromosome breakage and rejoining
    in Drosophila melanogaster: spontaneous chromosome
    aberrations in x-linked mutants defective in DNA metabolism,
    Proc. Natl. Acad. Sci. (U.S.), 76 (1979) 1377-1381.
40. Gatti, M., S. Pimpinelli, and G. Olivieri, The frequency and
    distribution of isolabeling in Chinese hamster chromosomes
    after exposure to x-rays, Mutat. Res., 23 (1974) 229-238.
41. Gatti, M., C. Tanzarella, and G. Olivieri, Variation with sex
    of irradiation-induced chromosome damage in somatic cells
    of Drosophila melanogaster. Nature, 247 (1974) 151-152.

42. Gautschi, J. R., and R. M. Kern, DNA replication in mammalian
    cells in the presence of cycloheximide, Exptl. Cell Res.,
    80 (1973) 15-26.

43. Geiger, L. E., and D. R. Morris, Polyamine deficiency reduces
    the rate of DNA replication fork movement in Escherichia
    coli, Nature, 272 (1978) 730-732.

44. German, J., Cytogenetical evidence for crossing over in vitro
    in human lymphoid cells, Science, 144 (1964) 298-301.

45. German, J., Chromosomal breakage syndrome. In: Birth Defects
    Original Article Series, Vol. 5, National Foundation-March
    of Dimes, New York, 1969, pp. 117-131.

46. German, J., R. Archibald, and D. Bloom, Chromosomal breakage
    in a rare and probably genetically determined syndrome of
    man, Science, 148 (1965) 506-507.

47. German, J., L. P. Crippa, and D. Bloom, Bloom's syndrome.
    III. Analysis of the chromosome aberration characteristic
    of this disorder, Chromosoma, 48 (1974) 361-366.

48. Gianelli, G., P. F. Benson, S. A. Pawsey, and P. E. Polani,
    Ultraviolet light sensitivity and delayed DNA chain
    maturation in Bloom's syndrome fibroblasts, Nature, 265
    (1977) 466-469.

49. Goth-Goldstein, R., Repair of DNA damaged by alkylating
    carcinogens is defective in xeroderma pigmentosum-derived
    fibroblasts, Nature, 267 (1977) 81-82.

50. Gropp, A., and G. Flatz, Chromosome breakage and blastic
    transformation of lymphocytes in ataxia telangiectasia,
    Humangenetik, 5 (1967) 77-79.

51. Hand, R., and J. German, A retarded rate of DNA chain growth
    in Bloom's syndrome, Proc. Natl. Acad. Sci. (U.S.), 72
    (1975) 758-762.

52. Harnden, D. G., Ataxia telangiectasia syndrome: cytogenetic
    and cancer aspects, In: Chromosomes and Cancer, J. German
    (Ed.), John Wiley & Sons, New York, 1974, pp. 619-636.

53. Hartley-Asp, B., The influence of caffeine on the mitomycin
    C-induced chromosome aberration frequency in normal human
    and xeroderma pigmentosum cells. Mutat. Res., 49 (1978)
    117-126.

54. Higgins, N. P., K. Kato, and B. Strauss, A model for
    replication repair in mammalian cells, J. Mol. Biol., 101
    (1976) 417-425.

55. Higurashi, M., and P. E. Conen, In vitro chromosomal radio-
    sensitivity in "chromosomal breakage syndrome," Cancer,
    32 (1973) 380-383.

56. Holliday, R., A mechanism for gene conversion in fungi, Genet.
    Res., 5 (1964) 282-304.

57. Holloman, W. K., and C. M. Radding, Recombination promoted by
    superhelical DNA and the recA gene of Escherichia coli,
    Proc. Natl. Acad. Sci. (U.S.), 73 (1976) 3910-3914.

58. Hyodo, M., H. Koyama, and T. Ono, Intermediate fragments of
    newly replicated DNA in mammalian cells. II. Effect of
    cycloheximide on DNA chain elongation, Exptl. Cell Res.,
    67 (1971) 461-463.
59. Ikushima, T., Role of sister chromatid exchanges in chromatid
    aberration formation, Nature, 268 (1977) 235-236.
60. Inoue, T., K. Kirano, A. Yokoiyama, T. Kada, and H. Kato, DNA
    repair enzymes in ataxia telangiectasia and Bloom's
    syndrome fibroblasts, Biochim. Biophys. Acta, 479 (1977)
    497-500.
61. Ishii, Y., and M. A Bender, Caffeine inhibition of prereplica-
    tion repair of mitomycin C-induced DNA damage in human
    peripheral lymphocytes, Mutat. Res., 51 (1978) 419-425.
62. Jacobs, A. J., R. L. O'Brien, J. W. Parker, and P. Paolilli,
    Abnormal DNA repair of 4-nitroquinoline-1-oxide-induced
    damage by lymphocytes in xeroderma pigmentosum, Mutat.
    Res., 16 (1972) 420-424.
63. Kaplan, J. C., G. B. Zamansky, P. H. Black, and S. A. Latt,
    Parallel induction of sister chromatid exchanges and
    infectious virus from SV40-transformed cells by alkylating
    agents, Nature, 271 (1978) 662-663.
64. Kato, H., Induction of sister chromatid exchange by ultraviolet
    light and its inhibition by caffeine, Exptl. Cell Res.,
    82 (1973) 383-390.
65. Kato, H., Possible role of DNA synthesis in formation of sister
    chromatid exchanges, Nature, 252 (1974) 739-741.
66. Kato, H., Induction of sister chromatid exchanges by chemical
    mutagens and its possible relevance to DNA repair, Exptl.
    Cell Res., 85 (1974) 239-247.
67. Kato, H., Spontaneous sister chromatid exchanges detected by
    a BUdR-labelling method, Nature, 251 (1974) 70-72.
68. Kato, H., Mechanisms for sister chromatid exchanges and their
    relation to the production of chromosome aberrations,
    Chromosoma, 59 (1977) 179-191.
69. Kato, H., Spontaneous and induced sister chromatid exchanges
    as revealed by the BUdR-labelling method, Int. Rev. Cytol.,
    49 (1977) 55-97.
70. Kato, H., and H. Shimada, Sister chromatid exchanges induced
    by mitomycin C: A new method of detecting DNA damage at
    chromosome level, Mutat. Res., 28 (1975) 459-464.
71. Kato, H., and H. F. Stich, Sister chromatid exchanges in ageing
    and repair-deficient human fibroblasts, Nature, 260 (1976)
    447-448.
72. Kavenoff, R., and B. H. Zimm, Chromosome-sized DNA molecules
    from Drosophila, Chromosoma, 41 (1973) 1-27.
73. Khilman, B. A., Molecular mechanisms of chromosome breakage
    and rejoining, In: Advances in Cell and Molecular Biology,
    Vol. 1, E. J. DuPraw (Ed.), Academic Press, New York, 1971,
    pp. 59-107.

74. Khilman, B. A., Caffeine and Chromosomes, Elsevier, Amsterdam, 1977.

75. Khilman, B. A., and S. Sturelid, Effects of caffeine on the frequency of chromosomal aberrations and sister chromatid exchanges induced by chemical mutagens in root tips of Vicis faba, Hereditas, 88 (1978) 35-43.

76. Kinsella, A. R., and M. Radman, Tumor promoter induced sister chromatid exchanges: relevance to mechanisms of carcino-genesis, Proc. Natl. Acad. Sci. (U.S.), 75 (1978) 6149-6153.

77. Laird, C. D., Chromatid structure: Relationship between DNA content and nucleotide sequence diversity, Chromosoma, 32 (1971) 378-416.

78. Lankas, G. R., Jr., C. S. Baxter, Jr., and R. T. Christian, Effect of tumor promoting agents on mutation frequencies in cultured V79 Chinese hamster cells, Mutat. Res., 45 (1977) 153-156.

79. Latt, S. A., Microfluorimetric detection of deoxyribonucleic acid replication in human metaphase chromosomes, Proc. Natl. Acad. Sci. (U.S.), 70 (1973) 3395-3399.

80. Latt, S. A., Sister chromatid exchanges, indices of human chromosome damage and induction by mitomycin C, Proc. Natl. Acad. Sci. (U.S.), 71 (1974) 3162-3166.

81. Latt, S. A., and K. S. Loveday, Characterization of sister chromatid exchange induction by 8-methoxypsoralen plus near UV light, Cytogenet. Cell Genet., 21 (1978) 184-200.

82. Latt, S. A., G. Stetten, L. A. Juergens, G. R. Buchanan, and P. S. Gerald, Induction by alkylating agents of sister chromatid exchanges and chromatid breaks in Fanconi's anemia, Proc. Natl. Acad. Sci. (U.S.), 72 (1975) 4066-4070.

83. Lehmann, A. R., Postreplication repair of DNA in ultraviolet-irradiated mammalian cells, J. Mol. Biol., 66 (1972) 319-337.

84. Lehmann, A. R., Postreplication repair of DNA in mammalian cells, Life Sci., 15 (1974) 2005-2016.

85. Lehmann, A. R., and S. Kirk-Bell, Effects of caffeine and theophylline on DNA synthesis in unirradiated and UV-irradiated mammalian cells, Mutat. Res., 26 (1974) 73-82.

86. Lehmann, A. R., S. Kirk-Bell, C. F. Arlett, M. C. Paterson, P. H. M. Lohman, E. A. De Weerd-Kastelein, and D. Bootsma, Xeroderma pigmentosum cells with normal levels of excision repair have a defect in DNA synthesis after UV-irradiation, Proc. Natl. Acad. Sci. (U.S.), 72 (1975) 219-223.

87. Maher, V. M., L. M. Ouellette, R. D. Curren, and J. J. McCormick, Frequency of ultraviolet-light induced mutations is higher in xeroderma pigmentosum variant cells than in normal human cells, Nature, 261 (1976) 533-535.

88. Marin, G., and D. M. Prescott, The frequency of sister chromatid exchanges following exposure to varying doses of H^3-thymidine or x-rays, J. Cell Biol., 21 (1964) 159-167.

89. Minyat, E. E., V. I. Ivanov, A. M. Kritzyn, L. E. Minchenkova,
     and A. K. Schyolkina, Spermine and spermidine-induced B̄ to
     Ā transition of DNA in solution, J. Mol. Biol., 128 (1979)
     397-409.

90. Meselson, M. S., and C. M. Radding, A general model for genetic
     recombination, Proc. Natl. Acad. Sci. (U.S.), 72 (1975)
     358-361.

91. Nagasawa, H., and J. B. Little, Effect of tumor promoters,
     protease inhibitors, and repair processes on x-ray-induced
     sister chromatid exchanges in mouse cells, Proc. Natl.
     Acad. Sci. (U.S.), 76 (1979) 1943-1947.

92. Nichols, W. W., C. I. Bradt, L. H. Toji, M. Godley, and M.
     Segawa, Induction of sister chromatid exchanges by trans-
     formation with simian virus 40, Cancer Res., 38 (1978)
     960-964.

93. Nilsson, K., and A. R. Lehmann, The effect of methylated
     oxypurines on the size of newly-synthesized DNA and on the
     production of chromosome aberrations after UV irradiation
     in Chinese hamster cells, Mutat. Res., 30 (1975) 255-266.

94. Paterson, M. C., Ataxia telangiectasia: A model inherited
     disease linking deficient DNA repair with radiosensitivity
     and cancer proneness. In: DNA Repair Mechanisms, P. C.
     Hanawalt, E. C. Friedberg, and C. F. Fox (Eds.), Academic
     Press, New York, 1978, pp. 637-650.

95. Paterson, M. C., B. P. Smith, P. H. M. Lohman, A. K. Anderson,
     and L. Fishman, Defective excision repair of γ-ray-damaged
     DNA in human (ataxia telangiectasia) fibroblasts, Nature,
     260 (1976) 444-447.

96. Pearson, P. L., J. D. Ellis, and H. J. Evans, A gross reduction
     in chiasma formation during meiotic prophase and a
     defective DNA repair mechanism associated with a case of
     human male infertility, Cytogenetics, 9 (1970) 460-467.

97. Perry, P., and H. J. Evans, Cytological detection of mutagen-
     carcinogen exposure by sister chromatid exchange, Nature,
     258 (1975) 121-125.

98. Perry, P., M. Jager, and H. J. Evans, Mutagen-induced sister
     chromatid exchanges in xeroderma pigmentosum and normal
     lymphocytes, In: Mutagen-Induced Chromosome Damage in Man,
     H. J. Evans and D. C. Lloyd (Eds.), Edinburgh University
     Press, Edinburgh, 1978, pp. 201-207.

99. Perry, P., and S. Wolff, New Giemsa method for the differential
     staining of sister chromatids, Nature, 251 (1974) 156-158.

100. Petes, T. D., R. A. Farber, G. M. Tarrent, and R. Holliday,
     Altered rate of DNA replication in ageing human fibroblast
     culture, Nature, 251 (1974) 434-436.

101. Politti, F., and A. Becchetti, Effect of caffeine on sister
     chromatid exchanges and chromosomal aberrations induced by
     mutagens in Chinese hamster cells, Mutat. Res., 45 (1977)
     157-159.

102. Popescu, N. C., S. C. Amsbaugh, and J. A. Dipaolo, The
     relevance of caffeine post-treatment to SCE incidence
     induced in Chinese hamster cells, Mutat. Res., 60 (1979)
     313-320.
103. Potter, H., and D. Dressler, On the mechanism of genetic
     recombination: Electron microscopic observation of
     recombination intermediates, Proc. Natl. Acad. Sci.
     (U.S.), 73 (1976) 3000-3004.
104. Regan, J. D., J. E. Trosko, and W. L. Carrier, Evidence for
     excision of ultraviolet-induced pyrimidine dimers from
     the DNA of human cells in vitro, Biophys. J., 8 (1968)
     319-325.
105. Riley, R., and T. E. Miller, The differential sensitivity of
     desynaptic and normal genotypes of barley to x-rays,
     Mutat. Res., 3 (1966) 355-359.
106. Robbins, J. H., W. R. Lewis, and A. E. Miller, Xeroderma
     pigmentosum epidermal cells with normal UV-induced
     thymine incorporation, J. Invest. Dermatol., 59 (1972)
     5402-5408.
107. Roberts, J. J., and K. N. Ward, Inhibition of post-replication
     repair of alkylated DNA by caffeine in Chinese hamster
     cells but not HeLa cells, Chem.-Biol. Interact., 7 (1973)
     241-264.
108. Rupp, W. D., and P. Howard-Flanders, Discontinuities in the
     DNA synthesis in an excision-defective strain of
     Escherichia coli following ultraviolet irradiation,
     J. Mol. Biol., 31 (1968) 291-304.
109. Rupp, W. D., C. E. Wilde III, D. L. Reno, and P. Howard-
     Flanders, Exchanges between DNA strands in ultraviolet-
     irradiated Escherichia coli, J. Mol. Biol., 61 (1971)
     25-44.
110. Sasaki, M. S., DNA repair capacity and susceptibility to
     chromosome breakage in xeroderma pigmentosum cells,
     Mutat. Res., 20 (1973) 291-293.
111. Sasaki, M. S., Is Fanconi's anaemia defective in a process
     essential to the repair of DNA cross links? Nature,
     257 (1975) 501-503.
112. Sasaki, M. S., Sister chromatid exchange and chromatid
     interchange as possible manifestation of different DNA
     repair processes, Nature, 269 (1977) 623-625.
113. Sasaki, M. S., Fanconi's anemia: A condition possibly
     associated with a defective DNA repair, In: DNA Repair
     Mechanisms, P. C. Hanawalt, E. C. Freidberg, and C. F.
     Fox (Eds.), Academic Press, New York, 1978, pp. 675-684.
114. Sasaki, M. S., unpublished data.
115. Sasaki, M. S., K. Toda, and A. Ozawa, Role of DNA repair in
     the susceptibility to chromosome breakage and cell killing
     in cultured human fibroblasts, In: Biochemistry of
     Cutaneous Epidermal Differentiation, M. Seiji and I. A.
     Bernstein (Eds.), University of Tokyo Press, Tokyo, 1977,
     pp. 167-180.

116. Sasaki, M. S., and A. Tonomura, A high susceptibility of Fanconi's anemia to chromosome breakage by DNA cross-linking agents, Cancer Res., 33 (1973) 1829-1836.
117. Sasaki, M. S., and A. Tonomura, Meiotic recombination and somatic recombination in man (abstr.), Japan. J. Genet., 52 (1977) 472-473.
118. Schneider, E. L., D. Kram, Y. Nakanishi, R. E. Monticone, R. R. Tice, B. A. Gilman, and M. L. Nieder, The effect of aging on sister chromatid exchange, Mech. Ageing Deve., 9 (1979) 303-311.
119. Schneider, E. L., and R. E. Monticone, Aging and sister chromatid exchange. II. The effect of the in vitro passage level of human fetal lung. fibroblasts on baseline and mutagen-induced sister chromatid exchange frequencies, Exptl. Cell Res., 115 (1978) 269-276.
120. Schönwald, A. D., and E. Passarge, U. V. light induced sister chromatid exchange in xeroderma pigmentosum lymphocytes, Hum. Genet., 36 (1977) 213-218.
121. Schroeder, T. M., Sister chromatid exchanges and chromatid interchanges in Bloom's syndrome, Humangenetik, 30 (1975) 317-323.
122. Schroeder, T. M., F. Auschütz, and A. Knopp, Spontane Chromosomen-Aberrationen bei familiärer Panmyelopathie, Humangentik, 1 (1964) 194-196.
123. Shaw, M. W., and M. M. Cohen, Chromosome exchanges in human leukocytes induced by mitomycin C, Genetics, 51 (1965) 181-190.
124. Sigal, N., and B. Albert, Genetic recombination: the nature of a crossed strand-exchange between two homologous DNA molecules, J. Mol. Biol., 71 (1972) 789-793.
125. Solomon, E., and M. Bobrow, Sister chromatid exchanges — A sensitive assay of agents damaging human chromosomes, Mutat. Res., 30 (1975) 273-278.
126. Sperling, K., R.-D. Wegner, H. Riehm, and G. Obe, Frequency and distribution of sister chromatid exchanges in a case of Fanconi's anemia, Humangenetik, 27 (1975) 227-230.
127. Stetka, D. G., and S. Wolff, Sister chromatid exchange as an assay for genetic damage induced by mutagen-carcinogens. II. In vitro test for compounds requiring metabolic activation, Mutat. Res., 41 (1976) 343-350.
128. Stich, H. F., and R. H. C. San, Reduced DNA repair synthesis in xeroderma pigmentosum cells exposed to the oncogenic 4-nitroquinoline 1-oxide and 4-hydroxyaminoquinoline 1-oxide, Mutat. Res., 13 (1971) 279-282.
129. Taylor, A. M. R., Unrepaired DNA strand breaks in irradiated ataxia telangiectasia lymphocytes suggested from cyto-genetic observations, Mutat. Res., 50 (1978) 407-418.

130. Taylor, A. M. R., D. G. Harnden, C. F. Arlett, S. A. Harcourt,
     A. R. Lehmann, S. Stevens, and B. A. Bridges, Ataxia
     telangiectasia: a human mutation with abnormal radiation
     sensitivity, Nature, 258 (1975) 427-429.
131. Taylor, A. M. R., J. A. Metcalfe, J. M. Oxford, and D. G.
     Harnden, Is chromatid-type damage in ataxia telangiectasia
     after irradiation at G_0 a consequence of defective repair?
     Nature, 260 (1976) 441-443.
132. Taylor, A. M. R., C. M. Rosney, and J. B. Campbell, Unusual
     sensitivity of ataxia telangiectasia cells to bleomycin,
     Cancer Res., 39 (1979) 1046-1050.
133. Taylor, J. H., P. S. Woods, and W. L. Hughes, The organization
     and duplication of chromosomes as revealed by autoradio-
     graphic studies using tritium-labeled thymidine, Proc.
     Natl. Acad. Sci. (U.S.), 43 (1957) 122-128.
134. Trosko, J. E., C. Chang, L. P. Yotti, and E. H. Y. Chu, Effect
     of phorbolmyristate acetate on the recovery of spontaneous
     and ultraviolet light-induced 6-thioguanine and ouabain-
     resistant Chinese hamster cells, Cancer Res., 37 (1977)
     188-193.
135. Trosko, J. E., and E. H. Y. Chu, Inhibition of repair of
     UV-damaged DNA by caffeine and mutation induction in
     Chinese hamster cells, Chem.-Biol. Interact., 6 (1973)
     317-332.
136. Trosko, J. E., P. Frank, E. H. Y. Chu, and J. E. Becker,
     Caffeine inhibition of postreplication repair of N-
     acetoxy-2-acetyl-aminofluorene-damaged DNA in Chinese
     hamster cells, Cancer Res., 33 (1973) 2444-2449.
137. Ueda, N., H. Uenaka, T. Akematsu, and T. Sugiyama, Parallel
     distribution of sister chromatid exchanges and chromosome
     aberrations, Nature, 262 (1976) 581-583.
138. Vogel, W., and T. L. Bauknecht, Effects of caffeine on sister
     chromatid exchanges (SCE) after exposure to UV light or
     triaziquone studied with a fluorescence plus Giemsa (FPG)
     technique, Human Genet., 40 (1978) 193-198.
139. Watson, A. W. F., Studies on a recombination-deficient mutant
     of Drosophila. II. Response to x-rays and alkylating
     agents, Mutat. Res., 14 (1972) 299-307.
140. Whitehouse, H. L. K., A theory of crossing-over by means of
     hybrid deoxyribonucleic acid, Nature, 199 (1963) 1034-1040.
141. Wolff, S., Relation between DNA repair, chromosome aberration,
     and sister chromatid exchanges, In: DNA Repair Mechanisms,
     P. C. Hanawalt, E. C. Friedberg, and C. F. Fox (Eds.),
     Academic Press, New York, 1978, pp. 751-760.
142. Wolff, S., and D. J. Bodycote, The induction of chromatid
     deletions in accord with the breakage-and-reunion
     hypothesis, Mutat. Res., 29 (1975) 85-91.

143. Wolff, S., D. J. Bodycote, and R. B. Painter, Sister chromatid
     exchanges induced in Chinese hamster cells by UV
     irradiation of different stages of the cell cycle: the
     necessity for cells to pass through S, Mutat. Res., 25
     (1974) 73-81.
144. Wolff, S., J. Bodycote, G. H. Thomas, and J. E. Cleaver,
     Sister chromatid exchanges in xeroderma pigmentosum cells
     that are defective in DNA excision repair or post-
     replication repair, Genetics, 81 (1975) 349-355.
145. Wolff, S., B. Rodin, and J. E. Cleaver, Sister chromatid
     exchanges induced by mutagenic carcinogens in normal and
     xeroderma pigmentosum cells, Nature, 265 (1977) 347-349.

CHAPTER 20

DNA REPAIR PROCESSES CAN ALTER THE FREQUENCY OF MUTATIONS

INDUCED IN DIPLOID HUMAN CELLS

J. JUSTIN McCORMICK and VERONICA M. MAHER

Department of Microbiology and Department of
Biochemistry, Carcinogenesis Laboratory, Fee Hall,
Michigan State University, East Lansing, Michigan
48824 (U.S.A.)

SUMMARY

The ability of DNA excision-repair processes in diploid human
fibroblasts to eliminate potentially cytotoxic and mutagenic lesions
induced by UV radiation or several chemical carcinogens, including
N-acetoxy-2-acetylaminofluorene or the "anti" 7,8-diol-9,10-epoxide
of benzo(a)pyrene, was investigated. Cells with normal rates of
excision were compared with cells with an intermediate rate of
excision (XP2BE or XP5BE) and cells with an excision rate $\sim$1% that
of normal (XP12BE) for sensitivity to the killing and mutagenic
action of these agents. The normal cells proved resistant to doses
which significantly reduced the survival of the XP cells and increased the frequency of mutations to 8-azaguanine resistance in the
XP cells 5- to 10-fold over background. Cells in confluence were
exposed to cytotoxic and mutagenic doses of these agents and allowed
to carry out excision repair. After various lengths of time they
were replated at lower densities to allow for expression of mutations to 6-thioguanine resistance and/or at cloning densities to
assay survival. Normal cells and XP cells with reduced rates of
excision repair (from complementation groups C or D) exhibited a
gradual increase in survival from an initial level of 15-20% to
80-100% if held in confluence. Recovery from UV irradiation was
complete in less than 24 hours, whereas after treatment with the
chemical agents, repair continued for several days and recovery followed similar kinetics. In contrast, XP12BE cells showed no excision
repair and no increase from an initial survival of 20%, even when
held for 7 days. Normal cells treated with these agents in confluence, but prevented from replicating for 7 days, exhibited background

or near background mutation frequencies, whereas the mutation frequency in XP12BE cells did not change with the time in confluence.

INTRODUCTION

Our studies with diploid human fibroblasts in culture can be summarized briefly by three questions: (1) Are somatic cell mutations causally involved in the carcinogenesis process? (2) Can excision repair processes protect human cells from the potentially mutagenic damage caused by carcinogens? (3) What is the role of DNA replication in causing the mutations in human cells which have been exposed to environmental carcinogens? If somatic cell mutations are causally involved in bringing about the malignant transformation of cells, then persons in the human population who have a genetic predisposition for cancer ought to have a genetic predisposition for mutation induction. The finding of a correlation between these two predispositions would not, of course, prove that the mechanism of carcinogenesis is somatic cell mutagenesis. However, a completely negative correlation would be significant in ruling out the somatic cell mutation hypothesis for the origin of cancer.

Xeroderma pigmentosum patients exhibit a greatly increased incidence of sunlight-induced skin cancer [11]. Cells from the majority of such patients are characterized by reduced rates of excision repair of pyrimidine dimers induced in DNA by UV radiation [1]. A few, designated XP variants, exhibit apparently normal or almost normal rates of excision repair of UV induced damage, but are abnormally slow at replicating UV-irradiated DNA [4]. If somatic cell mutations are causally involved in sunlight-induced cancer, one would expect cells from both classes of XP patients to exhibit a significantly greater sensitivity to the mutagenic action of sunlight than do cells derived from normal individuals. This is so because, even though cells from both kinds of patients exhibit different molecular defects, viz., abnormally slow excision repair or slow "post-replication repair," both classes of patients exhibit the clinical manifestations of the disease, i.e., are highly susceptible to skin cancer on areas of the body exposed to sunlight. To test this prediction, we developed methods for comparing the frequency of mutations induced in XP cells and normal human cells from low doses of UV radiation (254 nm). Although UV radiation below 290 nm does not reach the surface of the earth at sea level, exposure of human cells in culture to 2 hr of midsummer sunlight in midafternoon in Michigan has been shown to result in dimerization of 0.07% of the thymine [12]. Such a level of dimerization is comparable to that which we have induced in our cell cultures by exposing the cells to 15 J/m^2 of 254 nm radiation.

Because the XP cells are deficient in excision repair, they allow us to answer the question: can excision repair processes operating in normal human cells protect the cells from the potentially cytotoxic and mutagenic effect of exposure to UV radiation and/or chemical carcinogens? It is also possible with these diploid human fibroblasts, since they are very sensitive to contact inhibition of growth and will stop replicating upon reaching confluence, but continue to carry out DNA excision repair at the same rate as in the rapidly growing state, to ask the question: what is the role of replication in determining the mutagenic or cytotoxic effect of exposure to chemicals or radiation?

METHODS

Cell Strains, Media, and Exposure to Mutagens

The cell strains, media, and methods of UV irradiating or exposing the cells to chemical carcinogens for our studies have been described previously [5, 7-9].

Cytotoxicity

Cells were plated at cloning densities, allowed to attach, irradiated or treated with chemical carcinogens, and allowed to form colonies. Alternatively, cells were plated at higher densities or allowed to grow to confluence, and then treated and released from the dish by trypsinization and plated at cloning densities.

Mutagenicity

Two methods have been used: the in situ method for selection for resistance to AG and a replating method for selection for resistance to TG. They have been described elsewhere [6-8]. For selection in situ, $1-3 \times 10^6$ cells are plated into dishes, allowed to attach, exposed to carcinogen, and the survivors allowed a 5 to 8 days expression period in which to carry out at least three population doublings before being selected for AG resistance directly in the original dishes. This eliminates possible differences in cell doubling times between the resistant cells and the nonresistant cells in the populations, which would alter the observed mutation frequencies. When combined with the P(0) method of determining the chance of a random mutational event, selection in situ allows an accurate estimation of the mutation frequency per surviving target cell. However, because human cells are capable of strong metabolic cooperation it is necessary to keep the cell density low during selection. For selection by replating, a population of $1-5 \times 10^6$

exponentially growing cells is plated into 150-mm diameter dishes at
a density calculated to give 2.5×10^5 surviving cells/dish (and at
least 10^6 survivors in total), allowed to attach, treated, and
allowed to undergo an expression period of 6 to 9 days (> four population doublings). Alternatively, cells are grown to confluence,
treated 3 or 4 days after reaching confluence, and released immediately or at various times after treatment by plating at cloning
densities to assay survival and at densities adjusted to allow
2.5×10^5 surviving cells/150-mm dish for expression of mutations.
Cells are kept in rapid growth during expression by additional replating as necessary. At the end of the expression period, 1 to
10×10^6 cells are assayed for resistance to TG by replating into
dishes or into bulk cell culture vessels [7].

RESULTS

Evidence That Excision Repair Eliminates
Potentially Cytotoxic Lesions

     Our studies showed that normal cells are much more resistant
than the XP cells to low doses of UV light. For example, at a dose
of $0.6 \ J/m^2$, the XP12BE cells, a strain with less than 0.4% the
normal rate of excision repair of UV-induced DNA damage, show a
survival of 3%. In contrast, XP2BE cells, which have an excision
rate about 25% that of normal, show 20%, and the rapidly-excision
cells exhibit 100% survival. This differential survival was also
found when we compared these strains for their sensitivity to re-
active derivatives of aromatic amides and polycyclic hydrocarbons
[6, 9]. Recent biochemical studies in our laboratory show that the
survival is directly correlated with rate of excision of covalently
bound carcinogen residues from cellular DNA [2, 3].

     These results suggest that the rapid excision of potentially
cytotoxic carcinogen-induced DNA damage by the normal cells is responsible for the lack of cell death in this population as compared
to the XP cells and that the intermediate rate of excision by the
XP2BE cells allows them to excise about half of the potentially
cytotoxic lesions in the time allowed for repair following treatment. If so, then if one were able to lengthen the time allowed for
excision repair (i.e., the period between treatment and the "critical event(s)" responsible for cell death), human cells which
possess at least some excision capacity should be able to eliminate
all or most of the potentially cytotoxic lesions. We tested this
hypothesis by exposing replicate confluent cultures of cells to
cytotoxic levels of radiation and/or chemical carcinogens and then
releasing one set of cells immediately to measure survival, and
maintaining the rest for various periods of time to allow excision
repair to take place in the absence of DNA replication. The results
showed that normal cells, and also XP cells which can carry out

excision repair of DNA damage but at a slower than normal rate,
exhibit a gradual increase in survival from an initial level of 20%
to 40%, 60%, 80%, with time held in the nonreplicating state. In
contrast, no recovery was observed in cultures of XP12BE cells, even
when held confluent for 7 days [7]. For UV radiation, recovery is
complete in slightly less than 24 hr. In cells exposed to chemical
carcinogens, such as N-acetoxy-2-acetylaminofluorene, recovery requires several days [2, 6].

Evidence That Excision Repair Can Eliminate Potentially Mutagenic DNA Damage in Human Cells

When the frequencies of mutations induced in normal and XP
strains by exposure to low doses of UV were compared, we found that
the frequency of induced mutations to TG resistance is highest in
the XP12BE cells which are virtually unable to excise the DNA damage, somewhat lower in the XP cells with an intermediate level of
excision, and lowest in the excision repair-proficient normal cells.
These data suggest that the rate at which cells remove potentially
mutagenic DNA damage determines the frequency at which mutagenic
events are fixed in the population. Again, these results predict
that if one were able to lenghten the time allowed for treated cells
to remove potentially mutagenic damage, they might be able to exhibit
only background levels of mutations.

We tested this prediction for both UV radiation- and N-acetoxy-
2-acetylaminofluorene-induced DNA damage using the system outlined
above. Normal cells and XP12BE cells were exposed to doses adjusted
to kill 40 to 65% of the population and to induce significant increases in the frequency of mutations to TG resistance. After 7
days in confluence, normal fibroblasts exhibited near background
levels of mutations. In contrast, after 7 days in confluence, the
frequency of mutations induced in the excision repair-deficient
XP12BE cells was just as high as that observed in populations released immediately after treatment [2, 6]. These data indicate that
the excision repair capabilities of diploid human fibroblasts act
to decrease or eliminate the potentially harmful consequences of
exposure to low doses of UV radiation as well as chemically induced
DNA damage.

The survival of a treated cell depends upon the rate at which
it can excise DNA damage. Following exposure, there appears to be
a "critical time" in which a cell must manage to remove potentially
cytotoxic and/or mutagenic damage from its DNA. Excision repair
may be considered virtually "error-free," whereas DNA replication
appears to be causally involved in producing the mutagenic effect.
Earlier studies from our laboratory showed that cells from XP variant patients are also significantly more sensitive to the mutagenic
action of ultraviolet light [10]. The fact that both kinds of XP

patients, even though their molecular defects are not the same, show
the same clinical symptoms of the disease and similar sensitivities
to UV-induced mutations strengthens the correlation between mutagenesis and carcinogenesis and suggests that mutations might be involved
in the carcinogenesis process for skin cancer caused by exposure to
sunlight. However, many more studies are required before it will
be possible to determine exactly what kinds of DNA lesions are responsible for both of these processes.

ACKNOWLEDGEMENTS

These investigations were supported by grants CA 21247 and
CA 21253 awarded by the National Cancer Institute, DHEW, and contract
ER-78-S-02-4659 from the Department of Energy. The authors want to
acknowledge the invaluable contribution of B. Konze-Thomas, R. H.
Heflich, J. W. Levinson, L. Yang, D. J. Dorney, R. M. Hazard,
T. Kinney, and A. L. Mendrala to this research.

REFERENCES

1. Cleaver, J. E., Xeroderma pigmentosum: a human disease in which
       an initial stage of DNA repair is defective, Proc. Natl.
       Acad. Sci. (U.S.), 63 (1969) 428-435.
2. Heflich, R. H., R. M. Hazard, L. Lommel, J. D. Scribner, V. M.
       Maher, and J. J. McCormick, A comparison of the DNA binding,
       cytotoxicity, and repair synthesis induced in human
       fibroblasts by reactive derivatives of aromatic amide
       carcinogens, Chem.-Biol. Interact., 29 (1980) 43-56.
3. Heflich, R. H., et al., manuscript submitted.
4. Lehmann, A. R., S. Kirk-Bell, C. F. Arlett, M. C. Paterson,
       P. H. M. Lohmann, E. A. deWeerd-Kastelein, and D. Bootsma,
       Xeroderma pigmentosum cells with normal levels of excision
       repair have a defect in DNA synthesis after UV irradiation,
       Proc. Natl. Acad. Sci. (U.S.), 72 (1975) 219-223.
5. Maher, V. M., N. Birch, J. R. Otto, and J. J. McCormick, Cyto-
       toxicity of carcinogenic aromatic amides in normal and
       xeroderma pigmentosum fibroblasts with different DNA repair
       capabilities, J. Natl. Cancer Inst. 54 (1975) 1287-1294.
6. Maher, V. M., D. J. Dorney, B. Konze-Thomas, A. L. Mendrala,
       and J. J. McCormick, Biological relevance in diploid human
       cells of excision repair of lesions in DNA caused by ultra-
       violet light or N-AcO-AAF, Proc. Am. Assoc. Cancer Res.,
       19 (1978) 70.

7. Maher, V. M., D. J. Dorney, A. L. Mendrala, B. Konze-Thomas,
    and J. J. McCormick, DNA excision repair processes in human
    cells can eliminate the cytotoxic and mutagenic consequences
    of ultraviolet irradiation, Mutat. Res., in press.
8. Maher, V. M., and J. J. McCormick, Comparison of the mutagenic
    effect of ultraviolet radiation and chemicals in normal and
    DNA repair deficient human cells in culture. In: Chemical
    Mutagens, Vol. 6, F. J. deSerres and A. Hollaender, Ed.,
    Plenum Press, New York, 1980, pp. 309-329.
9. Maher, V. M., J. J. McCormick, P. L. Grover, and P. Sims, Effect
    of DNA repair on the cytotoxicity and mutagenicity of poly-
    cyclic hydrocarbon derivatives in normal and xeroderma pig-
    mentosum human fibroblasts, Mutat. Res., 43 (1977) 117-138.
10. Maher, V. M., L. M. Ouellette, R. D. Curren, and J. J.
    McCormick, The frequency of ultraviolet light-induced muta-
    tions is higher in xeroderma pigmentosum variants than in
    normal human cells, Nature, 261 (1976) 326-333.
11. Robbins, J. H., K. H. Kraemer, M. A. Lutzner, B. W. Festoff,
    and H. G. Coon, Xeroderma pigmentosum — an inherited
    disease with sun sensitivity, multiple cutaneous neoplasms,
    and abnormal DNA repair, Ann. Intern Med., 80 (1974) 221-
    248.
12. Trosko, J. E., D. Krause, and M. Isoun, Sunlight-induced pyri-
    midine dimers in human cells in vitro, Nature, 228 (1970)
    358-359.

CHAPTER 21

ULTRAVIOLET LIGHT INDUCTION OF DIPHTHERIA TOXIN-RESISTANT

MUTATIONS IN NORMAL AND DNA REPAIR-DEFICIENT HUMAN AND CHINESE

HAMSTER FIBROBLASTS

JAMES E. TROSKO, ROGER S. SCHULTZ, C. C. CHANG, and
TOM GLOVER

Department of Human Development, College of Human
Medicine, Michigan State University, East Lansing,
Michigan 48824 (U.S.A.)

SUMMARY

The role of unrepaired DNA lesions in the production of mutations is suspected of contributing to the initiation phase of
carcinogenesis. Since the molecular basis of mutagenesis is not
understood in eukaryotic cells, development of new genetic markers
for quantitative in vitro measurement of mutations for mammalian
cells is needed. Furthermore, mammalian cells, genetically deficient
for various DNA repair enzymes, will be needed to study the role of
unrepaired DNA lesions in mutagenesis. The results in this report
relate to preliminary attempts (1) to characterize the diphtheria
toxin resistance marker as a useful quantitative genetic marker in
human cells and (2) to isolate and characterize various DNA repair-
deficient Chinese hamster cells.

INTRODUCTION

On theoretical grounds, we have reason to believe that mutations
in either regulatory or structural genes of somatic cells in eukaryotes would lead to serious biological consequences, including cancer
[45, 82, 83], atherosclerosis [5], and "aging" [74, 84].

Consequently, it will be imperative that basic studies on the
molecular mechanisms of mutagenesis be undertaken. Experimentally,
the data that have been obtained, using a variety of bacterial

mutants, clearly implicate many genes affecting the repair of damaged DNA in the mutation process. Furthermore, the role of DNA damage in eukaryotic cells has been experimentally linked to cell killing [3, 50, 64, 80], mutagenesis in cells of certain cancer-prone human syndromes [28, 49], and transformation [4, 9, 36].

From another perspective, a large amount of data has implicated the role of DNA lesions as substrates for cell killing, mutations, transformation and cancer, when these lesions are not removed by "error-free" mechanisms before the DNA synthetic machinery reaches these lesions in the template DNA. It has been well documented that unrepaired DNA lesions, which enter the S-phase of the cell cycle, are substrates that lead to cytotoxic events [59, 63], mutations [6, 32, 43, 44, 62, 72, 88], in vitro transformed cells [7, 8, 18, 41, 42, 51, 53, 57, 61, 81], and tumors [1, 12, 23-25, 55, 58, 73, 86, 87].

In spite of both theoretical and experimental evidence for the role of mutations caused by unexcised DNA lesions in a various human disease states, very little is known about the molecular details in the mutation-fixation process. Bacterial studies have provided some information consistent with the postulation of constitutive and inducible error-free and error-prone DNA repair enzymes [11]. However, the exact nature of the genetic and molecular control of mutagenesis in bacteria is still not known.

Maher and McCormick [49] and Glover et al. [28] have data which indicate that the excision-repair mechanism in human cells is an error-free process, based on the observation that xeroderma pigmentosum cells (which lack excision repair functions) have higher induced mutation frequencies per unit dose (but similar frequencies per unit survival) than fibroblasts from normal individuals.

D'Ambrosio and Setlow [26], using a split-dose protocol based on bacterial studies [67], observed a cycloheximide-inhibitable enhancement of postreplication repair, which they interpret as evidence for an inducible DNA repair mechanism. Painter [56] has, however, challenged the interpretation of the data by D'Ambrosio and Setlow. Lytle [48], Sarasin and Hanawalt [66], DasGupta and Summers [27], and Jeeves and Rainbow [40] have presented evidence related to UV and chemical carcinogen reactivation of herpes simplex virus, simian virus 40 and adenovirus in monkey kidney or human cells. Other studies, designed to detect an inducible error-prone DNA repair system, have generated data which do not seem to be compatible with the postulation of an inducible error-prone repair system for mammalian cells [13, 21].

Progress in understanding mutagenesis in mammalian cells has lagged behind that of bacterial cells because (a) of the paucity of in vitro quantitative mutation assays for mammalian cells; and

(b) of the availability of known DNA repair-deficient mammalian cells which could be used for mutagenesis studies. The recent development of new in vitro markers for several genetic loci in mammalian cells have been reported [19, 71]. The advantages and limitations of each marker are only now becoming known by the detailed characterization and application of these systems.

The objective of this report is to outline the development of a method to create, isolate and characterize a variety of induced DNA repair-deficient mutants in Chinese hamster V79 cells and to characterize the effect on mutagenesis in DNA repair deficient human and Chinese hamster mutants by using the diphtheria toxin resistance marker. We report here initial progress in achieving these objectives.

SELECTION OF MUTAGEN-SENSITIVE OR PRESUMPTIVE REPAIR-DEFICIENT MUTANTS

The value of the use of mutants defective for one or more steps of the various DNA repair mechanisms has been demonstrated in understanding the mechanisms of mutagenesis in bacteria and yeast [31, 35, 75], as well as for screening purposes [2]. Recently, DNA repair-deficient mutants have been isolated for the purpose of delineating mechanisms of mutagenesis in Drosophila [76]. Although the use of drugs to modulate the repair of DNA damage has been used to study mutagenesis, the pleiotropic effects on the biochemistry and physiology of cells makes it difficult to interpret any observed modification of mutagenesis.

Recently, the use of cells derived from human syndromes known or suspected of having DNA repair deficiencies has given some insight to the role of some DNA repair enzymes in mutagenesis. However, for a variety of reasons (i.e., limited number of types of repair mutations; finite amount of cell material available from human sources; possible alteration of normal repair in viral-transformed human fibroblasts, etc.), techniques will be needed to select a wide variety of different types of DNA repair deficient mutants. Only a limited number of presumptive DNA repair mutants in various mammalian cells have been isolated and partially characterized [39, 47, 65, 70, 79]. However, some of the protocols have been too tedious for routine isolation of mutants; the mutants isolated do not maintain stable phenotypes; or the mutants isolated are not amenable for quantitative mutation assay studies. A variety of different protocols have been reported, including one which utilizes a viral suicide method [70].

We have developed a strategy to select for DNA repair mutants for Chinese hamster V79, primarily because these cells are extremely

adaptable for in vitro mutation studies related to both mechanisms
of mutagenesis and to mutagen screening [77, 78].

The basic procedures of the selection technique includes:
mutation induction by BrdU-black light and ultraviolet light treatments; incorporation of ^{3}H-thymidine in repair-proficient cells at
high temperature (38°C) following UV damage; cold holding (4°C) of
these cells to induce tritium killing; and recovery of repair-deficient mutants which could repair at low temperature (34°C). The
basic rationale behind these steps were: (a) assuming most DNA
mutants would be autosomal recessive and that the BrdU-black light
would induce many deletion-type mutants, survivors of this first
step would be UV-treated to induce point mutations, hopefully
opposite a deletion mutation; (b) survivors of this second mutagen
treatment were then exposed to a moderate dose of UV (10 J/m^2) to
induce sufficient amount of DNA damage to kill cells if they lacked
the ability to repair; (c) high specific activity ^{3}H-thymidine was
added to these UV-irradiated cells. If the cells excised the lesions,
radioactive residues were placed into the DNA. By holding the cells
at 4°C for 10 days, only those that were able to repair would die
of the tritium-induced killing. (d) After cold holding, those cells
that did not repair in the presence of the ^{3}H-thymidine survived
and were placed back at 34°C to recover from the original UV treatment.

This selection procedure allowed us to recover 72 clones of
cells. Each of these clones was isolated and propagated. Preliminary tests were performed on each clone to examine whether they were
either UV-sensitive or whether they lacked unscheduled DNA synthesis
after UV [78]. Approximately a dozen of these clones, when compared
to the parental strain, showed abnormal survival or unscheduled DNA
synthesis levels. On additional detailed testing, two of these
clones [UV^s-40; UV^s-44] were significantly sensitive to both UV and
x-rays (Figs. 1A and 1C), one was UV-resistant [UV^r-23] (Fig. 1A),
and one, which was very deficient in unscheduled DNA synthesis, was
slightly UV-sensitive (Fig. 1B) but not x-ray-sensitive (Fig. 1D).
The two UV-sensitive clones had normal levels of unscheduled DNA
synthesis. The UV-resistant clone appeared to have an enhanced level
of unscheduled DNA synthesis when compared to the control. The
clone, which was slightly UV-sensitive (UV^s-7), was almost completely
deficient in unscheduled DNA synthesis after UV irradiation (Fig.
2A). This observation is not too surprising since excision repair
levels in Chinese hamster is low when compared to human fibroblasts.
Chinese hamster cells appear to have a proficient "by-pass" or post-
replication repair mechanism, on which they depend for survival.
We are only now examining whether the two UV-sensitive clones have
a defect in a step of post-replication repair.

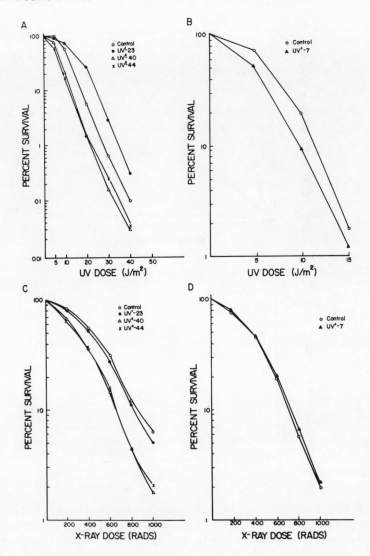

Fig. 1.   Survival curves for several presumptive DNA repair mutant
clones of Chinese hamster (V79) cells. Unpublished data is from
Schultz et al. [78].

A repeat of this selection protocol was performed. Additional
UV-sensitive clones have been isolated. However, no additional
characterization has been performed. Improvement of the selection
procedure can be made by maximizing the "expression time", as well
as by trying to place some of our mutants back through the selection
phases of the protocol (a reconstruction-type of experiment).

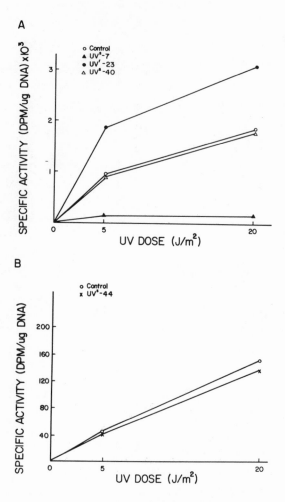

Fig. 2. UV-induced unscheduled DNA synthesis in the parental
and presumptive DNA repair mutant clones of Chinese hamster V79
cells.   Unscheduled DNA synthesis was measured in cells after they
were pretreated with arginine-deficient medium and hydroxyurea.
Cells were irradiated with various doses of UV light and incubated
with ^{3}H-thymidine (5 mCi/ml;   56 Ci/mmole) for 3 hr.   Unpublished
data from Schultz et al. [78].

     A variety of molecular techniques will be performed on these
presumptive DNA repair mutants to characterize the exact nature of
the genetic defect.   Assuming sister-chromatid exchanges (SCE'S)
can be induced by unexcised lesions in DNA [90], each of the clones
will be examined for SCE-induction.   If any, or all, of these prove

to be true DNA repair mutants, they all could be used in a variety of ways (i.e., somatic cell hybrid-complementation studies; screening, etc.), since they all have been shown to exhibit stable phenotypes.

MUTAGENESIS AT THE DIPHTHERIA-TOXIN RESISTANCE LOCUS IN MUTAGEN-SENSITIVE OR PRESUMPTIVE REPAIR-DEFICIENT HUMAN AND CHINESE HAMSTER MUTANTS

Since the original observation that certain strains of bacteria, which were both UV-sensitive and hypermutable because of they were deficient in excision repair enzymes [10, 68, 89], it was assumed that if such a genetic defect occurred in human beings, there would be drastic biological consequences. With the demonstration that cells from the classical type xeroderma pigmentosum were deficient in the ability to repair UV-induced DNA damage [20, 22, 69] when compared to fibroblasts from normal individuals [60], it was hypothesized that the predisposition to sunlight-induced skin carcinomas might be the result of their hypermutability due to a reduced ability to perform error-free repair of DNA damage. Maher et al. [49], using resistance to 8-azaguanine as a genetic marker, demonstrated that fibroblasts of several XP strains, when compared to normal fibroblasts, had increased cytotoxicity and mutation frequencies induced by UV irradiation or a number of chemical carcinogens.

Although one could assume that the hypermutability at the hypoxanthine-guanine phosphoribosyl transferase (HGPRT) locus holds for all other genetic loci in XP cells, we felt that it must and could be experimentally verified. We wished to examine, quantitatively, mutagenesis in DNA repair-deficient human and Chinese hamster cells using a genetic marker which did not have some of the problems associated with the HGPRT system (i.e., cell density or "metabolic cooperation" effects, drug concentration effects, the influence of serum components, and the possibility of epigenetic change resulting in the selected phenotype [52].

Recently, Moehring and Moehring demonstrated that one could isolate Chinese hamster ovary cells after selection with high concentrations of diphtheria toxin which were mutants with altered elongation factor-2 of protein synthesis [54]. Gupta and Siminovitch [29, 30] were able to show that diphtheria toxin-resistant mutants could be induced in normal human and Chinese hamster ovary cells by chemical mutagens. Glover et al. [28] later were able to measure, quantitatively, UV-induced mutations in normal and xeroderma pigmentosum fibroblasts. The detailed protocol for the use of the diphtheria toxin mutation assay for human fibroblasts is reported by Glover et al. [28] and for Chinese hamster lung fibroblasts (V79) by Chang et al. [14]. Having determined empirically the concentration of diphtheria toxin to use, the duration of exposure of the

cells to diphtheria toxin, maximum expression times for human and
Chinese hamster V79 cells, and the potential density effect on the
recovery of mutants, we wanted to examine whether XP cells and the
presumptive DNA repair mutants of Chinese hamster had altered UV-
induced mutation frequencies at the elongation-factor 2 locus.

It should be noted that there are at least two types of diphtheria toxin resistant (DT^r) mutants. One is a permeability variant,
in which uptake of toxin is impaired; the other is a translational
variant with altered EF-2. The translational mutants are cross-
resistant to Pseudomonas exotoxin A which has been shown to ADP-
ribosylate EF-2 in an identical fashion as diphtheria toxin [38],
but which enters the cell through a different mechanism [37]. By
using high concentrations of diphtheria toxin, one selects only for
presumptive EF-2 type mutants. These can then be cloned and cross
checked with Pseudomonas exotoxin A. Permeability-type diphtheria
toxin-resistant cells would be sensitive to Pseudomonas exotoxin A.

The results of an experiment, designed to compare the dose
response of UV-induced DT^r resistant mutants, which were presumptive
EF-2 type, in normal and XP fibroblasts are shown in Figure 3. The
experiments, from which these data were compiled, indicated that
the maximum expression times for the DT^r phenotype were approximately
10 days for normal fibroblasts and 14 days for XP fibroblasts. It
was noted that mutation frequencies at all UV doses for both normal
and XP cells declined after the maximum expression peak was achieved,
indicating a reduced fitness of the DT^r mutants. These results
indicate, within the dose range tested, the DT^r mutation frequency
increased linearly with increasing doses of UV-irradiation. These
results confirm the original observations of Maher and McCormick [49]
that XP cells have higher induced mutation frequencies per unit UV
dose than normal fibroblasts. Moreover, when the mutation frequencies of several of our experiments were plotted as a function of
UV survival (Fig. 4), they are shown to be overlapping and similar
in the normal and XP cell strains. Again, these results are consistent with the hypothesis that excision repair in human cells is
an error-free mechanism. Probably one of the most significant
implications of these results transcends the confirmation of the
somatic mutation hypothesis of carcinogenesis; namely, these results
are consistent with the somatic mutation theory of aging.

The reasoning behind that statement goes as follows. If we
assume that (a) aging is the result of a decrease in homeostatic
capacity of an organism on all levels [33], and (b) "since senescence
does occur in most living organisms, it is supposed that the genetic
program which orchestrates the development of an individual is in-
capable of maintaining it indefinitely" [34], then the accumulation
of lesions in DNA caused by a lack of excision repair should lead
either to induced mutations in daughter cells or to dysfunction of
the integrity of genes in nondividing cells [85]. We now know that

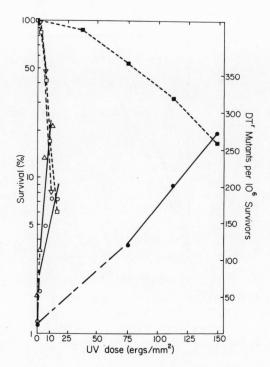

Fig. 3.   Dose-response of UV-induced cytotoxicity ($\square$, $\blacksquare$, $\triangledown$)
(left ordinate) and DT^r mutation frequencies ($\bullet$, $\circ$, $\triangle$) (right
ordinate in ($\blacksquare$, $\bullet$) 73-6NF and ($\square$, $\circ$ experiment 2; $\triangledown$, $\triangle$ experiment 3) XP7BE fibroblasts; (————) through induced mutation fre-
quencies determined by least-squares linear regression analysis.
Data from Glover et al. [28].

individual bacterial cells, which are deficient in excision repair,
are highly predisposed to cell death [70]. Those that do survive
have high mutation frequencies in their genes. In most cases, these
survivors are less able to cope with their environment. Similarly,
xeroderma pigmentosum cells, which lack an error-free excision repair
mechanism, are highly sensitive to cell killing [8, 50]. Those that
do survive have incurred large numbers of mutations, presumably at
any loci [including 6-TG^r, DT^r and the cancer locus(i)]. These
surviving cells in the xeroderma pigmentosum human individual are
associated, not only to skin carcinogenesis, but also to some neurological dysfunctions and to premature aging of the skin [86]. Although it might be argued that if this hypothesis were true, "why
don't organisms treated with chemical carcinogens which damage DNA
cause premature aging of animals?" As in the case of premature
aging of the exposed skin of xeroderma pigmentosum individuals, only

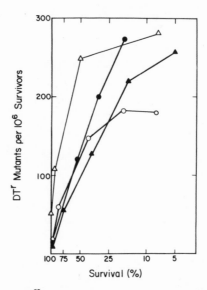

Fig. 4.   UV-induced DT^r mutation frequencies as a function of
cytotoxicity in (▲) 73-6NF fibroblasts, experiment 1; (●)
73-6NF fibroblasts, experiment 2; (o) XP7BE fibroblasts, experiment 2; (Δ) XP7BE fibroblasts, experiment 3.   Data from Glover
et al. [28].

exposed organs (where chemical carcinogens are either metabolized
or concentrated) would exhibit pre-mature aging symptoms.

Together with the original demonstration that higher mutation
frequencies are induced at the 6-TG locus in xeroderma pigmentosum,
these results seem to indicate any and all loci of xeroderma pigmentosum cells are potentially hypermutable due to the lack of an
error-free excision repair enzyme. The biological consequences of
this should be readily apparent. Since xeroderma pigmentosum is
only different in the rate at which it can repair DNA damage compared to normal cells, and since some DNA damage in normal cells can
act as substrates for mutations at any loci, the biological consequences of unrepaired DNA lesions, it seems to us, go beyond just
the induction of carcinogenesis and includes the disruption of the
genetic integrity to maintain homeostatic stability (i.e., senescence).

Preliminary studies on altered mutability in our persumptive
DNA repair deficient mutants have been performed on a couple of our
mutant clones. At this workshop, we wish to present unpublished
results on some of these presumptive DNA deficient mutants since
they seem to exhibit altered mutability [66].

TABLE 1

UV-INDUCED MUTAGENESIS IN THE PARENTAL CHINESE HAMSTER V79 LINE (743X)
AND THE UNSCHEDULED-DNA SYNTHESIS-DEFICIENT LINE (UV7)[a]

Cell line	UV dose (J/m^2)	Survival (%)	Expression time (days)	Mutation frequency/10^6 survivors		
				oua^r[b]	6TG^r	DT^r[c]
743X	0	100	2	8.5	—	—
UV7	0	100	4	2.6	—	—
743X	20	2.0	2.5	1,090	—	—
UV7	20	1.0	5	29,800	—	—
743X	0	100	7	—	13.7	1.6
743X	0	100	14	—	10.5	2.0
UV7	0	100	7	—	35.8	0.0
UV7	0	100	14	—	33.2	0.5
743X	10	17.7	7	—	130.8	41.4
743X	10	17.7	14	—	137.1	15.0
UV7	10	14.2	7	—	686.1	8.7
UV7	10	14.2	14	—	450.8	54.6

[a]Unpublished data from Schultz et al. [78].

[b]Expression time for oua^r permits development of 16 cell colonies before selection.

[c]Expression time for DT^r requires subculturing for indicated period plus development of 16 colonies before selection.

One of these clones, UV-7, which lacks almost all its excision repair as measured by unscheduled DNA synthesis, was examined for UV induced mutability at three different loci: resistance to 6-thioguanine (6-TG^r), resistance to ouabain (oua^r) and resistance to diphtheria toxin (DT^r). The quantitative characterization of the 6-TG^r and oua^r in Chinese hamster V79 has been reported [15]. Pre liminary quantitative characterization of DT^r for Chinese hamster V79 cells has been described [16] and will be reported in detail [14]. This UV-7 clone appears to be hypermutable at all three loci; however, the degree of mutability is vastly different between the loci (Table 1).

If we assume the diminished ability of unscheduled DNA synthesis in UV-7 reflects a true deficiency for excision repair, then these results are consistent with the hypothesis that, although excision repair is a minor repair mechanism in Chinese hamster cells, excision repair is an important mechanism to prevent mutation fixation. Its role in survival, however, seems to be minimal. At this stage, UV-7 appears to be a "xeroderma pigmentosum-like" cell line. As such, it has the potential to be a valuable mutant for screening environmental mutagens. Furthermore, since Chinese hamster V79 cells can be used to detect tumor promoters [91] and anti-tumor promoters [17], there is the possibility to use this mutant strain as a tester for environmental agents which either mutate genes or epigenetically alter cells, as well as to use it to study the mechanism of mutagenesis. Additional characterization with the other presumptive mutants should provide mammalian cell geneticists the tools to study the mutation process in higher organisms and to set the stage for comparative mutagenesis between species.

ACKNOWLEDGEMENTS

This research was supported by grants from the National Cancer Institute to J.E.T. (CA21104) and from the National Institute of Environmental Health Sciences to C.C.C. (Young Environmental Scientist Award, ESO1809).

REFERENCES

1. Albert, R. E., R. J. Burns, L. Bilger, D. Gardner, and W. Troll, Cell loss and proliferation induced by N-2-fluorenylacetemide in the rat liver in relation to hepatoma induction, Cancer Res., 32 (1972) 2172-2177.
2. Ames, B. N., W. E. Durston, E. Yamasaki, and F. D. Lee, Carcinogens are mutagens: A simple test system combining liver homogenates for activation and bacteria for detection, Proc. Natl. Acad. Sci. (U.S.), 70 (1973) 2281-2285.

3. Andrews, A. D., S. F. Barrett, and J. H. Robbins, Xeroderma pigmentosum neurological abnormalities correlate with colony-forming ability after ultraviolet radiation, Proc. Natl. Acad. Sci. (U.S.), 75 (1978) 1984-1988.
4. Barrett, C. J., T. Tsutsui, and P. O. P. Ts'o, Neoplastic transformation induced by a direct perturbation of DNA, Nature, 274 (1978) 229-232.
5. Benditt, E. P., The origin of atherosclerosis, Sci. American, 236 (1977) 74-85.
6. Berman, J. J., C. Tong, and G. M. Williams, Enhancement of mutagenesis during cell replication of cultured liver epithelial cells, Cancer Letters, 4 (1978) 277-283.
7. Bertram, J. S., A. P. Peterson, and C. Heidelberger, Chemical oncogenesis in cultured mouse embryo cells in relation to the cell cycle, In Vitro, 11 (1975) 97-106.
8. Berwald, Y., and L. Sachs, Transformation of normal cells to tumor cells by carcinogenic hydrocarbons, J. Natl. Cancer Inst., 35 (1965) 641-661.
9. Bouck, N., and G. diMayorca, Somatic mutations as the basis for malignant transformation of BHK cells by chemical carcinogens, Nature, 264 (1976) 722-725.
10. Boyce, R., and P. Howard-Flanders, Release of ultraviolet-induced thymine dimers from DNA in E. coli K-12, Proc. Natl. Acad. Sci. (U.S.), 51 (1964) 293-300.
11. Bridges, B. A., The involvement of E. coli DNA polymerase III in constitutive and inducible mutagenic repair, In: DNA Repair Mechanisms, P. Hanawalt, E. C. Friedberg, and C. F. Fox, Eds., Academic Press, New York, 1978, pp. 345-348.
12. Cayama, E., H. Tsuda, D. S. R. Sarma, and E. Farber, Initiation of chemical carcinogenesis requires cell proliferation, Nature, 275 (1978) 60-62.
13. Chang, C. C., S. M. D'Ambrosio, R. Schultz, J. E. Trosko, and R. B. Setlow, Modification of UV-induced mutation frequencies in Chinese hamster cells by dose fractionation, cycloheximide and caffeine treatments, Mutat. Res., 52 (1978) 231-245.
14. Chang, C. C., and J. E. Trosko, Induction and characterization of diphtheria toxin resistance Chinese hamster cells, in preparation.
15. Chang, C. C., J. E. Trosko, and T. Akera, Characterization of ultraviolet light-induced ouabain-resistant mutations in Chinese hamster cells, Mutat. Res., 51 (1978) 85-98.
16. Chang, C. C., J. E. Trosko, and T. W. Glover, Characterization of radiation-induced diphtheria toxin-resistant mutations in Chinese hamster V79 cells, Paper presented at 10th Annual Environmental Mutagen Society, (Abstract), March 8-12, 1979, New Orleans.
17. Chang, C. C., J. E. Trosko, and S. T. Warren, In vitro assay for tumor promoters and anti-promoters, J. Environ. Pathol. Toxicol., 2 (1978) 43-64.

18. Chen, T.T., and C. Heidelberger, Quantitative studies on
    malignant transformation of mouse prostate cells by
    carcinogenic hydrocarbons in vitro, Intern. J. Cancer, 4
    (1969) 166-178.
19. Chu, E. H. Y., and S. S. Powell, Selective systems in somatic
    cell genetics, In: Advances in Human Genetics, Vol. 7,
    H. Harris and K. Kirschhorn, Eds., Plenum Press, New
    York, 1976, pp. 189-258.
20. Cleaver, J. E., A human disease in which on initial stage of
    DNA repair is defective, Proc. Natl. Acad. Sci. (U.S.), 63
    (1969) 428-435.
21. Cleaver, J. E., Absence of interaction between x-rays and UV
    light in inducing ouabain- and thioguanine-resistant mutants
    in Chinese hamster cells, Mutat. Res., 52 (1978) 247-253.
22. Cleaver, J. E., and J. E. Trosko, Absence of excision of
    ultraviolet-induced cyclobutane dimers in xeroderma
    pigmentosum, Photochem. Photobiol., 11 (1970) 547-550.
23. Craddock, V. M., Liver carcinomas induced in rats by single
    administration of dimethylnitrosamine after partial
    hepatectomy, J. Natl. Cancer Inst., 47 (1971) 889-905.
24. Craddock, V. M., and J. V. Frei, Induction of liver cell
    adenomata in the rat by a single treatment with N-methyl-
    N-nitrosourea given at various times after partial
    hepatectomy, Brit. J. Cancer, 30 (1974) 503-511.
25. Craddock, V. M., and J. V. Frei, Induction of tumors in intact
    and partially hepatectomized rats with ethyl methane
    sulphonate, Brit. J. Cancer, 34 (1976) 207-209.
26. D'Ambrosio, S. M., and R. B. Setlow, Enhancement of post-
    replication repair in Chinese hamster cells, Proc. Natl.
    Acad. Sci. (U.S.), 73 (1976) 2396-2400.
27. DasGupta, U. B., and W. C. Summers, Ultraviolet-reactivation
    of herpes simplex virus is mutagenic and inducible in
    mammalian cells, Proc. Natl. Acad. Sci. (U.S.), 75 (1978)
    2378-2381.
28. Glover, T. W., C. C. Chang, J. E. Trosko, and S. S. Li,
    Ultraviolet light-induction of diphtheria toxin resistant-
    mutations in normal and xeroderma pigmentosum human fibro-
    blasts, Proc. Natl. Acad. Sci. (U.S.), 76 (1979) 3982-3986.
29. Gupta, R. S., and L. Siminovitch, Diphtheria toxin-resistant
    mutants of CHO cells affected in protein synthesis: a
    novel phenotype, Somat. Cell Genet., 4 (1978) 553-571.
30. Gupta, R. S., and L. Siminovitch, Isolation and characterization
    of mutants of human diploid fibroblasts resistant to
    diphtheria toxin, Proc. Natl. Acad. Sci. (U.S.), 75 (1978)
    3337-3340.
31. Hanawalt, P. C., P. K. Cooper, A. K. Ganesan, and C. A. Smith,
    DNA repair in bacteria and mammalian cells, Ann. Rev.
    Biochem., 48 (1979) 783-836.

32. Hanawalt, P., Repair models and mechanisms: overview, In: Molecular Mechanisms for Repair of DNA, Part B, P. Hanawalt and R. B. Setlow, Eds., Plenum Press, New York, 1975, pp. 421-430.

33. Hart, R. W., and R. B. Setlow, DNA repair and life-span of mammals, In: Molecular Mechanisms for the Repair of DNA, P. C. Hanawalt and R. B. Setlow, Eds., Plenum Press, New York, 1975, pp. 719-724.

34. Hayflict, L., Current theories of biological aging, Fed. Proc., 34 (1975) 9-13.

35. Haynes, R. H., DNA repair and the genetic control of radio-sensitivity in yeast, In: Molecular Mechanisms for Repair of DNA, Vol. 5B, P. C. Hanawalt, and R. B. Setlow, Eds., Plenum Press, New York, 1975, pp. 529-540.

36. Huberman, E., R. Mager, and L. Sachs, Mutagenesis and transformation of normal cells by chemical carcinogens, Nature, 264 (1976) 360-361.

37. Iglewski, B. H., and D. Kabat, NAD-dependent inhibition of protein synthesis by Pseudomonas aeurginosa toxin, Proc. Natl. Acad. Sci. (U.S.), 72 (1975) 2284-2288.

38. Iglewski, B. H., P. V. Liu, and D. Kabat, Mechanism of action of Pseudomonas aeurginosa exotoxin A: adenosine diphos-phate-ribosylation of mammalian elongation factor 2 in vitro and in vivo, Infect. Immunol., 15 (1977) 138-144.

39. Isomura, K., M. Nikaido, M. Houkaiwa, and T. Suguhara, Repair of DNA damage in ultraviolet-sensitive cells isolated from HeLa S3 cells, Radiat. Res., 53 (1973) 143-152.

40. Jeeves, W. P., and A. J. Rainbow, X-ray-enhanced reactivation of UV-irradiated adenovirus in normal human fibroblasts, Mutat. Res., 60 (1979) 33-41.

41. Kakunaga, T., Requirement for cell replication in the fixation and expression of the transformed state in mouse cells treated with 4-nitroquinoline 1-oxide, Intern. J. Cancer, 14 (1974) 736-742.

42. Kakunaga, T., Caffeine inhibits cell transformation by 4-nitro-quinoline-1-oxide, Nature, 258 (1975) 248-250.

43. Kimball, R. F., The relation between repair of radiation damage and mutation induction, Photochem. Photobiol., 8 (1969) 515-520.

44. Kondo, S., DNA repair and evolutionary considerations, In: Advances in Biophysics, Vol. 7, M. Kotani, Ed., Univ. of Tokyo Press, Tokyo, 1975, pp. 91-162.

45. Knudson, A. G., Jr., Mutations and childhood cancer: A probabilistic model for the incidence of retinoblastoma, Proc. Natl. Acad. Sci. (U.S.), 72 (1975) 5116-5120.

46. Kraemer, K. H., Progressive generative diseases associated with defective DNA repair: xeroderma pigmentosum and ataxia telangiectasia, In: DNA Repair Processes, W. W. Nichols and D. G. Murphy, Eds., Symposia Specialists Inc., Miami, 1977, pp. 37-71.

47. Kuroki, T., and S. Miyashita, Isolation of UV-sensitive clones
    from mouse cell lines by Lederberg Style replica plating
    J. Cell Physiol., 90 (1977) 79–90.
48. Lytle, C. D., and J. Copey, Enhanced survival of ultraviolet-
    irradiated herpes simplex virus in carcinogen-pretreat
    cells, Nature, 272 (1978) 60–62.
49. Maher, V. M., and J. J. McCormick, Effect of DNA repair on the
    cytotoxicity and mutagenicity of UV irradiation and of chem-
    ical carcinogens in normal and xeroderma pigmentosum cells,
    In: Biology of Radiation Carcinogenesis, J.M. Yuhas, R. W.
    Tennant, and J. D. Regan, Eds., Raven Press, New York,
    1976, pp. 129–145.
50. Maher, V. M., L. M. Ouelette, M. Mittlestat, and J. J.
    McCormick, Synergistic effect of caffeine on the cyto-
    toxicity of ultraviolet irradiation and of hydrocarbon
    epoxides in strains of xeroderma pigmentosum, Nature, 258
    (1975) 760–763.
51. Marquart, H., Cell cycle dependence of chemical induced
    malignant transformation in vitro, Cancer Res., 34 (1974)
    1612–1615.
52. Milman, G., E. Lee, G. S. Ghangas, J. R. McLaughlin, and M.
    George, Analysis of HeLa cell hypoxanthine phosphoribosyl-
    transferase mutants and revertants by two-dimensional
    polyacrylamide gel electrophoresis: Evidence for silent
    gene activation, Proc. Natl. Acad. Sci. (U.S.), 73 (1976)
    4589–4593.
53. Milo, G., and J. A. DiPaolo, Neoplastic transformation of human
    diploid cells in vitro after chemical carcinogen treatment,
    Nature, 275 (1978) 130–132.
54. Moehring, T. J., and J. M. Moehring, Selection and characteri-
    zation of cells resistant to diphtheria toxin and
    Pseudomonas exotoxin A: presumptive translational mutants,
    Cell, 11 (1977) 447–454.
55. Nagasawa, H., and R. Yanai, Frequency of mammary cell division
    in relation to age: Its significance in the induction of
    mammary tumors by carcinogens in rats, J. Natl. Cancer Inst.,
    52 (1974) 609–610.
56. Painter, R. B., Does ultraviolet light enhance postreplication
    repair in mammalian cells? Nature, 275 (1978) 243–245.
57. Peterson, A. R., J. S. Bertram, and C. Heidelberger, Cell cycle
    dependency of DNA damage and repair in transformable mouse
    fibroblasts treated with N-methyl-N'-nitro-N-nitrosoguani-
    dine, Cancer Res., 34 (1974) 1600–1607.
58. Pound, A. W., Carcinogenesis and cell proliferation, New
    Zealand Med. J., 67 (1968) 88–95.
59. Rauth, A. M., Evidence for dark-reactivation of ultraviolet
    light damage in mouse L cells, Rad. Res., 31 (1967) 121–
    128.
60. Regan, J. E., J. E. Trosko, and W. L. Carrier, Evidence for
    excision of ultraviolet-induced pyrimidine dimers from the
    DNA of human cells in vitro, Biophys. J., 8 (1968) 319–325.

61. Reznikoff, C. A., J. S. Bertram, D. W. Brankow, and C. Heidelberger, Quantitative and qualitative studies of chemical transformation of cloned C3H mouse embryo cells sensitive to post confluence inhibition of cell division, Cancer Res., 33 (1973) 3231-3238.

62. Riddle, J. C., and A. W. Hsie, An effect of cell-cycle position on ultraviolet-light induced mutagenesis in Chinese hamster ovary cells, Mutat. Res., 52 (1978) 409-420.

63. Roberts, J. J., and K. N. Ward, Inhibition of post-replication repair of alkylated DNA by caffeine in Chinese hamster cells but not HeLa cells, Chem.-Biol. Interact., 7 (1973) 241-264.

64. Roberts, J. J., The repair of DNA modified by cytotoxic, mutagenic and carcinogenic chemicals, In: Advances in Radiation Biology, Vol. 7, J. Lett and H. Adler, Eds., Academic Press, New York, 1978, pp. 211-436.

65. Rosenstein, B., and B. M. Ohlsson-Wilhelm, Isolation of UV-sensitive clones from a haploid frog cell line, Somatic Cell Genet., 5 (1979) 117-128.

66. Sarasin, A. R., and P. C. Hanawalt, Carcinogens enhance survival of UV-irradiated Simian virus 40 in treated monkey kidney cells: Induction of recovery pathway, Proc. Natl. Acad. Sci. (U.S.), 75 (1978) 346-350.

67. Sedgwick, S. G., Inducible error-prone repair in Escherichia coli, Proc. Natl. Acad. Sci. (U.S.), 72 (1975) 2753-2757.

68. Setlow, R. B., and W. L. Carrier, The disappearance of thymine dimers from DNA: An error-correcting mechanism, Proc. Natl. Acad. Sci. (U.S.), 51 (1964) 226-231.

69. Setlow, R. B., J. D. Regan, J. German, and W. L. Carrier, Evidence that xeroderma pigmentosum cells do not perform the first step in the repair of ultraviolet damage to the DNA, Proc. Natl. Acad. Sci. (U.S.), 64 (1969) 1035-1041.

70. Shiomi, T., and Sato, K., Isolation of UV-sensitive variants of human FL cells by a viral suicide method, Somat. Cell Genet., 5 (1979) 193-201.

71. Siminovitch, L., On the nature of hereditable variation in cultured somatic cells, Cell, 7 (1976) 1-11.

72. Simons, J. W. I. M., Development of a liquid holding technique for the study of DNA-repair in human diploid fibroblasts, Mutat. Res., 59 (1979) 273-283.

73. Sinard, A., and R. Daoust, DNA synthesis and neoplastic transformation in rat liver parenchyma, Cancer Res., 26 (1966) 1665-1672.

74. Sinex, F. M., The mutation theory of ageing, In: Theoretical Aspects of Ageing, M. Rickstein, M. L. Sussman, and J. Chesky, Eds., Academic Press, New York, 1974, pp. 23-32.

75. Smith, K. C., D. A. Youngs, E. Von der Schuren, K. M. Carlson, and N. J. Sargentini, Excision repair and mutagenesis are complex processes, In: DNA Repair Mechanisms, P. Hanawalt, E. G. Friedberg, and C. F. Fox, Eds., Academic Press, New York, 1978, pp. 247-250.

76. Smith, P. D., Mutagen sensitivity of <u>Drosophila</u> <u>melanogaster</u>,
    I. Isolation and preliminary characterization of a methyl
    methane-sulfonate-sensitive strain, Mutat. Res., 20 (1973)
    215-220.

77. Schultz, R., C. C. Chang, and J. E. Trosko, The mutation studies
    of mutagen sensitive and DNA repair mutants of Chinese
    hamster fibroblasts, submitted.

78. Schultz, R., J. E. Trosko, and C. C. Chang, Isolation and par-
    tial characterization of mutagen sensitive and DNA repair
    mutants of Chinese hamster fibroblasts, submitted.

79. Stamato, T. D., and C. A. Waldren, Isolation of UV-sensitive
    variants of CHO-KI by nylon cloth replica plating, Somat.
    Cell Genet., 3 (1977) 431-440.

80. Takebe, H., S. Nii, M. I. Ishii, and H. Utsumi, Comparative
    studies of host-cell reactivation, colony forming ability
    and excision repair after UV irradiation of xeroderma
    pigmentosum, normal human and some other mammalian cells,
    Mutat. Res., 25 (1974) 383-390.

81. Terzaghi, M., and J. Little, Repair of potentially lethal
    radiation damage in mammalian cells is associated with
    enhancement of malignant transformation, Nature, 253 (1975)
    548-549.

82. Trosko, J. E., and C. C. Chang, The role of mutagenesis in
    carcinogenesis, In: Photochemical and Photobiological
    Reviews, K. C. Smith, Ed., Plenum Press, New York, 1978,
    pp. 135-162.

83. Trosko, J. E., and C. C. Chang, Chemical carcinogenesis as a
    consequence of alterations in the structure and function
    of DNA, In: Chemical Carcinogens and DNA, P. Grover, Ed.,
    CRC Press, Boca Raton, 1979, pp. 181-200.

84. Trosko, J. E., and R. W. Hart, DNA mutation frequencies in
    mammals, Inter-discipl. Topics Geront., 9 (1976) 168-197.

85. Trosko, J. E., and C. C. Chang, Role of mutations and epigenetic
    changes in carcinogenesis: Correlations between chemical
    and radiation-induced carcinogenesis, In: Advances in
    Radiation Biology, J. T. Lett, Ed., in press.

86. Warwick, G. P., Effect of the cell cycle on carcinogenesis,
    Fed. Proc., 30 (1971) 1760-1765.

87. Williamson, R. C. N., F. L. R. Bauer, J. E. A. Oscarson,
    J. S. Ross, and R. A. Malt, Promotion of azoxymethane-
    induced colonic neoplasia by resection of the proximal
    small bowel, Cancer Res., 38 (1978) 3212-3217.

88. Witkin, E. M., Relationships among repair, mutagenesis and
    survival: overview, In: Molecular Mechanisms for Repair
    of DNA, Part A, P. Hanawalt and R. B. Setlow, Eds., Plenum
    Press, New York, 1975, pp. 347-355.

89. Witkin, E. M., Ultraviolet mutagenesis and inducible DNA repair
    in <u>Escherichia</u> <u>coli</u>, Bacteriol. Rev., 40 (1976) 869-907.

90. Wolff, S., Sister chromatid exchange, In: Annual Review of
        Genetics, Vol. II, H. L. Roman, A. Campbell, and L. M.
        Sandler, Eds., Annual Reviews Inc., Palo Alto, 1977, pp.
        183-202.
91. Yotti, L. P., C. C. Chang, and J. E. Trosko, Elimination of
        metabolic cooperation in Chinese hamster cells by a tumor
        promoter, Science, 206 (1979) 1089-1091.

CHAPTER 22

MUTATION INDUCTION IN A RADIATION-SENSITIVE VARIANT OF

MAMMALIAN CELLS

KOKI SATO

Division of Genetics, National Institute of Radiological
Sciences, 9-1, Anagawa 4, Chiba 260, Japan

SUMMARY

Ultraviolet light (UV)-induced mutations were compared between
a UV-sensitive variant and its parental mouse lymphoma cell line.
The variant was originally isolated for its sensitivity to 4-nitro-
quinoline-1-oxide by employing a replica plating method and proved
to be sensitive to the killing by UV as well. Caffeine potentiation
of UV killing was observed to a similar extent in the variant and
the parental cells, indicating that the caffeine-insensitive process
is responsible for UV sensitivity in the variant. The induced mutation frequency as determined by resistance to 6-thioguanine was
higher in the variant than in the parental cells per unit dose of
UV as well as at the comparable survival level.

It may be of great help for the elucidation of DNA repair
mechanisms to have a variety of repair-deficient mutants. In mammalian cells only those cells are available which have been derived from
hereditary human diseases such as xeroderma pigmentosum (XP),
Fanconi's anemia, Bloom's syndrome, ataxia telangiectasia, and
Cockayne's syndrome [8]. For the purpose of accumulating more
mutants of mammalian cells we have attempted to isolate radiation-
sensitive mutants, since radiation sensitivity is in many cases
related with repair deficiency. Mutants, if isolated, may be used
for studying such problems as excision versus postreplication repair,
constitutive versus inducible repair, error-free versus error-prone
repair, mutagenesis versus carcinogenesis, and the relationship
between the nature of damage and the mode of its repair.

The methods employed for mutant selection are bromouracil photolysis [3], tritium suicide [11], viral suicide [9], and replica
plating [4, 7, 10]. Some of the mutants isolated by these methods
were unstable in their phenotype of radiation sensitivity. This
phenotypic instability raises the question of genetic versus epigenetic mechanisms in mammalian cell mutagenesis. For the moment,
however, mutants with the stable phenotypes are easy to handle, and
we have tried to isolate stable ones.

Mouse lymphoma L5178Y cells were mutagenized by treatment with
N-methyl-N'-nitro-N-nitrosoguanidine and allowed to grow for a period
of expression. These cells were cloned, and individual clones were
examined for the sensitivity to 4-nitroquinoline-1-oxide (4NQO) by
replica plating. Of several thousand colonies tested, one clone
(designated Q31) failed to grow in the presence of 4NQO. Q31 cells
are 2.4 times as sensitive to 4NQO as the parental cells. This
phenotype has been stable for more than a year in culture.

It has been reported that 4NQO is classified as an ultraviolet
light (UV)-like agent on the basis of response of XP cells [1].
Hence, the survivals of Q31 and the parental cells were determined
as a function of UV dose (Fig. 1). The results show that Q31 cells
have little shoulder, a mean lethal dose (D_0) of 0.7 J/m^2, and an
extrapolation number (n) of 1.0, whereas the parental cells have a
wide shoulder, D_0 of 3.0 J/m^2, and n of 1.6. Thus Q31 cells appear
to be defective in repair of the DNA damage caused by 4NQO as well
as UV.

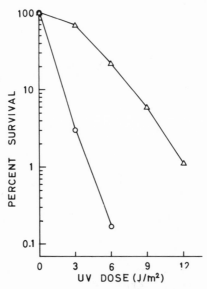

Fig. 1.   Survival curves for (△) L5178Y and (○) Q31 cells after UV
irradiation. Survival was determined by colony-forming ability.

Because response to ionizing radiation might be different from
that to UV, the killing effect of x-ray irradiation was investigated
in Q31 and the parental cells. The results demonstrated no difference in x-ray sensitivity between these two cell lines.

From the above findings it can be concluded that Q31 cells
resemble human XP cells which are deficient in excision repair. The
problem is that mouse cells in culture are reported to be very low
in the ability of removing pyrimidine dimers [2]. Hence Q31 cells
cannot be excision-deficient, since the parental cells are already
devoid of that ability.

Since the postreplication repair was assumed to be in operation
in rodent cells and this repair process was reported to be inhibited
by caffeine, the effect of caffeine on the killing by UV was compared
for Q31 and the parental cells. The results demonstrated that caffeine potentiated the killing effect by UV to almost the same extent
in Q31 cells as in the parental cells. Therefore, the process missing
in Q31 cells, if there is one, appears to be caffeine-insensitive.
In this connection there is a report that caffeine increases the
cytotoxicity of UV irradiation in the XP variant strains, whereas
caffeine exerts no measurable synergistic effect on the classical XP
strains [5].

The mutation frequencies induced with UV were compared between
Q31 and the parental cells. As shown in Fig. 2, higher frequency
of induced mutations is observed with the lower UV doses in Q31 cells.

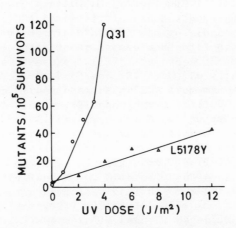

Fig. 2.   Induced mutation frequency in (△) L5178Y and (○) Q31
cells as a function of UV dose. Cells were irradiated with UV
(0.4 J/m^2/sec), allowed expression time of 10 days, and exposed to
6-thioguanine (5 µg/ml).

In order to see the relationship between the frequency of induced
mutations and the lethal effect of UV irradiation, we plotted the
mutation frequency against surviving fraction. In this figure (not
shown) again higher mutation frequencies are evident for Q31 cells
than for the parental cells at comparable cytotoxic UV doses.

These results together indicate that Q31 cells resemble XP
variants in many respects; intermediate UV sensitivity, caffeine
potentiation, and hypermutability [6]. However, they differ from
each other in the point that XP variants possess normal capacity of
excision repair but Q31 cells do not.

It will be interesting to see whether or not the postreplication repair system is operative in Q31 cells. A study along this
line is in progress.

REFERENCES

1. Cleaver, J. E., DNA repair with purines and pyrimidines in
        radiation- and carcinogen-damaged normal and xeroderma
        pigmentosum human cells, Cancer Res., 33 (1973) 362-369.
2. Fox, M., and B. W. Fox, Repair replication after U.V.-irradia-
        tion in rodent cell-lines of different sensitivity, Int. J.
        Radiat. Biol., 23 (1973) 359-376.
3. Isomura, K., O. Nikaido, N. Horikawa, and T. Sugahara, Repair
        of DNA damage in ultraviolet-sensitive cells isolated from
        HeLa S3 cells, Radiat. Res., 53 (1973) 143-152.
4. Kuroki, T., and S. Y. Miyashita, Isolation of UV-sensitive
        clones from mouse cell lines by Lederberg style replica
        plating, J. Cell. Physiol., 90 (1977) 79-90.
5. Maher, V. M., L. M. Ouellette, M. Mittlestat, and J. J.
        McCormick, Synergistic effect of caffeine on the cyto-
        toxicity of ultraviolet irradiation and of hydrocarbon
        epoxides in strains of Xeroderma pigmentosum, Nature, 258
        (1975) 760-763.
6. Maher, V. M., L. M. Ouellette, R. D. Curren, and J. J.
        McCormick, Frequency of ultraviolet light-induced mutations
        is higher in xeroderma pigmentosum variant cells than in
        normal human cells, Nature, 261 (1976) 593-595.
7. Sato, K., and N. Hieda, Isolation of a mammalian cell mutant
        sensitive to 4-nitroquinoline-1-oxide, Int. J. Radiat.
        Biol., 35 (1979) 83-87.
8. Setlow, R. B., Repair deficient human disorders and cancer,
        Nature, 271 (1978) 713-717.
9. Shiomi, T., and K. Sato, Isolation of UV-sensitive variants of
        human FL cells by a viral suicide method, Somat. Cell
        Genet., 5 (1979) 193-201.
10. Stamato, T. D., and C. A. Waldren, Isolation of UV-sensitive
        variants of CHO-K1 by nylon cloth replica plating, Somat.
        Cell Genet., 3 (1977) 431-440.

11. Trosko, J. E., R. S. Schultz, C. C. Chang, and T. Glover,
         Ultraviolét light induction of diphtheria-toxin resistant
         mutations in normal and DNA repair-deficient human and
         Chinese hamster fibroblasts, This volume.

CHAPTER 23

REPAIR OF HUMAN DNA IN MOLECULES THAT REPLICATE OR REMAIN

UNREPLICATED FOLLOWING ULTRAVIOLET IRRADIATION

RAYMOND WATERS

Genetics Department, University College
Singleton Park, Swansea SA2 8PP, U.K.

SUMMARY

The extent of DNA replication, the incidence of UV induced
pyrimidine dimers and the repair replication observed after their
excision was monitored in human fibroblasts UV irradiated with single
or split UV doses. The excision repair processes were measured in
molecules that remained unreplicated or in those that replicated
after the latter UV irradiation.

Less DNA replication was observed after a split as opposed to
single UV irradiation. Furthermore, a split dose did not modify the
excision parameters measured after a single irradiation, regardless
of whether the DNA had replicated or not.

INTRODUCTION

The fact that DNA replication can get past pyrimidine dimers
induced by the ultraviolet irradiation of mouse or Chinese hamster
cells has been unequivocally shown [3-5]. This conclusion is un-
avoidable because, although such cells excise few of these photo-
products after the UV doses employed [4-8], they are able to synthesize a considerable amount of daughter DNA larger than the interdimer
distance seen in parental strands [3-5]. The interpretation of
similar experiments in normal human cells [1] is, however, difficult
and has been the subject of some contention in recent years. Normal
human cells excise a far larger proportion of pyrimidine dimers than
do mouse cells [6, 8] and DNA replication in UV irradiated excision
deficient xeroderma pigmentosum cells is perturbed differently than
in similarly treated normal cells [7, 10]. The latter fact suggests

a close relationship between excision and DNA replication in human
cells. Thus the possibility that DNA replication in UV-irradiated
normal human cells rarely encounters pyrimidine dimers could not be
precluded. Experiments were, therefore, designed to monitor the
extent of DNA replication and the distribution of pyrimidine dimers
in the DNA of UV irradiated human cells at various times after
irradiation. In the light of recent inducible phenomena related to
UV-induced mutation in mammalian cells, the same events were also
measured in cells receiving a single UV dose, or in cells given a
smaller UV dose 24 hr prior to a larger one.

MATERIALS AND METHODS

Cell Culture

Normal human fibroblasts (HSBP) were routinely grown in
Dulbecco's modified medium plus 10% fetal calf serum at 37°C in an
atmosphere containing 5% CO_2. A monolayer of cells were subcultured
at a ratio of 1:3 for radioactive prelabeling. ^{3}H-Thymidine
(specific activity 3 Ci/mmole, 0.03 µCi/ml) or ^{32}P orthophosphate
(0.5 µCi/ml) was added to the medium. Once prelabeled for 24 hr,
cells were plated at 7×10^5 per 150 mm Petri dish and treated 40 hr
later. Density labeling was performed by the addition of 3 µg/ml
bromodeoxyuridine and 0.25 µg/ml fluorodeoxyuridine. For daughter
strand analyses, ^{32}P-prelabeled cells were incubated with ^{3}H-thymi-
dine (specific activity 3 Ci/mmole) at 5 µCi/ml in addition to
density label. Estimations of excision-resynthesis, extraction and
sedimentation of DNA and its subsequent analysis were performed as
previously described.

Experimental Approach

The experimental approach is outlined in Fig. 1.

RESULTS

Figure 2 shows a typical effect of UV irradiation on the amount
of DNA replicated in human fibroblasts. ^{3}H-Thymidine-prelabeled
cells were UV-irradiated and subjected to density labeling for
various times. The amount of DNA replication is determined by the
shift of radioactivity from a light/light to a heavy/light density.
Figure 3 summarizes data obtained by exposing cells to a UV "tickle"
24 hr prior to a larger UV dose. It can be seen that an irradiation
with 2.5 J/m^2 24 hr prior to a second dose of 5 or 10 J/m^2 resulted
in slightly less DNA replication than seen after the latter doses
alone. To investigate the nature of the replicated portions of DNA
in UV irradiated cells, ^{32}P-orthophosphate-prelabeled fibroblasts

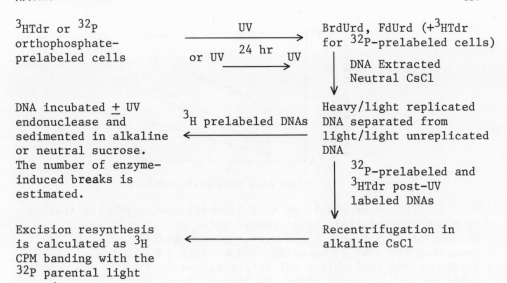

^{3}HTdr or ^{32}P orthophosphate-prelabeled cells	$\xrightarrow[\text{or UV}]{\text{UV}}$ $\xrightarrow[\text{UV}]{\text{24 hr}}$	BrdUrd, FdUrd ($+^3$HTdr for ^{32}P-prelabeled cells)

DNA incubated ± UV
endonuclease and
sedimented in alkaline
or neutral sucrose.
The number of enzyme-
induced breaks is
estimated.

^{3}H prelabeled DNAs

DNA Extracted
Neutral CsCl

Heavy/light replicated
DNA separated from
light/light unreplicated
DNA

^{32}P-prelabeled and
^{3}HTdr post-UV
labeled DNAs

Excision resynthesis
is calculated as ^{3}H
CPM banding with the
^{32}P parental light
strand

Recentrifugation in
alkaline CsCl

Fig. 1.   Experimental approach.

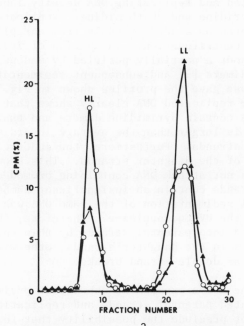

Fig. 2.   Isopynic sedimentation of ^{3}H-prelabeled human DNA (▲)
density-labeled after UV irradiation or (O) remaining unirradiated
HL and LL refer to DNA banding at heavy/light and light/light
densities of 1.695 and 1.745 g/cm^2, respectively.

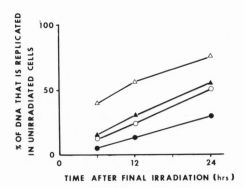

Fig. 3. Effect of single or dual irradiations on DNA replication
in human fibroblasts: open symbols refer to cells receiving a single
UV dose of ($\triangle$) 5 or ($\circ$) 10 J/m^2; closed symbols refer to cells
receiving 2.5 J/m^2 24 hr prior to ($\blacktriangle$) 5 or ($\bullet$) 10 J/m^2. The
extent of DNA replication was determined as in Fig. 2, and density
labeling was performed after the last UV dose.

were UV-irradiated and replicating DNA density labeled for 24 hr
with bromodeoxyuridine and ^{3}H-thymidine. Replicated DNA molecules
were then separated on a density basis from unreplicated ones by
cesium chloride centrifugation. Incubation of isolated replicated
DNA with or without a partially purified UV endonuclease specific
for pyrimidine dimers [9] and subsequent sedimentation in alkaline
or neutral sucrose gave the profiles shown in Fig. 4. Alkaline sedimentation of the replicated DNA clearly shows that the ^{32}P-labeled
parental strands contain pyrimidine dimers and that the ^{3}H-labeled
daughter strand is larger than the average interdimer distance seen
in the parental strands. Furthermore, the endonuclease does not
reduce the size of the daughter strands. This shows that the enzyme
preparation does not attack DNA containing bromodeoxyuridine and that
the daughter strands contain an insignificant number of pyrimidine
dimers. Neutral sedimentation of the same DNA was not modified by
incubation with the UV endonuclease. Therefore, the single-strand
breaks introduced into parental strands by this enzyme (Fig. 3) are
not opposite gaps in the daughter strands, otherwise they would have
been manifested as double-strand breaks.

Although the above experiment shows that pyrimidine dimers do
occur in replicated parental strands and replication can get past
them, it does not preclude the possibility that fewer dimers remain
in replicated as opposed to unreplicated DNA. The incidence of
dimers in both replicated and unreplicated strands has to be compared
directly in order to resolve this question. In addition to measuring
these parameters it was also decided to monitor the extent of excision

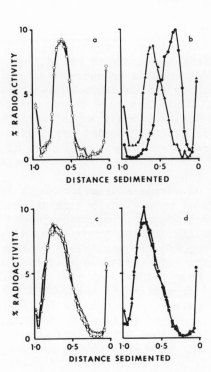

Fig. 4. Effect of UV endonuclease on the sucrose sedimentation of DNA replicated after the UV irradiation of human fibroblasts: (o , ●) ^{32}P parental strands and (△, ▲) ^{3}H-labeled daughter strands were obtained as described in text. The solid symbols in (b) and (d) denote DNA that was incubated with UV endonuclease prior to sedimentation. Upper frames (a) and (b) refer to sedimentation in 5–20% alkaline sucrose, and the lower frames (c) and (d) to sedimentation in 5–20% neutral sucrose.

resynthesis following the removal of pyrimidine dimers from the same DNAs. The experimental approach was as in Fig. 1 and the results are shown in Table 1. The frequencies of pyrimidine dimers found in parental replicated strands as opposed to unreplicated strands are the same from 6 to 24 hr after UV irradiation and immediate density labeling, regardless as to whether the cells received a smaller UV "tickle" one day prior to a second larger dose. The data for excision resynthesis after pyrimidine dimer repair generally substantiate this fact, in that the extent of repair observed is similar regardless of whether the DNA has replicated or not. However, an exception does occur when a UV "tickle" is given; it appears to reduce the amount of excision-resynthesis associated with replicated molecules by about 30%.

TABLE 1

PYRIMIDINE DIMER REMOVAL AND EXCISION RESYNTHESIS OF REPLICATED AND UNREPLICATED DNA[a]

Treatment[b]	Type of DNA	% of DNA that is replicated in unirradiated cells	Dimers/10^8 daltons	% Dimers repaired	$^3H/^{32}P$[c]
5 J/m²; 6 hr BU	LL	–	10 ± 1	33	–
5 J/m²; 6 hr BU	HL	20 ± 7	9 ± 1	40	–
5 J/m²; 12 hr BU	LL	–	7 ± 2	53	1.35
5 J/m²; 12 hr BU	HL	56 ± 2	8 ± 1	47	1.48
5 J/m²; 24 hr BU	LL	–	5 ± 1	67	1.98
5 J/m²; 24 hr BU	HL	76 ± 15	4 ± 1	73	2.11
10 J/m²; 12 hr BU	LL	–	14 ± 1	51	2.46
10 J/m²; 12 hr BU	HL	24 ± 6	12 ± 2	59	2.62
10 J/m²; 24 hr BU	LL	–	10 ± 1	67	3.48
10 J/m²; 24 hr BU	HL	50 ± 5	9 ± 2	68	3.37
2.5 J/m² 24 hr 5 J/m²; 24 hr BU	LL	–	4 ± 1	73	2.32
2.5 J/m² 24 hr 5 J/m²; 24 hr BU	HL	30 ± 8	5 ± 1	67	1.68
2.5 J/m² 24 hr 10 J/m²; 24 hr BU	LL	–	8 ± 1	71	3.63
2.5 J/m² 24 hr 10 J/m²; 24 hr BU	HL	16 ± 10	7 ± 2	76	2.68

[a] ^{3}HTdr-prelabeled cells were treated as described in text.

[b] x hr BU refers to the length of post-UV incubation in bromodeoxyuridine-containing medium. Dimers were induced at a rate $3.0/10^8$ daltons/J/m².

[c] $^3H/^{32}P$ denotes the degree of excision resynthesis associated with light DNA strands.

DISCUSSION

The data presented here clearly indicate that DNA replication can get past pyrimidine dimers induced in the DNA of normal human fibroblasts. As the same number of dimers is found in replicated parental strands as opposed to unreplicated ones at times of 6 to 24 hr after irradiation, and excision mechanism operating preferentially on DNA that is (or is about to be) replicated does not operate to any visible extent.

The inability to isolate sufficient replicated molecules at times prior to 6 hr renders it impossible to determine whether the same is true for earlier times after irradiation. However, if a preferential repair of replicating molecules does occur at such early times, it will not operate on a large proportion of the DNA and could not be considered a major means employed by human fibroblasts to deal with the UV damage induced in replicating molecules. The application of a small UV dose 24 hr before a larger dose and density labeling did not greatly influence any of the parameters measured, except that a 30% reduction in the amount of excision-resynthesis occurs only in the replicated DNA isolated from cells receiving the UV "tickle." As the UV "tickle" did not significantly influence the number of dimers remaining in parental replicated DNA versus unreplicated DNA, the significance of the reduction in excision-resynthesis remains to be determined.

ACKNOWLEDGEMENTS

R. Waters would like to thank J. D. Regan for the cell line used in these experiments, W. L. Carrier for the UV endonuclease, and Mrs. J. Meredith for her expert technical assistance.

REFERENCES

1. Buhl, S. N., R. B. Setlow, and J. D. Regan, Steps in DNA chain elongation and joining after ultraviolet irradiation of human cells, Int. J. Radiat. Biol., 22 (1972) 417-424.
2. Carrier, W. L., and R. B. Setlow, Endonuclease from <u>Micrococcus</u> <u>luteus</u> which has activity toward ultraviolet-irradiated deoxyribonucleic acid: purification and properties, J. Bacteriol., 102 (1970) 178-186.
3. Lehmann, A. R., Postreplication repair of DNA in ultraviolet-irradiated mammalian cells, J. Mol. Biol., 66 (1972) 319-337.
4. Meyn, R. E., D. L. Vizard, R. R. Hewitt, and R. M. Humphrey, The fate of pyrimidine dimers in the DNA of ultraviolet-irradiated Chinese hamster cells, Photochem. Photobiol., 20 (1974) 221-226.

5. Meyn, R. E., R. R. Hewitt, L. F. Thomson, and R. M. Humphrey,
    Effects of ultraviolet irradiation on the rate and sequence
    of DNA replication in synchronized Chinese hamster cells,
    Biophys. J., 16 (1976) 517-525.

6. Paterson, M. C., P. H. M. Lohman, and M. L. Sluyter, Use of a
    UV endonuclease from _Micrococcus luteus_ to monitor the
    progress of DNA repair in UV irradiated human cells, Mutat.
    Res., 19 (1973) 245-256.

7. Rude, J. M., and E. C. Friedberg, Semi-conservative deoxyribo-
    nucleic acid synthesis in unirradiated and ultraviolet-
    irradiated xeroderma pigmentosum and normal human skin
    fibroblasts, Mutat. Res., 42 (1977) 433-442.

8. Setlow, R. B., J. D. Regan, and W. L. Carrier, Different levels
    of excision repair in mammalian cell lines, 16th Annual
    Meeting Biophysical Society (1972) 19a (Abstr.).

9. Waters, R., Repair of DNA in replicated and unreplicated
    portions of the human genome, J. Mol. Biol., 127 (1979)
    117-127.

10. Waters, R., O. Hernandez, H. Yagi, D. M. Jerina, and J. D. Regan,
    Postreplication repair of DNA in human fibroblasts after UV
    irradiation or treatment with metabolites of benzo(a)pyrene,
    Chem.-Biol. Interact., 20 (1978) 289-297.

CHAPTER 24

DNA REPAIR IN NUCLEI ISOLATED FROM HELA CELLS

UMBERTO BERTAZZONI, CARMEN ATTOLINI,
and MIRIA STEFANINI

Laboratorio CNR di Genetica Biochimica ed
Evoluzionistica and Istituto di Genetica
dell'Universita' di Pavia, 27100 Pavia, Italy

SUMMARY

We have studied the DNA repair synthesis in HeLa cell isolated
nuclei in presence of aphidicolin, which selectively inhibits DNA
polymerase α but not DNA polymerases β and γ. The drug strongly
depresses the DNA synthesis rate both in vivo and in the subcellular
system but seems not to interfere with DNA repair. The enhancement
in nucleotide incorporation by isolated nuclei after UV-irradiation
is observed only in the presence of ATP.

INTRODUCTION

During the past few years we have been studying the function of
eukaryotic DNA polymerases α, β, and γ in DNA replication and repair.
There is mounting evidence for a role of α-polymerase in DNA replication, β-polymerase in DNA repair, and γ-polymerase in the replication of mitochondrial DNA [9]. However a final assessment of the
biology of these enzymes has not been obtained, and further experiments are needed to prove directly their functions in the metabolism
of DNA, particularly in the case of the DNA repair, for its complexity
and the inherent difficulties in measuring it.

We have tried recently to develop a subcellular system which
could be used for studying DNA repair in vitro and possibly yield an
integrated repair complex similar to what has been already obtained
for DNA replication [3]. We have chosen HeLa cell nuclei which are
convenient to prepare and store and incorporate nucleotides very
efficiently. The problem in measuring DNA repair in nuclei is that

the background incorporation is very high, and it becomes difficult
to evaluate any increase of it after UV-irradiation.

We have tested the possibility of depressing DNA synthesis
without interfering with DNA repair by treating the nuclei with a
compound, aphidicolin, which has been shown recently to be a potent
inhibitor of DNA synthesis by blocking specifically the activity of
DNA polymerase α, but not DNA polymerases β and γ [5, 7, 8].
Aphidicolin is a tetracyclic diterpenoid extracted from Cephalosporium
aphidicola.   A summary of its action on cellular processes and enzyme
activities is given in Table 1.   It is evident that its selective
inhibition of DNA synthesis and of α-polymerase makes it particularly
suitable for DNA repair studies.

TABLE 1

EFFECT OF APHIDICOLIN ON CELLULAR PROCESSES AND ENZYME ACTIVITIES

	Process or enzyme activity	References
Inhibition	Cellular DNA synthesis	[5, 7, 8]
	DNA polymerase α	[5, 6, 8]
	Herpes simplex virus DNA polymerase	[8]
	Vaccinia virus DNA polymerase	[8]
No Effect	RNA synthesis	[5]
	Protein synthesis	[5]
	Meiotic maturation	[5]
	Deoxyribonucleotide pool	[5]
	DNA polymerase β	[5, 8]
	DNA polymerase γ	[5, 8]
	E. coli DNA polymerase I	[5]
	E. coli RNA polymerase	[5]
	Reverse transcriptase	[5]
	Thymidine kinase	[5]
	Terminal deoxynucleotidyl transferase	[1]

METHODS

Isolation of Nuclei

HeLa S_3 cell suspensions containing from 2 to 5×10^8 cells
were used for the preparation of nuclei following the method of

Krokan et al. [6]. The isolated nuclei were immediately resuspended
for use in incubation experiments.

Assay of DNA Synthesis

The kinetics of dTTP incorporation by isolated nuclei were performed essentially as described by Brun and Weissbach [3]. A 10 µl
portion of isolated nuclei (about 2.3×10^6) resuspended in 120 mM
N-2 hydroxyethylpiperazine-N'-2-ethanesulfonic acid (Hepes), pH 7.5,
2 mM [ethylenebis(oxyethylenenitrilo)]tetraacetic acid (EGTA), 3 mM
$MgCl_2$, 1 mM dithiothreitol (DTT), and 50 mM glucose was incubated at
37°C (0.13 ml) in 50 mM Tris-HCl, pH 8.0, 8 mM $MgCl_2$, 6.5 mM ATP,
2 mM DTT, 50 mM NaCl, 60 µM (each) of the four dNTPs containing
[^{3}H] dTTP (600 cpm/pmole). Aliquots (0.040 ml) of the incubation
mixture were taken at different times, spotted on GF/C filters, and
treated for acid insoluble radioactivity as described by Bollum [12].

Assay of DNA Repair

Isolated nuclei, resuspended as described above, were placed in
plastic capsules and given a UV-irradiation dose of 45 J/m^2 over a
period of 20-30 sec. The irradiated nuclei were immediately
recovered from the capsule and, after 10 min in ice, incubated at
37°C in a reaction mixture containing (in 0.13 ml) 2.5×10^6 nuclei,
100 mM Hepes, pH 7.5, 0.15 mM each of dATP, dGTP and dCTP, 1 µm dTTP
(about 20,000 cpm/p mole), 2 to 4 mM ATP and 9 mM $MgCl_2$. Aliquots
of the reaction were spotted at different times on GF/C and treated
as described [2].

Unscheduled DNA Synthesis

HeLa S3 cells were incubated for 3 hr in the presence of [^{3}H]-
thymidine. Aphidicolin, when needed, was added to the incubation
medium at the concentration of 10 µg/ml. UV irradiation and autoradiographic procedures were carried out as already described [10].

RESULTS

We measured first the effect of aphidicolin on DNA synthesis in
nuclei isolated from dividing cells (Fig. 1). An aphidicolin concentration of 10 µg/ml gives 80 to 90% inhibition and increasing it to
30 µg/ml does not further depress DNA synthesis rate; this residual
incorporation can be ascribed in part to DNA repair synthesis but
also to a lack of access of aphidicolin to its target. The extent
of inhibition obtained in vivo is much higher than that obtained in
vitro on DNA polymerase α [5] and HeLa synchronized nuclei [11].

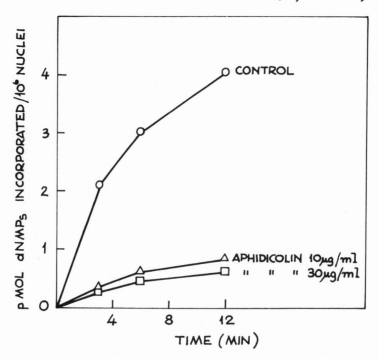

DNA SYNTHESIS IN HELA NUCLEI (60μM dTTP)

Fig. 1.   Effect of aphidicolin on rate of DNA synthesis in nuclei
isolated from HeLa cells.   The assay of nucleotide incorporation was
performed as described in the Methods Section.

This discrepancy is difficult to understand and is possibly related
to some compartmentalization of the drug within the cell.

      In order to measure DNA repair synthesis in isolated nuclei we
harvested HeLa cells when cultures approached saturation and we
lowered the concentration of dTTP in the assay incubation mixture by
about a factor of 50.   We irradiated the isolated nuclei with UV
light (at 45 J/m^2) and compared the kinetics of nucleotide incorporation with the untreated control nuclei.   The results are shown in
Fig. 2.   The reaction was carried out in the presence of aphidicolin,
both for irradiated and control nuclei.   It is evident that the UV-
treated nuclei show a 2- to 3-fold increase in nucleotide incorporation over the control.   The reaction is linear for about 60 min.

      We attempted a partial characterization of the DNA repair system
and we found that it is completely dependent on the addition of Mg^{2+}
and is reduced to about 50% by omitting other deoxynucleoside

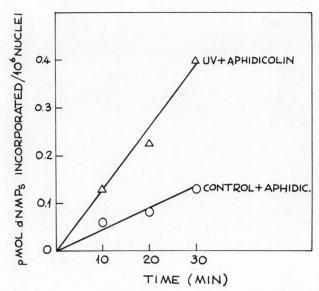

Fig. 2.   DNA repair incorporation following UV irradiation in HeLa
nuclei.   Control and UV-irradiated nuclei were incubated in presence
of aphidicolin, as described in Methods.

triphosphates (Table 2).   The addition of salt does not seem to
affect the rate of the reaction.   If ATP is omitted, a considerable
increase in nucleotide incorporation is observed, as if the overall
inhibitory effect of aphidicolin on DNA synthesis were not operating.

To understand this effect of ATP more clearly we studied the
effect of ATP concentration on the nucleotide incorporation by isolated nuclei both in the presence and in the absence of aphidicolin
and with control and UV-irradiated nuclei.   The results are reported
in Fig. 3.   Untreated control nuclei show a sharp increase in nucleotide incorporation at 2 mM ATP, and the reaction tends to decrease
rapidly at higher ATP concentration.   The nucleotide incorporation
of control nuclei in the presence of aphidicolin presents a different
pattern, showing its maximal activity at zero ATP concentration and
declining to low levels at high ATP concentration.   The incorporation
by UV-treated nuclei in presence of aphidicolin shows a curve similar
to control untreated nuclei with a maximum at 2 mM ATP.   It is evident that the absence of ATP tends to minimize the aphidicolin effect
as if the action of the drug is mediated by ATP.

TABLE 2

CHARACTERIZATION OF DNA REPAIR SYNTHESIS BY UV
IRRADIATED NUCLEI IN PRESENCE OF APHIDICOLIN

Addition	dNMPs incorporated (pmole/10^6 nuclei)[a]
Complete reaction	0.064
$-Mg^{2+}$	0.003
$-dNTPs$	0.032
$+NaCl$, 50 mM	0.054
$-ATP$	0.159

[a]The data represent the average of two
separate experiments.

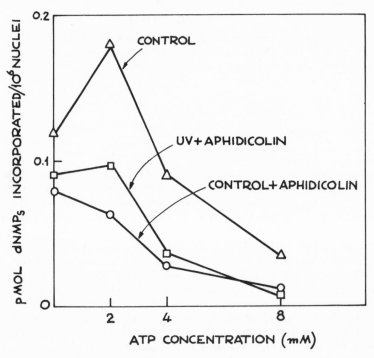

Fig. 3.   Effect of ATP concentration on nucleotide incorporation by
control, UV-treated, and aphidicolin-treated nuclei. Reaction mixtures containing different concentrations of ATP were used to measure
incorporation of nucleotides by control nuclei, nuclei incubated with
aphidicolin, and UV-irradiated nuclei incubated in presence of
aphidicolin.

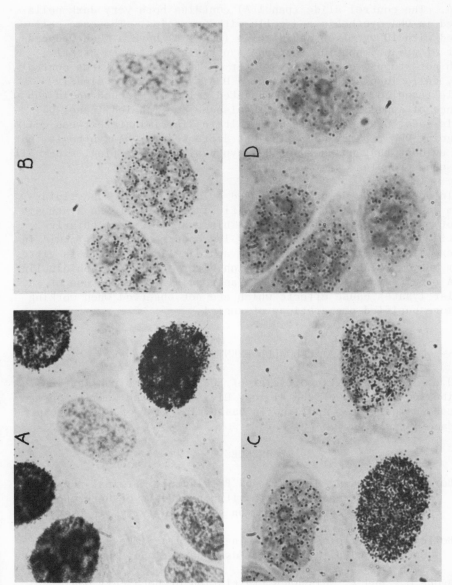

Fig. 4. Unscheduled DNA synthesis of HeLa cells in presence of aphidicolin: (A) control cells;
(B) control cells incubated in presence of 10 µg/ml of aphidicolin; (C) UV-irradiated cells;
(D) UV-irradiated cells incubated in the presence of 10 µg/ml of aphidicolin.

In order to understand if aphidicolin is interfering in vivo with unscheduled DNA synthesis we have performed a few autoradiographic experiments on HeLa cells. The results are reported in Fig. 4. The control slide (panel A) contains both very dark cells engaged in DNA synthesis and cells with no grains. The same cells treated with 10 µg/ml of aphidicolin (panel B) have a much reduced number of grains, showing that DNA synthesis is reduced greatly, though not stopped completely. After UV irradiation of the control cells, cells involved in unscheduled DNA synthesis are clearly visible (panel C). When the irradiated cells are incubated in the presence of aphidicolin, all cells also become labeled (panel D). In this case, however, it is difficult to discriminate between cells undergoing DNA repair and cells just depressed in DNA synthesis, but it is evident that unscheduled DNA synthesis is operating, since all cells show granules.

In conclusion, we have presented evidence that a subcellular system can be devised in which specific inhibition of DNA synthesis but not of DNA repair takes place. This system is particularly sensitive to the presence of ATP for its occurrence. This could in part explain why other authors using aphidicolin in a semi-in vitro system but omitting ATP observe an inhibitory effect of aphidicolin on DNA repair systems [4]. It is also possible that the use of cellular lysates cause effects which are not observed when working with more purified preparations of nuclei.

ACKNOWLEDGEMENTS

U.B. is a scientific official of EURATOM. This publication is contribution No. 1618 of the Biology Division of the Commission of European Communities. Aphidicolin was a kind gift of Dr. B. Hesp, ICI, Macclesfield, U.K.

REFERENCES

1. Bertazzoni, U., E. Ginelli, and P. Plevani, Terminal deoxynucleotidyl transferase: in vitro synthesis of heteropolymers and effect of aphidicolin on enzyme activity, in preparation.
2. Bollum, F. J., In: Procedures in Nucleic Acid Research, G. L. Cantoni and D. R. Davies, Eds., Harper and Row, New York, 1966, p. 296.
3. Brun, G., and A. Weissbach, Initiation of HeLa cell DNA synthesis in a subnuclear system, Proc. Natl. Acad. Sci. (U.S.), 75 (1978) 5931-5935.
4. Hanaoka, F., H. Kato, S. Ikegami, H. Ohashi and M. Yamada, Aphidicolin does inhibit repair replication in HeLa cells, Biochim. Biophys. Res. Commun., 87 (1979) 575-580.

5. Ikegami, S., T. Taguchi, M. Ohashi, M. Oguro, and Y. Mano,
    Aphidicolin prevents mitotic cell division by interfering
    with the activity of DNA polymerase α, Nature, 275 (1978)
    458-460.
6. Krokan, H., E. Bjørklid, and H. Prydz, DNA synthesis in isolated
    HeLa cell nuclei. Optimalization of the system and
    characterization of the product, Biochemistry, 14 (1975)
    4227-4232.
7. Ohashi, M., T. Taguchi and S. Ikegami, Aphidicolin: a specific
    inhibitor of DNA polymerases in the cytosol of rat liver,
    Biochem. Biophys. Res. Commun., 82 (1978) 1084-1090.
8. Pedrali-Noy, G., and S. Spadari, Effect of aphidicolin on viral
    and human DNA polymerases, Biochem. Biophys. Res. Commun.,
    88 (1979) 1194-1202.
9. Stefanini, M., A. I. Scovassi, and U. Bertazzoni, Function of
    DNA polymerases α, β and γ in DNA replication and repair,
    In: Lymphocyte Stimulation: Biochemical and Immunological
    processes; Differential Sensitivity to Radiation,
    A. Castellani and F. Celada, Eds., Plenum Press, New York,
    in press.
10. Stefanini, M., E. Ascari, and F. Nuzzo, UV-induced DNA repair
    in hairy cell leukemia patients, Cancer Letters, 7 (1979)
    235-241.
11. Wist, E., and H. Prydz, The effect of aphidicolin on DNA syn-
    thesis in isolated HeLa cell nuclei, Nucleic Acids Res., 6
    (1979) 1583-1590.

CHAPTER 25

REPAIR AND INDUCTION OF CHROMOSOME ABERRATIONS AND POINT

MUTATIONS IN MAMMALIAN SOMATIC CELLS: A SUMMARY AND PERSPECTIVE

SHELDON WOLFF

Laboratory of Radiobiology and Department of Anatomy
University of California at San Francisco
San Francisco, California 94143 (U.S.A.)

It is now somewhat over 50 years since the discovery of the first agent, x-rays, with which we were able to "transmutate" the gene. This discovery, which allowed us to obtain genetic variants, was invaluable in enabling us to gain insights about the organization of genetic material. From the first it was noted that the mutations seemed to fall into two classes, those that were changes in the gene itself, so-called point mutations, and those that were the result of gross chromosomal changes, including deletions. One particular point of controversy concerned whether or not spontaneous mutations were "gene" mutations, whereas radiation-induced mutations were mainly chromosomal. Largely because the gene was an abstraction in the sense that its chemical nature was unknown, the problem was intractable.

Today we possess very sophisticated knowledge about the chemical nature of the genetic material, its organization into chromosomes, and the chemistry of its repair, replication, and control. We now have far more tools with which it is possible to induce mutations. We now know that mutations can be caused not only by physical agents such as radiation, but by a whole variety of different chemicals that can interact with DNA. We know that many of the mutations are not necessarily induced or fixed at the time of the initial insult, but can develop later as a result of perturbations in the cells' ability to repair and replicate modified DNA. We have been aided in these studies not only by a judicious choice of agents that induce a variety of different lesions in DNA, but also by the use of mutant lines of cells that are deficient in rather well circumscribed steps necessary for DNA repair and replication.

Interestingly enough, in our advanced state of sophistication we are just now coming to grips with the problems that were so difficult 50 years ago. For instance, it was early recognized that radiation-induced recessive mutations were mainly chromosomal mutations that, unlike spontaneous mutations, were in large part deleterious or lethal when homozygous, and that excellent correlations could be made between cell killing and the induction of chromosome aberrations. As a matter of fact, at low doses of ionizing radiation virtually all cell killing could be attributed to a nuclear effect upon the genes and chromosomes of the cell. The development of cell culture methods now has given us more degrees of freedom in the types of mutation studies we can carry out. We are no longer restricted to morphological studies with whole organisms, but can work with the chemical phenotypes of the cells themselves. Studies at this chemical level have underscored the reasons for the original controversy of 50 years ago. For instance, most mutation studies involved the induction of mutants that have lost the ability to carry out an essential enzymatic step in DNA metabolism. Frequently, the locus studied is the HGPRT locus. HGPRT$^-$ mutants are resistant to such purine analogs as 8-azaguanine. Loss of enzyme activity could be caused either by a point mutation that leads to production of an inactive enzyme or to a deletion that leads to no enzyme. X-rays have been found capable of inducing HGPRT$^-$ (azaguanine-resistant) mutations, but not ouabain-resistant mutations. Since the ouabain locus controls the production of the Na$^+$/K$^+$ ATPase that functions in the cell membrane, deletions of this locus are lethal. The differing results with these two loci support the Stadlerian point of view that x-rays induce deletions rather than point mutations.

With ultraviolet radiation and with certain chemicals, however, both kinds of mutation can be formed. The papers presented in the session, Repair and Induction of Chromosome Aberrations and Point Mutations in Mammalian Somatic Cells, in this meeting underscore the advances that we are now making in our understanding of "mutation" and how induced mutation rates are affected by the repair enzymes in the cells.

In cells of higher organisms, mutagenic chemicals can be studied by cytogenetic methods as well as studies in somatic cell genetics. The classical cytogenetic studies dealt with the induction of chromosome aberrations. Although ionizing radiations can break DNA directly and induce large numbers of double-strand breaks that result in aberrations, chemical mutagens differ in that they are mainly S-dependent substances that (like UV) induce lesions that can lead to chromatid breaks only in S when DNA replicates. The resultant aberrations are thought to be caused by misreplication of DNA, rather than direct breakage as caused by the few S-independent chemicals and ionizing radiation. Models to account for this were presented by Bender, who has been one of the pioneers in developing models by which enzymes involved in DNA repair and replication could attack lesions in DNA and translate them into broken chromatids. Additionally, Bender presented evidence from ataxia telangiectasia cells showing that in these cells, even with x-ray damage, aberrations can be produced by such mechanisms.

In recent years another type of cytogenetic endpoint, which is very sensitive to S-dependent agents and is very easy to score, has been studied extensively. This is the sister chromatid exchange (SCE). Dr. Sasaki proposed that aberrations, SCEs, and mutagenicity are reflections of DNA damage and repair. Thus, all are indices of mutation. Because there are many ways in which SCEs differ from ordinary chromosome aberrations, he has proposed two different repair pathways that enable the cell to tolerate damage. One of the indications that SCEs and aberrations are different comes from experiments with caffeine, which has been found to increase aberrations and cell killing but, with the exception of his experiments with endoreduplicated chromosomes, not SCEs. Sasaki suggests that SCEs are produced by a replicative bypass mechanism of the type first proposed by Strauss and his co-workers, whereas aberrations are caused by a post-replication type of repair.

One of the differences between SCEs and aberrations (which cause cell death) can be seen in experiments on potentially lethal damage recovery as carried out in Fornace's and Little's laboratory; they found that if after exposure they hold the cells before plating them, the SCEs increase whereas aberrations and cell death decrease. The SCEs, however, unlike aberrations and killing, are correlated with malignant transformation, which has already been correlated with viable mutations by Huberman. Fornace has now presented evidence from alkaline elution experiments that repair of single strand breaks can be correlated with both a decrease in aberrations and killing. He pointed out, however, that the single-strand breaks observed might have been derived from original double-strand breaks of the type that leads to aberrations.

Both Sasaki and Maher and McCormick have pointed out that even with chemicals, mutations at the HGPRT locus could be deletions. One mechanism by which these could be brought about has been postulated by Roberts to be the saturation of repair mechanisms that results in incomplete DNA synthesis. This would lead to chromosomal damage seen mainly as deletions.

Such a mechanism could account for the apparent paradoxes seen when one considers seemingly conflicting results from various types of experiments. Thus, although aberrations are related to cell death, and mutations often are not, Maher has clearly shown a direct correlation between cytotoxicity and mutations at the HGPRT⁻ locus

indicating that the mutagenic lesion and the lethal lesion both
increase linearly with dose. Thus, it now behooves us to be more
specific when we use the word "mutation." As a catch-all phrase to
refer to all heritable damage it has been very useful in the past.
In the future it still might be useful when one makes risk estimates
for mutagens. When, however, one deals with experiments designed to
determine fundamental mechanisms and correlations, it soon becomes
apparent that the catch-all phrase is too imprecise and covers so
many genetic changes brought about by different molecular mechanisms
that it leads not only to ambiguity, but to apparent contradictory
results.

The papers in this meeting clearly show that as we become more
knowledgeable, we don't solve all our problems but merely raise new
questions. We realize that our previous models, like our new models,
are naive. For instance, the discovery that UV-sensitive xeroderma
pigmentosum cells are excision-defective led to the hypothesis that
UV-induced cell killing was caused by the repair defect. In contrast, Chinese hamster cell lines, such as B14FAF and several of
those isolated by Trosko, are defective in repair but are not sensitive to killing. At least one of his mutants, however, is sensitive
to mutation induction, leading him to postulate that excision repair
in Chinese hamster prevents mutation fixation, but has a minimal
effect on survival. Furthermore, it has been long known that even
excision repair-proficient cells often do not excise all dimers,
indicating that the cells are able to survive with dimers (and also
with some chemically-induced lesions). The reasons for the uncoup-
ling between excision repair and cell death are as yet unclear and
point to the unknown complexities in the ways in which cells can
cope with damaged DNA.

It has been pointed out that not only are there many repair
mechanisms and enzymes, many of which presumably are still unknown,
but also that each chemical mutagen can induce a whole spectrum of
lesions, the proportions of which may vary from mutagen to mutagen.
As Strauss showed, the lesions can vary in their repairability and
the way in which they affect replication. With chemicals, some of
the lesions are major products that are measurable, but these may
or may not be mutagenic. Other products, however, are minor products
that are more difficult to deal with. If they are measurable, then,
of course, it can be determined if they are mutagenic. In some
instances, however, minor lesions that have yet to be measured must
be invoked to account for the experimental results.

Consequently, it has become increasingly clear that as a result
of our progress in chemical mutagenesis and its dependence on DNA
repair mechanisms, we have reached the stage where we should refine
our models and test them to see if they still have heuristic value
or are ready to be discarded. To do this, we should in the future
define the chemical nature of the mutation as precisely as possible

and discriminate between deletions, base changes, and frameshifts.
Attempts should be made to determine the spectrum of lesions made
by a mutagen and to discriminate between the various lesions in
order to ascertain which ones are responsible for the particular
genetic endpoint. Attempts also need to be made to determine the
relation between the mutant cells defective in repair and the
lesions in whose repair they are defective.

It is hoped that the added precision obtained in defining the
lesions, their repair, and the genetic endpoint will lead to the
grand synthesis of all the types of information presented at this
conference, including that which seems to be somewhat contradictory.

CHAPTER 26

RELATIONSHIP BETWEEN UNSCHEDULED DNA SYNTHESIS AND MUTATION

INDUCTION IN MALE MICE

GARY A. SEGA

Biology Division, Oak Ridge National Laboratory
Oak Ridge, Tenn. 37830 (U.S.A.)

SUMMARY

Unscheduled DNA synthesis (UDS) induced in the germ cells of
male mice by chemical and physical agents can be studied in vivo by
making use of the timing of spermatogenesis and spermiogenesis. In
meiotic and postmeiotic germ-cell stages, UDS occurs from leptotene
through midspermatid stages but is not detected in later stages. No
consistent correlation has been seen between the occurrence of UDS
in the germ cells and reduced dominant lethal frequencies or reduced
specific-locus mutation frequencies. It is suggested that the UDS
observed in the germ cells may be principally involved in the removal
of DNA lesions which, if left, could give rise to subtle genetic
damage that current mammalian genetic tests may not be able to detect.
Characterization of mouse stocks with reduced UDS capability in their
germ cells plus the development of biochemical genetic markers that
can measure single amino acid substitutions will likely be necessary
before the relationship between UDS in mammalian germ cells and repair
of genetic damage can be clearly established.

INTRODUCTION

The first evidence for unscheduled DNA synthesis (UDS) in
mammalian somatic cells was provided by Rasmussen and Painter [17]
when they demonstrated that UV radiation induced the uptake of labeled
thymidine into the DNA of cultured HeLa and Chinese hamster cells
grown in culture. Later, Kofman-Alfaro and Chandley [11], also using
in vivo procedures, were able to demonstrate UDS in spermatogenic
cells of the mouse after exposure to x-rays or UV. Similar findings

were observed in rat germ cells after in vitro UV exposure [10] and
in human germ cells after in vitro UV exposure [5].

The induction of UDS in mammalian germ cells can also be studied
by in vivo procedures. In the male mouse it is possible to study UDS
in vivo in meiotic and postmeiotic germ-cell stages by making use of
the sequence of events that occur during spermatogenesis and spermiogenesis. In developing male germ cells, the last DNA synthesis takes
place during a 14-hr period [14] in preleptotene spermatocytes.
After DNA synthesis, these spermatocytes continue to develop through
a series of germ cell stages for about a 28-30 day time period [15,
16, 24] before late spermatids leave the testes and enter the caput
epididymides. Two to three days later, the developing sperm reach
the caudal epididymides, and in 2-3 days more they enter the vas.
If the DNA from any meiotic or postmeiotic germ-cell stage is damaged
by a physical or chemical agent and UDS is induced, it can be
detected by an unscheduled incorporation of [3H]thymidine ([3H]dT)
into the germ cell. The unscheduled uptake of [3H]dT can be measured
either directly by examining the affected germ-cell stages by use of
autoradiography [31] or indirectly by waiting until the germ cells
have matured into sperm in the caudal epididymides and vasa deferentia and then assaying the [3H]dT activity contained in several
million of these sperm by liquid scintillation counting (LSC) [23,
26, 27].

SIGNIFICANCE OF UDS IN GERM CELLS

The ability of a chemical agent or any of its metabolites to
induce a UDS response in mouse germ cells indicates that DNA lesions
have been induced and the germ cells are presumably attempting to
restore the integrity of the damaged DNA. Although the term "DNA
repair" has at times been used synonymously for UDS, it can be mis-
leading. There is no way currently available to know for certain
that "repaired" DNA has been restored to its original condition
through the process of UDS. We can only say that it does not seem
likely that UDS induced in mouse germ cells represents terminal
addition of deoxynucleotides to broken ends of DNA, since no terminal
transferase has been detected in mouse testes [1, 2].

Also, unpublished data we have collected suggest that excision
of alkylated DNA bases is associated with the UDS response. At
various times after i.p. injection of [3H]MMS, testes and vas sperm
heads were recovered and DNA was extracted and then hydrolyzed under
mild conditions similar to those described by Lawley [12]. The
hydrolysates were analyzed on Sephadex G-10 columns to determine
guanine and 7 methylguanine (MeG) content.

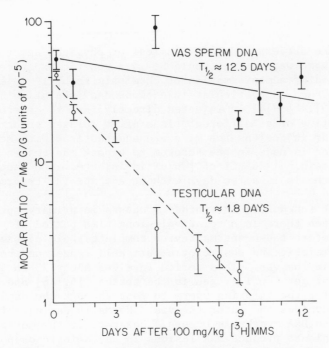

Fig. 1. Comparison of the rates of loss of 7 MeG from (●) vas
sperm DNA and (○) testicular DNA after a single IP injection of
100 mg/kg of [³H]MMS. The error bars represent ± 1 standard devia-
tion. The least-squares fits are indicated.

        The half-life of 7 MeG in testicular DNA was found to be ∿2 days
(Fig. 1), which is considerably shorter than its reported half-life
of ∿6 days in DNA in vitro [13]; this implies that 7 MeG may be
enzymatically excised from testicular DNA in vivo. At the same time
the half-life of 7 MeG in sperm DNA is ∿12 days, if it is assumed
that the initial level of DNA alkylation in all of the stages is
approximately the same. We have previously noted [25] that 4 hr after
exposure to EMS the alkylations per deoxynucleotide in testicular
DNA were about the same as those in sperm DNA; recent results with
MMS have been similar [24]. It therefore does appear that the initial
level of DNA alkylation is about the same in different germ-cell
stages. The long half-life of 7 MeG in sperm DNA compared with its
in vitro half-life of ∿6 days may be related to the highly condensed
state of the sperm nucleus in which the chromatin is packaged almost
as a crystalline structure. The very different half-lives of 7 MeG
in sperm and testicular DNA fit in well with our observation that a
UDS response can be measured in meiotic and post-meiotic stages found
in the testes but not in maturing sperm during a 2-week sampling
period following treatment.

GENERAL PROCEDURES FOR MEASURING UDS IN MOUSE GERM CELLS

Male mice are exposed to a chemical or physical agent in
exactly the same way as they would be in a genetic experiment. The
general method of administration of chemicals is by IP injection, but
other routes such as testicular injections and inhalation have also
been used [29]. [^{3}H]dT is injected directly into the testes either
at the same time or at different times after mutagen treatment. For
the testicular injections the mice are anesthetized with Metofane, a
small incision is made in the scrotum to expose the testes and 36 µl
of water containing ∿36 µCi of [^{3}H]dT is injected into each testis.
The incision heals in a few days without any special treatment.

The last scheduled DNA synthesis occurs in primary spermatocytes, and then there is a relatively long time period of about 33
to 36 days before these spermatocytes complete their passage through
a series of meiotic and postmeiotic germ cell stages and become mature
spermatozoa in the vas. This period involves about 28 to 30 days for
development of germ cell stages in the testes [15, 16] and another
4 to 6 days for the maturing sperm to pass through the caput and
caudal epididymides and enter the vas. Normally during this extended
time period no DNA synthesis occurs. However, if the mutagen being
studied is able to produce DNA lesions in any meiotic or postmeiotic
germ-cell stages, UDS if induced, can be detected by the unscheduled
uptake of the [^{3}H]dT into the affected germ cells. UDS occurring in
any stage can be studied indirectly by making use of the timing of
spermatogenesis and spermiogenesis in the mouse and recovering sperm
from the caudal epididymides or vasa deferentia at the appropriate
times after treatment of the males. For example, sperm recovered
from the caudal epididymides 16 days after treatment represent germ
cells that were mostly in early spermatid stages at the time of
treatment.

If a mutagen exposure–UDS response curve is desired for a particular germ-cell stage, then at the appropriate time after treatment
the males are killed and sperm are recovered from the caudal epididymides or vasa deferentia. If it is desired to study all of the
germ-cell stages undergoing a UDS response to a particular agent,
then every few days for 5 to 6 weeks after treatment sperm samples
are recovered from the treated males.

In the recovery of the sperm, the caudal epididymides or vasa
deferentia are dissected from the animals, diced, and sonicated to
destroy all cell types except for the sperm heads. The tails and
midpieces (with their associated mitochondria) are sheared off in
this process. After several washes in a Ficoll–SDS solution, a pure
population of sperm heads is obtained free of sperm tails, midpieces,
somatic cells, or cellular debris [23, 26]. One male typically
yields ∿7 × 10^6 sperm heads from the vasa deferentia and about twice
that number from the caudal epididymides. Several million of these

sperm are then assayed by LSC to determine [3H]dT activity, and the
number of sperm present in each scintillation vial is determined by
hemacytometer counts of a diluted sample of the same sperm stock.
Finally, the [3H]dT disintegrations per minute (dpm) per 10^6 sperm
heads is calculated. Although LSC is an indirect means of measuring
the UDS that had occurred in earlier germ-cell stages, it has the
advantage that it is sensitive to low levels of induced UDS, since
millions of sperm heads are sampled.

To make direct observations of the germ-cell stages undergoing
UDS we use autoradiographic procedures [29, 31]. This also provides
information on the uniformity of the UDS response within a particular
germ cell stage in a single testis and can be used to study the distribution of [3H]dT labeling from UDS throughout the chromosomes in
diakinesis. However, autoradiographs are hard to quantitate and are
not as sensitive as LSC for detecting low levels of induced UDS.

GERM CELL STAGES THAT UNDERGO UDS WHEN EXPOSED TO MUTAGENIC AGENTS

We have made a detailed study of the meiotic and postmeiotic
germ-cell stages undergoing UDS when exposed to mutagenic agents
using MMS, EMS, cyclophosphamide (CPA), mitomen (DMO), and x-rays
[23, 27, 30, 31]. Gonial cells have not yet been thoroughly studied
because of the difficulty in distinguishing UDS from the scheduled
DNA synthesis occurring in these germ-cell stages. Other workers
studying UDS have used x-rays and UV in an in vitro system with mouse
germ cells [11], UV in vitro with rat germ cells [10], and MMS and
procarbazine in vivo with the rabbit [4, 21]. In all of these
studies the basic finding is that mutagens can induce UDS in meiotic
stages and in postmeiotic stages up to about midspermatids. No UDS
is detected in late spermatids and sperm cells.

Figure 2 shows the pattern of the UDS response induced by a
250 mg/kg IP injected dose of EMS in different germ cell stages of
the mouse. (The [3H]dT was given at the same time as the EMS.) Note
that for about the first two weeks after treatment there is no unscheduled presence of [3H]dT label in the sperm recovered from the
vas. These sperm represent germ cell stages that were treated as
mature spermatozoa to late spermatids. In weeks 3 and 4 after EMS
treatment, the vas sperm show the unscheduled presence of [3H]dT.
These sperm represent germ cell stages that were treated as midspermatids to early meiotic stages.

The absence of UDS in the mature spermatozoa to late spermatid
stages is not due to failure of EMS to ethylate DNA in these stages.
In our chemical dosimetry studies we found that the DNA in these germ
cell stages is being alkylated [25, 28]. As we have discussed in an
earlier paper [23], the germ-cell stages exhibiting no UDS are those

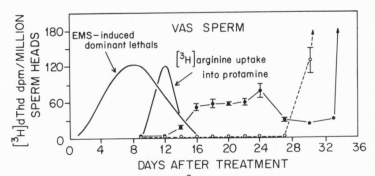

Fig. 2.   Unscheduled uptake of [³H]dT into meiotic and postmeiotic
germ cell stages of male mice after testicular injection of [³H]dT
and IP injection of 250 mg/kg of EMS, measured in sperm passing
through the vasa deferentia;   (●) [³H]dT activity in sperm heads
from EMS-treated animals;   (o) [³H]dT activity in sperm heads from
control animals.   Also indicated is the dominant lethal frequency
pattern obtained with EMS (the peak in dominant lethals is around
50–60% with 250 mg/kg of EMS [7, 9]) and the time period where protamine is synthesized.   Data from Sega [23].

in which protamine has either replaced, or is in the process of
replacing, the usual chromosomal histones. At the time of protamine
synthesis an extensive condensation of the spermatid nucleus begins.
It is possible that the DNA lesions present in these cells have
become inaccessible to the enzymatic system which gives rise to UDS
in the earlier germ cell stages. Also, much of the cytoplasm is lost
from the spermatids as they develop from mid to late spermatid stages,
and the enzymatic system which produces the UDS response may be lost
at this time.

RELATIONSHIP BETWEEN GENETIC EFFECTS AND UNSCHEDULED
DNA SYNTHESIS INDUCED BY MUTAGENS

When EMS was first found to induce UDS in specific germ-cell
stages of male mice, it was noted that these stages showed no detectable dominant-lethal mutations [23]. This led to an initial hypothesis that UDS might be important in removing dominant-lethal mutations
from the germ cells. However, other mutagens, including isopropyl
methanesulfonate (IMS) [26], CPA [30], and x-rays [27] were then
found that produced UDS in germ cell stages that also showed dominant
lethal mutations [3, 6, 8, 22].

Figure 3 shows the patterns of dominant-lethal frequencies seen
after treatment of male mice with EMS [7, 9] and x-rays [6, 22] and
how they are related to UDS. While the germ-cell stages showing UDS
after EMS treatment (and sampled as sperm in the vas during weeks 3
and 4 after treatment) do not give rise to dominant-lethal mutations,

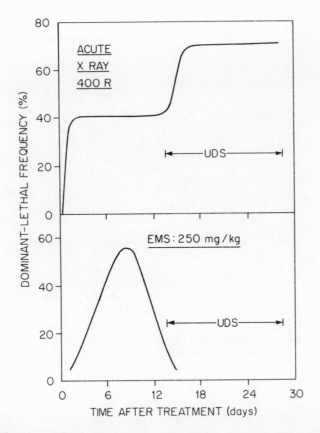

Fig. 3.   Relationship between the dominant lethal frequency patterns induced by EMS [7, 9] and x-rays [6, 22], and the occurrence of unscheduled DNA synthesis (UDS) in the germ cells of male mice [23, 27].

these same germ-cell stages also undergo UDS after x-ray treatment but show nearly twice as high a dominant-lethal frequency as the germ cells sampled in the vas during the first two weeks of mating after x-ray treatment, when no UDS was detected.

The absence of dominant lethals in germ-cell stages showing a UDS response when exposed to EMS may be fortuitous. Figure 4, taken from a recent paper of ours [28] shows that after an IP injection of 200 mg/kg of [³H] EMS, the level of ethylations per vas sperm head closely parallels the dominant-lethal frequency curve produced by EMS (Fig. 3). However, the ethylations per deoxynucleotide in the sperm DNA do not correlate with the dominant lethal curve.

Using sperm from the caudal epididymides of the same treated males we again measured sperm head ethylation and then extracted

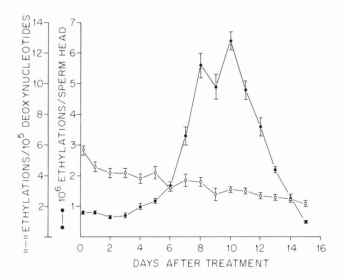

Fig. 4.   Ethylation of sperm heads and sperm DNA taken from the
vasa deferentia during a 2-week period following IP injection of
200 mg/kg [³H]EMS: (●) 10^6 ethylations per sperm head;   (o)
ethylations per 10^5 deoxynucleotides.   Standard deviations are
indicated.   From Sega and Owens [28].

sperm protamine (a basic protein that replaces the usual histones in
maturing sperm) and measured the extent of its ethylation (Fig. 5).
Taking into account the 2- to 3-day shift toward earlier germ-cell
stages recovered from the caudal epididymides as compared to those
recovered from the vasa deferentia [23], the ethylations per sperm
head and the ethylations per OD_{206} unit of protamine both closely
parallel the dominant-lethal curve obtained with EMS.

These results have led us to suggest a model for the induction
of dominant lethals by EMS which is shown in Fig. 6.   After protamine
synthesis (in maturing spermatid stages), but before cysteine disulfide bonds are formed, EMS could ethylate the sulfhydryl groups and
thus effectively block normal disulfide-bond formation.   This in turn
would prevent normal chromatin condensation in the sperm nucleus,
leading to stresses in the chromatin structure that eventually result
in a lethal chromosome break.   Some of our recent work [24] using
[³H]MMS has, in fact, shown that S-methyl-L-cysteine is a major
alkylation product recovered from mouse sperm protamine.

Our findings suggest to us that, even in the absence of a UDS
response, EMS would probably not be effective in producing dominant
lethals in meiotic and postmeiotic stages where no protamine is

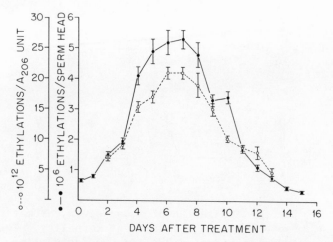

Fig. 5.   Ethylation of sperm heads and sperm protamine from the
caudal epididymides at various times after IP injection of mice with
200 mg/kg of [^{3}H]EMS.   (●) 10^6 ethylations per sperm head;   (o)
10^{12} ethylations per A_{206} unit of purified protamine recovered from
the sperm heads.   From Sega and Owens [28].

present.   We feel the UDS response observed in these stages likely
involves the restoration of altered deoxynucleotides which might
otherwise give rise to subtle genetic damage such as recessive point
mutations, but not necessarily to chromosomal aberrations or dominant
lethals.

Data on specific-locus mutation frequencies in each of the first
four mating weeks following treatment with chemical mutagens is not
extensive enough to determine if a difference in mutation frequency
exists between germ-cell stages showing UDS (sampled in weeks 3 and
4 of mating after treatment) and those not showing UDS (sampled in
the first two weeks of mating).   However, more data are available
for x-rays.

With an acute x-ray exposure of 300 R, specific-locus mutation
frequencies have been determined by W. L. Russell for each of the
first four weeks of mating after treatment and were reported elsewhere [27](Table I).   The mutation frequency in each of the four
weeks is at least an order of magnitude higher than the spontaneous
frequency, and there is no reduction in the frequency in weeks 3 and
4 as compared with weeks 1 and 2.   In fact, the mutation frequency
is higher (at a 90% confidence level) in week 3 than it is in the
first two weeks.   There is no indication UDS results in a reduced
specific-locus mutation frequency after x-ray treatment.

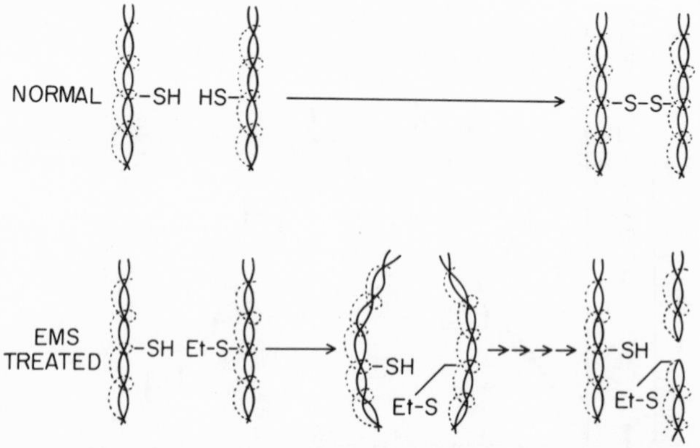

Fig. 6. Model for the ethylation of mouse sperm chromatin by EMS, leading to chromosome breakage and dominant lethality. The double helices represent double-stranded DNA and the dashed lines represent the associated sperm protamine. The sulfhydryl (-SH) groups are part of the cysteine residues in the protamine, and the ethylated sulfhydryl group is represented as Et-S-. In normal nuclear condensation (a), the sulfhydryl groups of cysteine cross-link to form disulfide bridges in the chromatin. However, if EMS ethylates a nucleophilic sulfhydryl group before a disulfide bond forms (b), crosslinking of the sulfhydryl groups may not take place. This could lead to stresses in the chromatin structure and eventually produce a chromosome break either near the region of ethylation (as shown) or away from this region, where stresses in the chromatin might be greater.

L. B. Russell has shown that among the specific-locus mutations induced by x-rays at the "dilute" and "short ear" loci [18] and the albino locus [19] there are a number representing intragenic changes. However, those mutations induced in the stages considered in this paper, namely the post-spermatogonial stages, could all be small deficiencies. Thus, in the case of x-rays, the UDS response we measure in the meiotic and post-meiotic stages may represent restoration of damaged deoxynucleotides and/or single-strand breaks but may have no effect on the removal of specific-locus mutations in the mouse in which small deletions are involved. By the same reasoning, the occurrence of x-ray-induced dominant lethals in germ-cell stages showing a UDS response may indicate that the enzymatic system giving rise to the UDS can handle some types of DNA lesions but not those which could generally give rise to dominant lethals as, for example, double-strand breaks.

TABLE 1

SPECIFIC-LOCUS MUTATION FREQUENCIES INDUCED IN MEIOTIC AND
POSTMEIOTIC GERM-CELL STAGES OF MALE MICE AFTER EXPOSURE TO 300 R
OF ACUTE X-RAYS[a]

Week after 300 R[b]	Progeny scored	Mutants[c]	Mutation frequency/[d] locus/gamete
First	9,281	13	$2.0 \left(\begin{matrix}3.3\\1.0\end{matrix}\right) \times 10^{-4}$
Second	9,412	12	$1.8 \left(\begin{matrix}3.1\\1.0\end{matrix}\right) \times 10^{-4}$
Third	4,266	10	$3.4 \left(\begin{matrix}5.9\\1.8\end{matrix}\right) \times 10^{-4}$
Fourth	3,499	4	$1.6 \left(\begin{matrix}3.9\\0.6\end{matrix}\right) \times 10^{-4}$
Control	531,500	28	$0.075 \left(\begin{matrix}0.107\\0.051\end{matrix}\right) \times 10^{-4}$

(Third and Fourth are bracketed together as UDS)

[a] Data of W. L. Russell cited by Sega [27].

[b] Treated males were (101 × C3Hf)F_1 hybrids, 12–21 weeks old.

[c] Seven loci were scored for mutation. See Russell [20] for
description of mutations.

[d] Upper and lower 95% confidence limits of the observed
mutation frequencies are shown in parentheses.

DEVELOPMENT AND CHARACTERIZATION OF MOUSE STOCKS
WITH REDUCED UDS LEVELS

A total of 22 mouse stocks have been tested for the UDS response
of their germ cells to MMS [24]. Males from each of the stocks were
given the usual testicular injections of [^{3}H]dT followed immediately
by an IP injection of 75 mg/kg of MMS, which was known to induce a
high level of UDS in several germ cell stages of the (C3Hf × 101)F_1
hybrid males that we ordinarily use. Sperm from the caudal epididymides, representing early spermatid stages at the time of treatment, were recovered 16 days after treatment and assayed for unscheduled [^{3}H]dT incorporation.

Within the experimental uncertainties, most of the 22 stocks
showed about the same UDS response in the early spermatids (Fig. 7).
However, there was a significant difference between the stocks
showing the highest UDS response and those showing the lowest. The

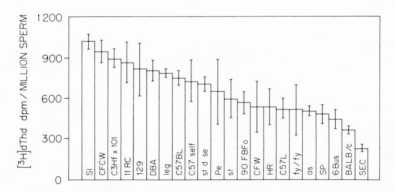

Fig. 7.   Unscheduled DNA synthesis occurring in early spermatid
stages of 22 different mouse stocks following exposure to 75 mg/kg
of MMS.   Sperm from the caudal epididymides were assayed for the
unscheduled presence of [^{3}H]dT 16 days after treatment.   These sperm
represent early spermatid stages at the time of treatment.   Standard
deviations are indicated.

(C3Hf × 101)F_1 hybrids showed one of the highest responses, while
SEC and BALB/c males were the two stocks showing the lowest UDS
responses, being only one-third to one-fourth of that for the
(C3Hf × 101)F_1 males.

    BALB/c males were chosen for further studies since their body
and testis weights are very similar to (C3Hf × 101)F_1 males of the
same age.   With other doses of MMS there was a consistent reduction
in the UDS levels induced in BALB/c germ cells compared to that
observed in the germ cells of (C3Hf × 101)F_1 males.   This effect is
not due to reduced levels of DNA methylation in BALB/c germ cells,
because recent chemical dosimetry studies by us [24] have shown that
the testicular DNA and sperm DNA of both stocks are alkylated to the
same extent by equimolar injected doses of [^{3}H]MMS.   Such data at
least suggest that the germ cells of BALB/c males may be less efficient than those of (C3Hf × 101)F_1 males in the removal of DNA
methylation products.   The eventual characterization of mouse stocks
with reduced UDS capability in their germ cells plus the development
of biochemical genetic markers that can measure single amino acid
substitutions will likely be necessary before the relationship
between UDS in mammalian germ cells and repair of genetic damage can
be clearly established.

ACKNOWLEDGEMENT

This research was sponsored by the Office of Health and Environmental Research, U.S. Department of Energy, under contract W-7405-eng-26 with the Union Carbide Corporation.

REFERENCES

1. Bollum, F. J., personal communication.
2. Bollum, F. J., Terminal deoxynucleotidyl transferase: biological studies, in: Advances in Enzymology, Vol. 47, A. Meister, Ed., Wiley, New York, 1978, pp. 347-373.
3. Brittinger, D., Die mutagene Wirkung von Endoxan bei der Maus, Humangenetik, 3 (1966) 156-165.
4. Bürgin, H., B. Schmid, and G. Zbinden, Assessment of DNA damage in germ cells of male rabbits treated with isoniazid and procarbazine, Toxicology, 12 (1979) 251-257.
5. Chandley, A. C., and S. Kofman-Alfaro, "Unscheduled" DNA synthesis in human germ cells following UV irradiation, Exptl. Cell Res., 69 (1971) 45-48.
6. Ehling, U. H., Comparison of radiation and chemically-induced dominant lethal mutations in male mice, Mutat. Res., 11 (1971) 35-44.
7. Ehling, U. H., R. B. Cumming, and H. V. Malling, Induction of dominant lethal mutations by alkylating agents in male mice, Mutat. Res., 5 (1968) 417-428.
8. Ehling, U. H., D. G. Doherty, and H. V. Malling, Differential spermatogenic response of mice to the induction of dominant-lethal mutations by n-propyl methanesulfonate and isopropyl methanesulfonate, Mutat. Res., 15 (1972) 175-184.
9. Generoso, W. M., and W. L. Russell, Strain and sex variations in the sensitivity of mice to dominant-lethal induction with ethyl methanesulfonate, Mutat. Res., 8 (1969) 589-598.
10. Gledhill, B. L., and Z. Darzynkiewicz, Unscheduled synthesis of DNA during mammalian spermatogenesis in response to UV irradiation, J. Exptl. Zool., 183 (1973) 375-382.
11. Kofman-Alfaro, S., and A. C. Chandley, Radiation-initiated DNA synthesis in spermatogenic cells of the mouse, Exptl. Cell Res., 69 (1971) 33-44.
12. Lawley, P. D., Methylation of DNA by carcinogens: some applications of chemical analytical methods, in: Screening Tests in Chemical Carcinogenesis, R. Montesano, H. Bartsch, L. Tomatis, and W. Davis, Eds., IARC Sci. Publ. No. 12, Lyon, 1976, pp. 181-210.
13. Margison, G. P., M. J. Capps, P. J. O'Connor, and A. W. Craig, Loss of 7-methylguanine from rat liver DNA after methylation in vivo with methylmethanesulphonate or dimethylnitrosamine, Chem. Biol. Interact., 6 (1973) 119-124.

14. Monesi, V., Autoradiographic study of DNA synthesis and the cell cycle in spermatogonia and spermatocytes of mouse testis using tritiated thymidine, J. Cell Biol., 14 (1962) 1-18.

15. Oakberg, E. F., A description of spermiogenesis in the mouse and its use in analysis of the cycle of the seminiferous epithelium and germ cell renewal, Am. J. Anat., 99 (1956) 391-414.

16. Oakberg, E. F., Duration of spermatogenesis in the mouse and timing of stages of the cycle of the seminiferous epithelium, Am. J. Anat., 99 (1956) 507-516.

17. Rasmussen, R. E., and R. B. Painter, Evidence for repair of ultraviolet damaged deoxyribonucleic acid in cultured mammalian cells, Nature, 203 (1964) 1360-1362.

18. Russell, L. B., Definition of functional units in a small chromosomal segment of the mouse and its use in interpreting the nature of radiation-induced mutations, Mutat. Res., 11 (1971) 107-123.

19. Russell, L. B., W. L. Russell and E. M. Kelly, Analysis of the albino-locus region of the mouse. I. Origin and viability, Genetics, 91 (1978) 127-139.

20. Russell, W. L., X-ray induced mutations in mice, Cold Spring Harbor Symp. Quant. Biol., 16 (1951) 327-336.

21. Schmid, B., I. P. Lee, and G. Zbinden, DNA repair processes in ejaculated sperms of rabbits treated with methyl methane-sulfonate, Arch. Toxicol., 40 (1978) 37-43.

22. Schröder, J. H., and O. Hug, Dominante Letalmutationen in der Nachkommenschaft bestrahlter männlicher Mäuse. I. Unter-suchung der Dosiswirkungsbeziehung und des Unterschiedes zwischen ganz-und Teilkorperbestrahlung bei metiotischen und postmeiotischen Keimzellenstadien, Mutat. Res., 11 (1971) 215-245.

23. Sega, G. A., Unscheduled DNA synthesis in the germ cells of male mice exposed in vivo to the chemical mutagen ethyl methanesulfonate, Proc. Natl. Acad. Sci. (U.S.), 71 (1974) 4955-4959.

24. Sega, G. A., Unpublished data.

25. Sega, G. A., R. B. Cumming, and M. F. Walton, Dosimetry studies on the ethylation of mouse sperm DNA after in vivo exposure to ^{3}H ethyl methanesulfonate, Mutat. Res., 24 (1974) 317-333.

26. Sega, G. A., J. G. Owens, and R. B. Cumming, Studies on DNA repair in early spermatid stages of male mice after in vivo treatment with methyl-, ethyl-, propyl-, and isopropyl methanesulfonate, Mutat. Res., 36 (1976) 193-212.

27. Sega, G. A., R. E. Sotomayor, and J. G. Owens, A study of unscheduled DNA synthesis induced by x-rays in the germ cells of male mice, Mutat. Res., 49 (1978) 239-257.

28. Sega, G. A., and J. G. Owens, Ethylation of DNA and protamine by ethyl methanesulfonate in the germ cells of male mice and the relevancy of these molecular targets to the induction of dominant lethals, Mutat. Res., 52 (1978) 87-106.

29. Sega, G. A., and R. E. Sotomayor, Unscheduled DNA synthesis in mammalian germ cells - its potential use in mutagenicity testing, in: Chemical Mutagens: Principles and Methods for their Detection, Vol. 7, F. J. de Serres, Ed., Plenum Press, New York, 1979, in press.

30. Sotomayor, R. E., G. A. Sega, and R. B. Cumming, Unscheduled DNA synthesis in spermatogenic cells of mice treated in vivo with the indirect alkylating agents cyclophosphamide and mitomen, Mutat. Res., 50 (1978) 229-240.

31. Sotomayor, R. E., G. A. Sega, and R. B. Cumming, An autoradiographic study of unscheduled DNA synthesis in the germ cells of male mice treated with x-rays and methyl methanesulfonate, Mutat. Res., 62 (1979) 293-309.

CHAPTER 27

RADIATION- AND DRUG-INDUCED DNA REPAIR IN MAMMALIAN OOCYTES

AND EMBRYOS

ROGER A. PEDERSEN and BRIGITTE BRANDRIFF

Laboratory of Radiobiology and Department of Anatomy
University of California, San Francisco, California
94143   (U.S.A.)

SUMMARY

A review of studies showing ultraviolet- or drug-induced unscheduled DNA synthesis in mammalian oocytes and embryos suggests
that the female gamete has an excision repair capacity from the
earliest stages of oocyte growth. The oocyte's demonstrable excision repair capacity decreases at the time of meiotic maturation
for unknown reasons, but the fully mature oocyte maintains a repair
capacity, in contrast to the mature sperm, and contributes this to
the zygote. Early embryo cells maintain relatively constant levels
of excision repair until late fetal stages, when they lose their
capacity for excision repair.

These apparent changes in excision repair capacity do not have
a simple relationship to known differences in radiation sensitivity
of germ cells and embryos.

INTRODUCTION

There is now direct and inferential evidence that male and
female germ cells of mammals are capable of repairing DNA damage
during gametogenesis. In males, repair has been demonstrated directly after ultraviolet (UV) or x-irradiation and after mutagen
treatment of early spermatogenic stages but has not been detected
in mature spermatozoa [12, 33, 43, 73, 74]. In females, repair of
UV damage has been observed at all stages of germ cell maturation.
We will review the evidence for repair in female mammalian germ cells
and in early embryos, with particular emphasis on the mouse, the
species used in most studies. Indirect evidence for repair

capability in oocytes comes from dose-fractionation studies of
specific locus mutations and dominant lethal effects. However, we
will primarily consider cases in which direct observations of unscheduled DNA synthesis after UV or drug treatment indicate a capacity for excision repair. We will also consider how changing repair
capacities compare to sensitivity for mutation induction or cell
killing in mammalian oocytes and embryos.

In classical work, Muller [57] determined that x-ray-damaged
chromosomes in Drosophila spermatozoa did not rejoin broken ends
before fertilization. Using similar split-dose studies, Dempster
[18], Kaufmann [40] and others [53] confirmed Muller's discovery
and concurred in suggesting that x-ray-induced breaks are rejoined
after fertilization; this has been further demonstrated by Würgler
and Maier [87]. In other early work Henshaw [37] showed that sea
urchin eggs recovered from x-ray-induced cleavage delay in proportion
to the time between irradiation and insemination with unirradiated
sperm. Failla [26] extended this work by showing that the similar
cleavage delay caused by irradiating sperm could be reduced exponentially by allowing sperm to reside in the egg for 20-100 min
before cleavage began. Failla [26, 27] concluded that a radiation
repair process occurs during sperm and egg recovery.

The initial evidence that mammalian oocytes were capable of
radiation repair was the discovery that mouse oocytes exposed to
chronic γ- or x-irradiation at low dose rates incurred substantially
fewer specific locus mutations than those exposed to equivalent acute
doses of x-rays [50, 70, 71]. Because there were no specific locus
mutations induced in mouse oocytes exposed to neutron radiation more
than 7 weeks before fertilization, Russell [69] suggested that early
oocytes may have a more efficient repair mechanism than later-stage
oocytes and spermatogonia [70, 72]. These early observations stimulated attempts to detect repair processes by direct observation of
mouse oocytes and early embryos.

                          OOGENESIS AND EMBRYOGENESIS

The general features of oogenesis and early embryogenesis are
similar in most mammalian species that have been studied. Primordial
germ cells differentiate in the extraembryonic mesoderm and are then
seen in yolk sac endoderm during early organogenesis [13]. They
subsequently migrate to the genital ridges via the hind gut endoderm
and mesentery, where they proliferate until the entire cohort of
spermatogonia or oogonia is produced. In female mice and rats,
these enter meiotic prophase relatively synchronously (after com-
pleting their last premeiotic S phase) at 15-16 days of gestation.
In males, initiation of meiosis occurs after birth. At birth,
mammalian ovaries contain the female's lifetime supply of oocytes.
In the mouse, these are initially "resting" or primordial dictyate

oocytes, but beginning in the first neonatal week and increasing
until the third week, large numbers of oocytes begin growth [63].
The resting oocytes continue to be recruited into growth as follicles
mature throughout the reproductive lifespan, although this occurs at
a lower rate with increasing age. In immature and pregnant mice,
the growing oocytes are not ovulated, but instead they degenerate
in large follicles (stage 5b); the time required for an oocyte to
develop from its recruitment into a growing follicle until ovulation
has been estimated at 19 days by labeling follicle cells [63] and at
6 weeks by labeling the zona pellucida [58]. In immature mice (0-35
days) there is extensive atresia, illustrated by the observation that
4,000-5,000 oocytes leave the resting pool but only about 850 develop
into oocytes in growing follicles [63]. By comparison, during the
period from 1 to 12 months, 4000-5000 oocytes leave the resting
oocyte pool and most of these enter the growth phase, although only
700-800 are actually ovulated in cycling mice [63]. In mature mice,
there are 100-300 growing oocytes at any time before 2 years of age,
when oocytes are depleted and ovulation ceases.

At ovulation, meiotic maturation occurs. The germinal vesicle,
which is about one-third the diameter of the oocyte, breaks down,
chromosomes condense into metaphase I of meiosis, and the first polar
body is emitted, with separation of homologous chromosomes; oocytes
progress to metaphase II, where they are arrested until fertilization. Oocytes acquire the capacity for spontaneous maturation in
chemically defined medium after they reach approximately 60 μm in
diameter [80]. During the entire growth period until meiotic maturation, the oocyte is capable of extensive RNA and protein synthesis
[55]. Despite a report that some oocyte DNA synthesis occurs after
birth [17], it seems likely that scheduled DNA synthesis in oocytes
occurs only before the beginning of meiosis [48].

Upon fertilization the fully grown oocyte, arrested in metaphase
II, emits the second polar body, separating chromatids. Male and
female pronuclei form within 10 hr, and DNA synthesis occurs [44,
49]. First cleavage takes place 18-24 hr after fertilization. In
the mouse, subsequent cleavages occur at approximately 10-hr intervals in vivo or slightly longer intervals in vitro, with asynchrony
appearing at the second cleavage [8, 41]. In late 8-cell-stage
embryos, cell boundaries become less distinct as the process of
compaction begins, coincident with the differentiation of cell contact and junctions [21]. This process continues at the morula (12-
to 16-cell) stage. Development of the blastocyst is apparent when
trophectoderm (outer cells) begin to secrete the blastocoel fluid.
At this stage the inner cell mass, which gives rise to the fetus,
can be clearly distinguished by light microscopy from the trophectoderm, which gives rise to the placenta. When placed in a suitable
nutritional environment in vitro the blastocyst attaches to the
substrate, and the trophectoderm transforms into a sheet of giant
trophoblast cells. This grows out on the substratum, leaving the

inner cell mass derivatives exposed directly to the culture medium
[86]. Both fetal and placental cells continue to proliferate and
differentiate in culture for approximately 1 week beyond the blastocyst stage and can develop into early organogenesis-stage embryos
with a beating heart and active circulatory system [39].

EVIDENCE FOR EXCISION REPAIR

UV irradiation can result in autoradiographically detectable
DNA synthesis in cells that are not in S phase. This "unscheduled"
DNA synthesis appears to reflect the removal and replacement of damaged bases, particularly thymine dimers [59]. The excision repair
system includes at least four enzyme activities, an endonuclease, an
exonuclease, a polymerase, and a ligase, to accomplish the repair
replication that is observed [77]. Because UV light and certain
mutagenic drugs induce substantial ("long-patch") repair reactions,
they have generally been used to determine the excision repair capacity of mouse oocytes and embryos. Evidence for unscheduled DNA synthesis in the mouse has been obtained by exposing various stages of
oocytes and embryos to 15-450 J/m^2 UV light from germicidal mercury
lamps (254 nm) and then culturing the cells in ^{3}H-thymidine and exposing them to autoradiographic emulsion for grain counting. We have
carried out a regression analysis of published data in order to estimate the response of various stages of oocytes and embryos to a UV
dose of 60 J/m^2 (Table 1). This procedure allowed a rough comparison
of data obtained with various dose regimens and autoradiographic exposure times, even though the small number of data points in each
study (one to six) limited the confidence that could be placed on
estimates from regression analysis. In this comparison we disre-
garded differences in labeling conditions, thymidine permeability,
and pool sizes because there were few data regarding the effect of
these parameters on grain counts in the stages of cells examined.
It is important to bear in mind that an accurate quantitative comparison of repair capacity between stages would require such information, and that the present comparisons are based only on available
data for grain counts, dose, and autoradiographic exposure time.

The earliest stage of oocyte that has been studied, and the
most important one from a genetic standpoint, is the resting or primordial oocyte. Pedersen and Mangia [62] obtained resting oocytes
from newborn female mice and irradiated them with 15-60 J/m^2 UV
light at a dose rate of 1.3 J/m^2/sec. The normalized value obtained
by regression analysis of their data was approximately 14 grains/day
of autoradiographic exposure for a dose of 60 J/m^2 (Fig. 1a; Fig.
2a-c). Growing oocytes (approximately 65 μm diameter) irradiated
with 60 J/m^2 showed much higher ^{3}H-thymidine incorporation, approximately 118 grains/day of autoradiographic exposure (Fig. 1b; Fig.
2d-f). Seeking an explanation for this large difference in incorporation between stages, Pedersen and Mangia [62] determined the

TABLE 1

UV-INDUCED DNA SYNTHESIS[a]

Stage	Response at 60 J/m^2			
	Observed grains	Grains from regression analysis[a]	Grains/Day[b]	Reference
Resting oocyte	216 ± 38	198	14	[62]
Growing oocyte	855 ± 53	827	118	[62]
Germinal vesicle stage	605 ± 114	544	39	[54]
	240 ± 12[c,d]		17	[10]
Metaphase I	77 ± 11	63	5	[54]
	100 ± 10[c,d]		7	[10]
Metaphase II	37 ± 11	36	3	[54]
	120[d]	77	5	[45]
	100 ± 10[c,d]		7	[10]
Morula	91 ± 7		4	[61]
Blastocyst	76 ± 6		4	[61]
Trophoblast	94 ± 7		5	[61]
Inner cell mass	46 ± 5		2	[61]

[a]To compare data in these studies we computed grain counts/day of autoradiographic exposure, based where possible on the regression of grains with dose. The correlation coefficient (r) was calculated for both linear (grains = m[dose] + b) and nonlinear (grains = b[dose]^m) regression to determine the best fit. A dose of 60 J/m^2 was used for comparison because this was the dose most commonly used.

[b]Data normalized to 1 day of autoradiographic exposure.

[c]Dose = 50 J/m^2.

[d]Data estimated from figures.

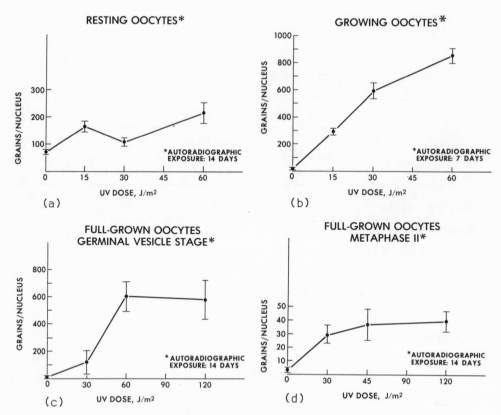

Fig. 1.   UV-induced unscheduled DNA synthesis in mouse oocytes:
(a) resting stage from [62];   (b) growing stage from [62];   (c) fully
grown germinal vesicle stage from [54];   (d) fully grown metaphase I
stage from [54].

Fig. 2.   Unscheduled DNA synthesis in mouse oocytes: (a) resting
oocyte (12-14 μm diameter), differential interference contrast
microscopy;   (b) autoradiograph of control resting oocyte, with
arrow indicating boundary of nucleus;   (c) autoradiograph of resting
oocyte exposed to 60 J/m² UV light;   (d) growing oocyte (60 μm
diameter), differential interference contrast microscopy;   (e) autoradiograph of control growing oocyte;   (f) autoradiograph of growing
oocyte exposed to 60 J/m² UV light.   Magnifications: a,d = 400×;
b,c,e,f = 512×.   Reprinted with permission from Pedersen and Mangia
[62].

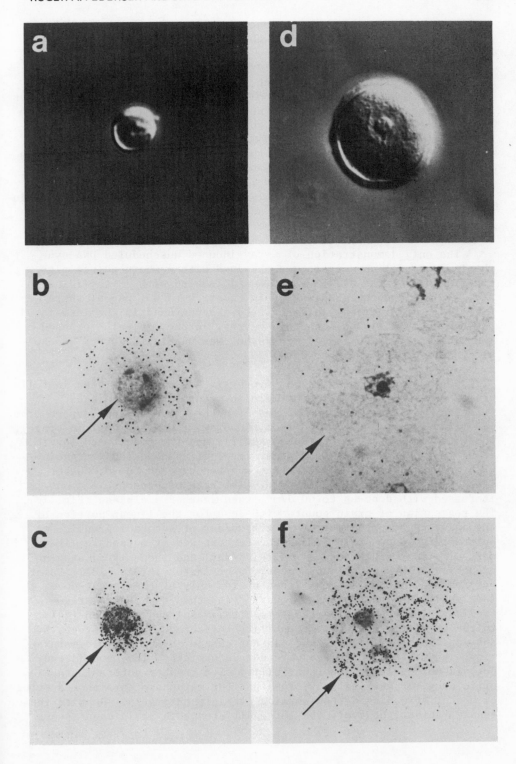

relative autoradiographic efficiency in the two stages by labeling oocytes with ^{3}H-thymidine during their premeiotic S phase. They found a 2.2-fold higher efficiency in the autoradiography of growing oocytes than of resting oocytes. Even correcting for this difference, however, they concluded that there was approximately a 6-fold greater ^{3}H-thymidine incorporation into UV-irradiated growing oocytes than in resting oocytes. Other factors that may have contributed to the observed difference, such as thymidine permeability, precursor pool size, and the extent of UV damage to DNA, were not evaluated. The most obvious changes between the resting and the growing oocytes are the large increases in cytoplasmic and nuclear radii. These changes may affect the dose of UV light received, and the 10-fold increase in nuclear volume probably reflects changes in the chromatin configuration and may affect the accessibility of DNA to repair enzymes, as discussed later.

The only demonstration of x-ray-induced unscheduled DNA synthesis in mammalian oocytes was obtained with newborn guinea pigs exposed to 5000 rad at 385 rad/min and labeled with ^{3}H-thymidine in vivo [16]. Although absolute grain counts were not given, there was a 2- to 3-fold increase in grains above background in the irradiated oocytes, but not in the control oocytes. Crone [16] also exposed mouse oocytes to 200 rad of x-rays but was unable to detect unscheduled DNA synthesis at that dose.

UV-induced unscheduled DNA synthesis has also been seen in fully grown mouse oocytes undergoing meiotic maturation. Masui and Pedersen [54] studied three stages of naturally ovulated oocytes from ICR mice, those just removed from the ovary (germinal vesicle stage), those cultured for 6-8 hr (metaphase I), and those cultured for 16-18 hr (metaphase II). The highest level of unscheduled synthesis occurred in germinal vesicle-stage oocytes exposed to 30, 60, or 120 J/m^2 UV light at 1.3 J/m^2/sec. In these oocytes grain count increased with dose up to 60 J/m^2, then reached a plateau (Fig. 1c). The regression of grain counts with dose for the linear portion of the curve gave approximately 39 grains/day of autoradiographic exposure for a dose of 60 J/m^2. Oocytes exposed at metaphase I had markedly lower grain counts (5 grains/day) and those irradiated at metaphase II had even lower counts (3 grains/day) (Fig. 1d). Polar body chromatin showed significant grains only at the lowest dose (30 J/m^2), and even then had fewer grains than any oocyte stage studied. In interpreting these results, Masui and Pedersen [54] ruled out differences in permeability to isotope between stages by showing that thymidine uptake did not change during meiotic maturation; thymidine pool sizes were not determined. They considered, but did not evaluate, the possibility of a greater autoradiographic efficiency for germinal vesicles than for metaphase chromosomes owing to better spreading of the germinal vesicle chromatin. Despite these considerations, however, the large difference in grain count seems

to indicate a substantial decrease in the oocyte's capacity for unscheduled DNA synthesis at the time of germinal vesicle breakdown.

In another study, Ku et al. [45] irradiated metaphase II oocytes
obtained by superovulation of (C3H × DBA 2) F_1 mice. Oocytes were
exposed to 30-450 J/m^2 at 2, 5.2, or 15 J/m^2/sec and cultured in
^3H-thymidine of unspecified concentration or specific activity. At
the lowest dose rate they found 5 grains per oocyte chromosome set/
day of exposure (estimated for a dose of 60 J/m^2 from doses 1-120
J/m^2 in their figure). They carried out DNAse controls to show that
grains were indeed contained in the DNA. At the higher dose rates
they found significantly lower grain counts but could not account
for this difference.

Recently, Brazill and Masui [10] studied UV- and drug-induced
unscheduled DNA synthesis in random-bred CBL mouse oocytes using an
experimental design that reduced the variation due to autoradiographic efficiency. After exposing oocytes at the germinal vesicle,
metaphase I, or metaphase II stage, they cultured them for 2 hr in
^3H-thymidine followed by a cold thymidine chase and then continued
the incubation in unlabeled medium until the oocytes reached metaphase II, when they were fixed for autoradiography. Oocytes exposed
at the germinal vesicle stage to a single UV dose (50 J/m^2, dose rate
not given) had 17 grains/day; when exposed at metaphase I or metaphase II they had 7 grains/day. This confirmed Masui and Pedersen's
finding [54] of a decrease in unscheduled DNA synthesis during
meiotic maturation. Brazill and Masui [10] showed that this change
was not due to differential autoradiographic efficiency because they
performed all grain counts on metaphase II chromosomes, regardless
of the stage exposed. They also confirmed the very low level of
unscheduled DNA synthesis when the first polar body was irradiated
(at metaphase II) but showed that the polar body had grain counts
comparable to the oocyte when irradiation and ^3H-thymidine incorporation occurred before polar body formation (germinal vesicle or
metaphase I stage).

Further insight into the polar body's deficiencies came from
Brazill and Masui's data [10] on oocytes treated with drugs. They
exposed germinal vesicle, metaphase I, or metaphase II oocytes to
either 10^{-5} M 4-nitroquinoline 1-oxide (4NQO) or 10^{-3} M methyl
methanesulfonate (MMS). The 4NQO treatment of germinal vesicle-
stage oocytes induced 6 grains/day of autoradiographic exposure and
induced fewer grains at metaphase I and II stages and in the polar
body. The MMS treatment, however, induced approximately the same
level of grains at all oocyte stages and in the polar body, 1 grain/
day of autoradiographic exposure. There were essentially no grains
on control oocytes after correction for background. Citing unpublished data that showed similar grain counts in oocytes and polar
bodies when eggs were irradiated at the germinal vesicle stage and
labeled with ^3H-thymidine at metaphase II, they proposed that the

decreased capacity for unscheduled DNA synthesis in polar bodies
treated with UV or 4NQO is due to loss of an endonuclease activity.
Although there is no direct evidence that oocytes are deficient for
this enzyme activity, their observation that MMS induced similar
levels of unscheduled DNA synthesis in both oocytes and polar bodies
indicates that the polar body is deficient for an early step in excision repair. In this regard the polar body resembles xeroderma
pigmentosum cells, which cannot repair UV damage but can carry out
unscheduled DNA synthesis in response to damage by MMS and other
agents that induce short-patch repair [14, 65, 76].

A change in capacity for carrying out early steps in excision
repair may also account for the large decrease in oocyte unscheduled
DNA synthesis between the germinal vesicle stage and metaphase I or
II. This interpretation is supported by the observation that MMS-
induced repair in oocyte DNA remains unchanged during oocyte maturation [10]. This point could be resolved with additional data from
other agents that induce short-patch repair, such as x-rays or ethyl
methanesulfonate [65].

The change in oocyte organization at the time of germinal
vesicle breakdown could also contribute to the observed differences
in repair activity. The contents of the germinal vesicle, which
occupy approximately 1/27 the volume of the oocyte, may be correspondingly diluted or redistributed upon germinal vesicle breakdown.
Despite the observed decrease in unscheduled DNA synthesis during
meiotic maturation, the remaining capacity in the meiotically mature
metaphase II oocyte, or unfertilized egg, raises the possibility that
egg cytoplasm may confer a repair capacity on the repair-incompetent
male gamete after fertilization.

Our own recent work has revealed a capacity for unscheduled DNA
synthesis in pronuclear-stage mouse embryos irradiated with UV light
[9]. Embryos from ICR mice were exposed to 15–60 J/m^2 UV light
several hours after sperm penetration, then labeled with ^{3}H-thymidine
and fixed for autoradiography at the pronuclear stage. After a
2-week exposure to emulsion, both pronuclei showed dose-dependent
increases in grain counts similar to the grain numbers of irradiated,
unfertilized metaphase II oocytes (approximately 3 grains/day at
60 J/m^2). These results indicate a capacity for excision repair
during the interval between sperm penetration and the first embryonic
S phase.

In an earlier attempt to determine whether mouse egg cytoplasm
was able to repair drug-induced damage to sperm DNA, Sega et al.
[75] examined eggs fertilized by sperm of MMS-treated males but found
no autoradiographic evidence for unscheduled DNA synthesis. Differences in procedures, including mode of damage and strain of mice,
may account for our different findings. Using another approach,
Generoso et al. [31, 32] have inferred that repair of alkylation

damage in sperm DNA occurs after fertilization in some strains of mice (see below).

The excision repair capacity of other preimplantation and early postimplantation-stage mouse embryos was studied by Pedersen and Cleaver [61] (Fig. 3). They irradiated embryos with 60 J/m^2 UV light at 1.3 J/m^2/sec and found the following grain counts/day of exposure: morula, 4; blastocyst, 4; postimplantation trophoblast, 5; and postimplantation inner cell mass, 2. Unlike oocytes, embryos had S phase nuclei at all stages studied, particularly in the early cleavage stages. The preponderance of S phase nuclei in 8-cell and earlier stages made it difficult to analyze cleavage-stage embryos for their repair capability [60]. Nevertheless, because similar levels of unscheduled DNA synthesis were observed in pronuclear embryos and morulae, it seems likely that early cleavage-stage embryos also have an excision repair capacity.

In their study of mouse fetal stages, Peleg et al. [64] assessed excision repair and unscheduled DNA synthesis in primary cultures initiated at 13-15 or 17-19 days of gestation. At the first and second transfers 13- to 15-day fetal cells excise 50% of UV-induced thymine dimers within 24 hr; this decreased to 4% of dimers by the ninth transfer. Autoradiographically detected unscheduled DNA synthesis showed similar decreases during successive transfers. Cells grown from 17- to 19-day fetuses did not show excision repair in the first or subsequent transfers and had low levels of unscheduled DNA synthesis. These observations suggest that the low levels of excision repair seen in adult mouse cells, as compared with other mammalian species, are the result of a developmentally regulated decline, rather than an inherently low level of excision repair in mice [7, 36, 47, 59].

OTHER EVIDENCE FOR REPAIR

In addition to the dose-rate effects for mutation induction cited earlier, inferential evidence for repair in oocytes and embryos comes from studies of chromosome aberrations, dominant lethality, and embryo radiosensitivity. Brewen et al. [11] measured aberrations in metaphase I chromosomes of CD1/CR mouse oocytes irradiated 8-14 days earlier with different x-ray dose regimens and found a clear dose-rate effect for deletions and exchanges. They concluded that the different rates of aberrations caused by similar doses of chronic and acute x-rays indicate a 2-track process. Furthermore, by fractionating the acute dose they demonstrated recovery within 135 min after exposure to 200 rad of x-rays; they also concluded that this recovery or repair process was not significantly altered by increasing the initial dose from 100 to 300 rad.

Fig. 3.   Unscheduled DNA synthesis in mouse embryos: (a) morula
stage of a pre-implantation mouse embryo cultured from the 2-cell
stage, differential interference contrast;   (b) autoradiographs of
S phase and interphase nuclei of control morula;   (c) autoradiographs of S phase and interphase nuclei of a UV-irradiated morula;
(d) blastocyst stage preimplantation mouse embryo cultured from the
2-cell stage, differential interference contrast;   (e) autoradiographs of S phase and interphase nuclei of control blastocyst;
(f) autoradiographs of S phase and interphase nuclei of UV-irradiated
blastocyst.   Magnifications: a,d = 600×; b,c,e,f, = 720×.   Reprinted with permission from Pedersen and Cleaver [61].

Using another approach Generoso et al. [31] combined cytogenetic
analysis of metaphase I chromosomes and dominant lethal analysis of
embryos obtained from matings between mutagen-treated (101 × C3H) F_1
males and various strains of females. They found that matings with
T stock females produced higher rates of isopropyl methanesulfonate-
induced dominant lethality and chromatid aberrations than matings
with other strains. They concluded that these differences were due
to strain differences in capacity for repair of alkylation damage in
pronuclear stage embryos. Interestingly, there were no strain differences with x-ray-induced damage and less obvious differences with
ethyl methanesulfonate, triethylenemelamine, and benzo(a)pyrene,
suggesting that if repair is responsible for the maternal species-
specific response, then different lesions have unique effects in
the oocyte and early embryo and may be handled by different repair
enzymes [32].

In an attempt to detect postreplication repair in early embryos
Eibs and Spielmann [25, 81] treated UV-irradiated NMRI mouse embryos
with 0.1-0.5 mM caffeine. Although these concentrations of caffeine
had no detrimental effect on control mouse embryo development in
vitro to the blastocyst stage, caffeine potentiated the inhibitory
effects of UV irradiation. The authors concluded that there is a
capacity for postreplication repair in the preimplantation mouse
embryo. This is the only report of such a capability in mammalian
germ cells or embryos.

The ability of rat blastocysts to recover from damage induced
by x-rays, γ-rays, and helium ions has been deduced from studies of
delayed-implanting embryos. In these studies there was a reduction
in embryo killing when delayed-implanting embryos were irradiated
2 days or more before implantation was induced; the survival rates
returned to normal levels, although fetal weights (and, in some
cases, placental weights) were reduced [38, 82-85]. Because these

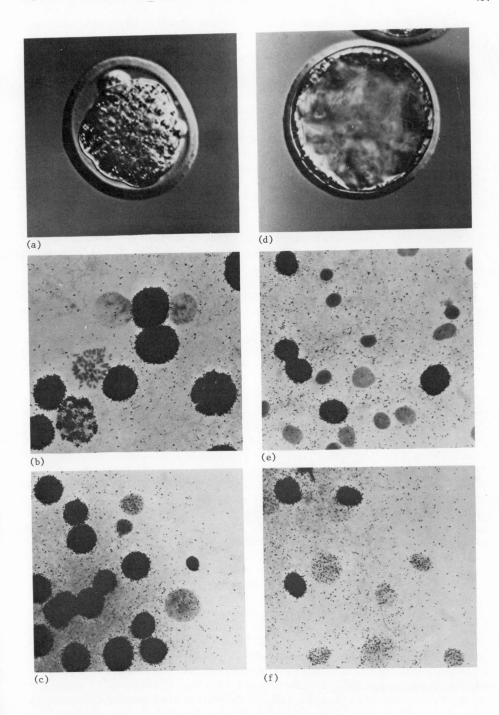

(a)

(d)

(b)

(e)

(c)

(f)

studies were carried out in utero, the recovery phenomenon may include maternal tissues as well as embryonic cells.

RADIATION SENSITIVITY OF OOCYTES AND EMBRYOS

The effects of radiation on mammalian oocytes and embryos are
complex. They vary between species and between strains and depend
on age and stage of meiosis or mitosis. In addition, physical factors such as temperature, oxygen tension, and type and method of
irradiation influence the outcome of exposure. For a meaningful
discussion of radiosensitivity, it is important to specify which
criterion is used for assessing effects [2, 4, 53].

Primordial oocytes are more sensitive to killing by x-irradiation than later stages of oocytes in the juvenile and adult rat and
mouse. Degenerative changes become apparent 3-6 hr after exposure,
and by 18 hr most affected oocytes have died. Exposure to 300 rad
destroyed nearly the entire population of primordial oocytes in
adult rats [52]. The greatest sensitivity to radiation killing of
mouse oocytes occurs during the third week after birth, when a dose
of 20 rad leaves only 1% of the oocytes intact. In addition to
x-rays, tritium and aromatic hydrocarbons also have lethal effects
on primordial mouse oocytes [3, 19], with a peak sensitivity at 2-3
weeks after birth [20, 28].

With dominant lethality as the criterion of damage, oocytes are
most sensitive during metaphase I of meiosis [24, 51, 68]. Mouse
oocytes are more sensitive for specific locus mutation induction at
growing and fully grown stages than at resting stages, as discussed
previously.

Irradiation of pregnant mice during preimplantation stages results in extensive embryo death, but no malformations are induced in
embryos that survive to birth [67]. As judged by comparing subsequent preimplantation development, pronuclear stages of the mouse
are more sensitive than 2-cell stages to UV and x-irradiation [23,
25, 46]. One possible explanation for the considerable variability
in studies of early mouse embryos might be the differential sensitivity of embryos as they progress through the cell cycle [22, 35,
66]. Sensitivity is high shortly after fertilization and at early
pronuclear stages and becomes lower in later pronuclear stages;
early 2-cell stages are relatively resistant compared to 2-cell
stages just before the second cleavage [66]. It seems likely that
similar variations in radiosensitivity occur also at later stages,
when cleavage is asynchronous and the contribution of the cell cycle
differences to overall radiosensitivity cannot be readily determined.
Irradiation at later stages indicates decreasing sensitivity to UV
at the 8-cell stage [25] and complex changes in the sensitivity to
x rays [1, 29, 34, 42]. Cells giving rise to the inner cell mass

are more susceptible to tritium and x-ray damage than precursors of trophoblast [34, 79].

Given the large number of variables in the studies described here it is difficult to ascertain the role of DNA repair in the radiation sensitivity in mammalian oocytes and embryos. The extreme sensitivity of early oocytes to cell killing occurs at a time of moderate excision repair capacity. The increase in sensitivity to specific locus mutation induction, which occurs as oocytes develop, coincides with an apparent increase in excision repair capacity. A change in opposite directions would be expected if repair capacity alone accounted for the mutation data. The increase in dominant lethal induction that occurs during meiotic maturation coincides with an apparent decrease in excision repair. Before attributing causality to this coincidence, however, we should consider the possibility that both excision repair and dominant lethality are regulated by other properties in the maturing oocyte. Finally, the changes in radiation sensitivity during early embryo development occur during a time of relatively constant excision repair capability.

CONCLUSIONS

A review of studies showing UV- or drug-induced unscheduled DNA synthesis in mammalian oocytes and embryos suggests that the female gamete has an excision repair capacity from the earliest stages of oocyte growth. The oocyte's demonstrable excision repair capacity decreases at the time of meiotic maturation for unknown reasons, but the fully mature oocyte maintains a repair capacity in contrast to the mature sperm and contributes this to the zygote. Early embryos maintain relatively constant levels of excision repair until late fetal stages, when primary fibroblast cultures, at least, lose their capacity for excision repair.

It must be borne in mind that this comparison between stages rests on several unverified assumptions, including constant thymidine pool sizes, permeability, and a constant relationship between autoradiographically demonstrated unscheduled DNA synthesis and excision repair. Furthermore, because unscheduled DNA synthesis is usually measured after UV irradiation, there is little information about the oocyte or embryo's ability to repair other types of lesions, such as those induced by drugs or ionizing radiation. Thus it is not surprising that oocyte and embryo radiosensitivity appears not to be related to repair capacity. Sega et al. [75] recently came to a similar conclusion about the relationship between excision repair and radiosensitivity in male germ cells.

Although the role of repair processes in mutation induction and cell killing is unclear, some avenues for further research are open. The analysis of different types of excision repair processes and even specific enzyme activities is imperative if we are to understand the role of repair in the quantitative relationship between damage and mutation induction. Long-patch and short-patch repair involve different enzyme activities [65], and additional enzymes are involved in repairing base damage [30].

In addition, the role of chromatin compaction in repair needs to be clarified, particularly for germ cells. Recent reports [6, 15, 78] indicate that the excision repair that occurs after UV irradiation or treatment with alkylating agents is in the linker regions between nucleosomes at early times after treatment. The inaccessibility of DNA to repair enzymes may also be involved in some complementation groups of xeroderma pigmentosum because repair-deficient cell lines can remove thymine dimers from purified DNA but not from chromatin [56]. It is interesting in this regard that mouse oocyte chromatin is organized into nucleosomes [5].

Our ultimate concern is the relevance of repair in model mammalian systems to human cells. This is important for establishing risks of environmental radiation and chemical exposure of human beings. A thorough understanding of agent-specific and strain-specific variability in repair processes in model rodent systems will go a long way toward determining the effectiveness of DNA repair in alleviating human genetic hazards.

ACKNOWLEDGEMENTS

We thank Ms. Mary McKenney and Ms. Naomi Sinai for assistance with the manuscript, and Dr. William Bodell for his comments. This work was supported by the U.S. Department of Energy.

REFERENCES

1. Alexandre, H. L., Effects of x-irradiation on preimplantation mouse embryos cultured in vitro, J. Reprod. Fert., 36 (1974) 417-420.
2. Baker, T. G., Radiosensitivity of mammalian oocytes with particular reference to the human female, Am. J. Obstet. Gynecol., 110 (1971) 746-761.
3. Baker, T. G., and A. McLaren, The effect of tritiated thymidine on the developing oocytes of mice, J. Reprod. Fert., 34 (1973) 121-130.

4. Baker, T. G., and P. Neal, Action of ionizing radiations on the
    mammalian ovary, In: The Ovary, Ed. 2, Vol. 3, Regulation of
    Oogenesis and Steroidogenesis, L. Zuckerman and B. J. Weir,
    Eds., Academic Press, New York, 1977, pp. 1-58.
5. Bakken, A., Unpublished data.
6. Bodell, W. J., and M. R. Banerjee, The influence of chromatin
    structure on the distribution of DNA repair synthesis studied
    by nuclease digestion, Nucl. Acids Res., 6 (1979) 359-370.
7. Bowden, G. T., J. E. Trosko, B. G. Shapas, and R. K. Boutwell,
    Excision of pyrimidine dimers from epidermal DNA and non-
    semiconservative epidermal DNA synthesis following ultra-
    violet irradiation of mouse skin, Cancer Res., 35 (1975)
    3599-3607.
8. Bowman, P., and A. McLaren, Cleavage rate of mouse embryos in
    vivo and in vitro, J. Embryol. Exptl. Morphol., 24 (1970)
    203-207.
9. Brandriff, B., and R. A. Pedersen, Unpublished data.
10. Brazill, J. L., and Y. Masui, Changing levels of UV light and
    carcinogen-induced unscheduled DNA synthesis in mouse oocytes
    during meiotic maturation, Exptl. Cell Res., 112 (1978)
    121-125.
11. Brewen, J. G., H. S. Payne, and I. D. Adler, X-ray-induced
    chromosome aberrations in mouse dictyate oocytes, II. Frac-
    tionation and dose rate effects, Genetics, 87 (1977) 699-708.
12. Chandley, A. C., and S. Kofman-Alfaro, "Unscheduled" DNA syn-
    thesis in human germ cells following UV irradiation, Exptl.
    Cell Res. 69 (1971) 45-48.
13. Chiquoine, A. D., The identification, origin, and migration of
    the primordial germ cells in the mouse embryo, Anat. Rec.
    118 (1954) 135-146.
14. Cleaver, J. E., DNA repair with purines and pyrimidines in
    radiation- and carcinogen-damaged normal and xeroderma
    pigmentosum human cells, Cancer Res., 33 (1973) 362-369.
15. Cleaver, J. E., Nucleosome structure controls rates of excision
    repair in DNA of human cells, Nature, 270 (1977) 451-453.
16. Crone, M., Radiation stimulated incorporation of ^{3}H-thymidine
    into diplotene oocytes of the guinea-pig, Nature, 228 (1970)
    460.
17. Crone, M., and H. Peters, Unusual incorporation of tritiated
    thymidine into early diplotene oocytes of mice, Exptl. Cell
    Res., 50 (1968) 664-668.
18. Dempster, E. R., Absence of a time factor in the production of
    translocations in Drosophila sperm by x-irradiation, Am.
    Naturalist, 75 (1941) 184-187.
19. Dobson, R. L., and M. F. Cooper, Tritium toxicity: effect of
    low-level ^{3}HOH exposure on developing female germ cells in
    the mouse, Rad. Res., 58 (1974) 91-100.

20. Dobson, R. L., C. G. Koehler, J. S. Felton, T. C. Kwan, B. J.
    Wuebbles, and D. C. L. Jones, Vulnerability of female germ
    cells in developing mice and monkeys to tritium, gamma rays,
    and polycyclic aromatic hydrocarbons, In: Developmental
    Toxicology of Energy-Related Pollutants, U.S. Department of
    Energy Symposium Series, 47 (1978) 1-14.

21. Ducibella, T., D. F. Albertini, E. Anderson, and J. D. Biggers,
    The preimplantation mammalian embryos: characterization of
    intercellular junctions and their appearance during develop-
    ment, Dev. Biol., 45 (1975) 231-250.

22. DuFrain, R. J., The effects of ionizing radiation on preimplan-
    tation mouse embyros developing in vitro. In: Workshop on
    Basic Aspects of Freeze Preservation of Mouse Strains,
    O. Mühlbock, Ed., Gustav Fischer Verlag, Stuttgart, 1976,
    pp. 73-84.

23. DuFrain, R. J., and A. P. Casarett, Response of the pronuclear
    mouse embryo to x-irradiation in vitro, Rad. Res., 63 (1975)
    494-500.

24. Edwards, R. G., and A. G. Searle, Genetic radiosensitivity of
    specific post-dictyate stages in mouse oöcytes, Genet. Res.,
    4 (1963) 389-398.

25. Eibs, H.-G., and H. Spielmann, Differential sensitivity of pre-
    implantation mouse embryos to UV irradiation in vitro and
    evidence for post-replication repair, Rad. Res., 71 (1977)
    367-376.

26. Failla, P. M., Recovery from radiation-induced delay of cleavage
    in gametes of Arbacia punctulata, Science, 138 (1962)
    1341-1342.

27. Failla, P. M., Recovery from division delay in irradiated
    gametes of Arbacia punctulata, Rad. Res., 25 (1965) 331-340.

28. Felton, J. S., T. C. Kwan, B. J. Wuebbles, and R. L. Dobson,
    Genetic differences in polycyclic-aromatic-hydrocarbon
    metabolism and their effects on oocyte killing in developing
    mice, In: Developmental Toxicology of Energy-Related Pollu-
    tants, U.S. Department of Energy Symposium Series, 47 (1978)
    15-26.

29. Fisher, D. L., and M. Smithberg, In vitro and in vivo x-irrad-
    iation of preimplantation mouse embryos, Teratology, 7
    (1973) 57-64.

30. Reynolds, R. J., and E. C. Friedberg, Molecular mechanism of
    pyrimidine dimer excision in Saccharomyces cerevisiae.
    I. Studies with intact cells and cell-free systems, This
    volume, p. 121.

31. Generoso, W. M., Repair in fertilized eggs of mice and its
    role in the production of chromosomal aberrations, This
    volume, p. 411.

32. Generoso, W. M., K. T. Cain, M. Krishna, and S. W. Huff, Genetic lesions induced by chemicals in spermatozoa and spermatids of mice are repaired in the egg, Proc. Natl. Acad. Sci. (U.S.), 76 (1979) 435-437.

33. Gledhill, B. L., and Z. Darzynkiewicz, Unscheduled synthesis of DNA during mammalian spermatogenesis in response to UV irradiation, J. Exptl. Zool., 183 (1973) 375-382.

34. Goldstein, L. S., A. I. Spindle, and R. A. Pedersen, X-ray sensitivity of the preimplantation mouse embryo in vitro, Rad. Res., 62 (1975) 276-287.

35. Hamilton, L., The influence of the cell cycle on the radiation response of early embryos, In: The Cell Cycle in Development and Differentiation, M. Balls and F. S. Billett, Eds., Cambridge University Press, 1973.

36. Hart, R. W., and R. B. Setlow, Correlation between deoxyribonucleic acid excision-repair and life-span in a number of mammalian species, Proc. Natl. Acad. Sci. (U.S.), 71 (1974) 2169-2173.

37. Henshaw, P. S., Studies of the effect of roentgen rays on the time of the first cleavage in some marine invertebrate eggs. I. Recovery from roentgen-ray effects in Arbacia eggs, Am. J. Roentgenol., 27 (1932) 890-898.

38. Hooverman, L. L., R. K. Meyer, and R. C. Wolf, Recovery from x-ray irradiation injury during delayed implantation in the rat, J. Endocrinol., 41 (1968) 75-84.

39. Hsu, Y.-C., In vitro development of individually cultured whole mouse embryos from blastocyst to early somite stage, Dev. Biol. 68 (1979) 453-461.

40. Kaufmann, B. P., The time interval between x-radiation of sperm of Drosophila and chromosome recombination, Proc. Natl. Acad. Sci. (U.S.), 27 (1941) 18-24.

41. Kelly, S. J., J. G. Mulnard, and C. F. Graham, Cell division and cell allocation in early mouse development, J. Embryol. Exptl. Morphol., 48 (1978) 37-51.

42. Kirkpatrick, J. F., Radiation induced abnormalities in early in vitro mouse embryos, Anat. Rec., 176 (1973) 397-403.

43. Kofman-Alfaro, S., and A. C. Chandley, Radiation-initiated DNA synthesis in spermatogenic cells of the mouse, Exptl. Cell Res., 69 (1971) 33-44.

44. Krishna, M., and W. M. Generoso, Timing of sperm penetration, pronuclear formation, pronuclear DNA synthesis, and first cleavage in naturally ovulated mouse eggs, J. Exptl. Zool., 202 (1977) 245-252.

45. Ku, K. Y., L. A. Moustafa, and P. Voytek, Induced DNA repair synthesis by ultraviolet radiation in mature mouse oocytes arrested in metaphase, II, IRCS Med. Sci., 3 (1975) 607.

46. Ku, K. Y., and P. Voytek, The effects of U.V.-light, ionizing radiation and the carcinogen N-acetoxy-2-fluorenylacetamide on the development in vitro of one- and two-cell mouse embryos, Intern. J. Rad. Biol., 30 (1976) 401-408.

47. Lieberman, M. W., and P. D. Forbes, Demonstration of DNA repair
     in normal and neoplastic tissues after treatment with proxi-
     mate chemical carcinogens and ultraviolet radiation, Nature,
     241 (1973) 199-201.
48. Lima-de-Faria, A., and K. Borum, The period of DNA synthesis
     prior to meiosis in the mouse, J. Cell Biol., 14 (1962)
     381-388.
49. Luthardt, F. W., and R. P. Donahue, Pronuclear DNA synthesis
     in mouse eggs: an autoradiographic study, Exptl. Cell Res.,
     82 (1973) 143-151.
50. Lyon, M. F., and R. J. S. Phillips, Specific locus mutation
     rates after repeated small radiation doses to mouse oocytes,
     Mutat. Res., 30 (1975) 375-382.
51. Lyon, M. F., and B. D. Smith, Species comparisons concerning
     radiation-induced dominant lethals and chromosome aberra-
     tions, Mutat. Res., 11 (1971) 45-58.
52. Mandl, A. M., A quantitative study of the sensitivity of oocytes
     to x-irradiation, Proc. Roy. Soc. (London), B150 (1959)
     53-71.
53. Mandl, A. M., The radiosensitivity of germ cells, Biol. Rev.,
     39 (1964) 288-371.
54. Masui, Y., and R. A. Pedersen, Ultraviolet light-induced un-
     scheduled DNA synthesis in mouse oocytes during meiotic
     maturation, Nature, 257 (1975) 705-706.
55. Moor, R. M., and G. M. Warnes, Regulation of meiosis in mammal-
     ian oocytes, Brit. Med. Bull., 35 (1979) 99-103.
56. Mortelmans, K., E. C. Friedberg, H. Slor, G. Thomas, and J. E.
     Cleaver, Defective thymine dimer excision by cell-free ex-
     tracts of xeroderma pigmentosum cells, Proc. Natl. Acad.
     Sci. (U.S.), 73 (1976) 2757-2761.
57. Muller, H. J., An analysis of the process of structural change
     in chromosomes of Drosophila, J. Genet., 40 (1940) 1-66.
58. Oakberg, E. F., Timing of oocyte maturation in the mouse and
     its relevance to radiation-induced cell killing and muta-
     tional sensitivity, Mutat. Res., 59 (1979) 39-48.
59. Painter, R. B., and J. E. Cleaver, Repair replication, un-
     scheduled DNA synthesis, and the repair of mammalian DNA,
     Rad. Res., 37 (1969) 451-466.
60. Pedersen, R. A., Unpublished data.
61. Pedersen, R. A., and J. E. Cleaver, Repair of UV damage to DNA
     of implantation-stage mouse embryos in vitro, Exptl. Cell
     Res., 95 (1975) 247-253.
62. Pedersen, R. A., and F. Mangia, Ultraviolet-light-induced un-
     scheduled DNA synthesis by resting and growing mouse oocytes,
     Mutat. Res., 49 (1978) 425-429.
63. Pedersen, T., Follicle growth in the mouse ovary, In: Oogenesis,
     J. D. Biggers and A. W. Schuetz, Eds., University Park Press,
     Baltimore, 1972, pp. 361-376.

64. Peleg, L., E. Raz, and R. Ben-Ishai, Changing capacity for DNA excision repair in mouse embryonic cells in vitro, Exptl. Cell Res., 104 (1976) 301-307.

65. Regan, J. D., and R. B. Setlow, Two forms of repair in the DNA of human cells damaged by chemical carcinogens and mutagens, Cancer Res., 34 (1974) 3318-3325.

66. Russell, L. B., and C. S. Montgomery, Radiation-sensitivity differences within cell-division cycles during mouse cleavage, Intern. J. Rad. Biol., 10 (1966) 151-164.

67. Russell, L. B., and W. L. Russell, An analysis of the changing radiation response of the developing mouse embryo, J. Cell Comp. Physiol., 43 (Suppl. 1) (1954) 103-149.

68. Russell, L. B., and W. L. Russell, The sensitivity of different stages in oogenesis to the radiation induction of dominant lethals and other changes in the mouse, In: Progress in Radiobiology, Proceedings of the Fourth International Conference on Radiobiology, J. S. Mitchell, B. E. Holmes, and C. L. Smith, Eds., Oliver and Boyd, Edinburgh, 1956, pp. 187-192.

69. Russell, W. L., Effect of the interval between irradiation and conception on mutation frequency in female mice, Proc. Natl. Acad. Sci. (U.S.), 54 (1965) 1552-1557.

70. Russell, W. L., L. B. Russell, and E. M. Kelly, Radiation dose rate and mutation frequency, Science, 128 (1958) 1546-1550.

71. Russell, W. L., L. B. Russell, and E. M. Kelly, Dependence of mutation rate on radiation intensity, In: Symposium on the Immediate and Low Level Effects of Ionizing Radiations, A. A. Buzzati-Traverso, Ed., Taylor and Francis, London, 1960, pp. 311-319.

72. Searle, A. G., Mutation induction in mice, In: Advances in Radiation Biology, Vol. 4, J. T. Lett, H. Adler, and M. Zelle, Eds., Academic Press, New York, 1974, pp. 131-207.

73. Sega, G. A., Unscheduled DNA synthesis in the germ cells of male mice exposed in vivo to the chemical mutagen ethyl methanesulfonate, Proc. Natl. Acad. Sci (U.S.), 71 (1974) 4955-4959.

74. Sega, G. A., Relationship between unscheduled DNA synthesis and mutation induction in male mice, This volume, p. 373.

75. Sega, G. A., R. E. Sotomayor, and J. G. Owens, A study of unscheduled DNA synthesis induced by x-rays in the germ cells of male mice, Mutat. Res., 49 (1978) 239-257.

76. Setlow, R. B., Repair deficient human disorders and cancer, Nature, 271 (1978) 713-717.

77. Setlow, R. B., DNA repair pathways, This volume, p. 45.

78. Smerdon, M. J., T. D. Tlsty, and M. W. Lieberman, Distribution of ultraviolet-induced DNA repair synthesis in nuclease sensitive and resistant regions of human chromatin, Biochemistry, 17 (1978) 2377-2386.

79. Snow, M. H. L., Abnormal development of pre-implantation mouse
     embryos grown in vitro with [^{3}H]thymidine, J. Embryol.
     Exptl. Morphol., 29 (1973) 601-615.
80. Sorensen, R. A., and P. M. Wassarman, Relationship between
     growth and meiotic maturation of the mouse oocyte, Dev.
     Biol., 50 (1976) 531-536.
81. Spielmann, H., and H.-G. Eibs, Recent progress in teratology:
     a survey of methods for the study of drug actions during
     the preimplantation period, Arzneim. Forsch., 28 (1978)
     1733-1742.
82. Ward, W. F., H. Aceto, Jr., and M. Sandusky, Repair of sublethal
     and potentially lethal radiation damage by rat embryos ex-
     posed to gamma rays or helium ions, Radiology, 120 (1976)
     695-700.
83. Ward, W. F., R. K. Meyer, and R. C. Wolf, Recovery from lethal
     x-ray damage during delayed implantation in the rat,
     J. Endocrinol., 51 (1971) 657-663.
84. Ward, W. F., R. K. Meyer, and R. C. Wolf, Differential radio-
     sensitivity of rat blastocysts during delayed implantation,
     Proc. Soc. Exptl. Biol. Med., 140 (1973) 797-801.
85. Ward, W. F., R. K. Meyer, and R. C. Wolf, DNA synthesis in rat
     blastocysts x-irradiated during delayed implantation, Rad.
     Res., 55 (1973) 189-196.
86. Wiley, L. M., and R. A. Pedersen, Morphology of mouse egg
     cylinder development in vitro: a light and electron micro-
     scopic study, J. Exptl. Zool., 200 (1977) 389-402.
87. Würgler, F. E., and P. Maier, Genetic control of mutation
     induction in Drosophila melanogaster, I. Sex-chromosome
     loss in x-rayed mature sperm, Mutat. Res., 15 (1972) 41-53.

CHAPTER 28

REPAIR IN FERTILIZED EGGS OF MICE AND ITS ROLE IN THE

PRODUCTION OF CHROMOSOMAL ABERRATIONS

WALDERICO M. GENEROSO

Biology Division, Oak Ridge National Laboratory
Oak Ridge, Tennessee   37830 (U.S.A.)

SUMMARY

The fertilized egg may influence the yield of dominant-lethal
mutations produced from chemical treatment of male postmeiotic germ
cells to a small or large extent depending upon the mutagen used and
the competence of the egg to repair the premutational lesions induced.
The strain of females has little influence on the yield of dominant-
lethal mutations induced by triethylenemelamine or ethyl methanesulfonate in spermatids and spermatozoa, but it has a large influence
in the case of isopropyl methanesulfonate. In addition to this difference, triethylenemelamine and ethyl methanesulfonate induce high
levels of heritable translocations at these germ cell stages whereas
isopropyl methanesulfonate is practically ineffective, even though
doses of these chemicals produced comparable levels of dominant-lethal
mutations. These differences between ethyl methanesulfonate and triethylenemelamine on one hand and isopropyl methanesulfonate on the
other were hypothesized to be a function of the types of chromosomal
lesions present at the time of repair activity and whether or not
chromosomal aberrations were already fixed at the time of postfertilization pronuclear DNA synthesis.

INTRODUCTION

Repair has long been recognized as an important factor in mutagenesis studies with eukaryotic organisms. Evidence is accumulating
which clearly demonstrates that increased sensitivity to induction
of point mutations and chromosomal aberrations is correlated with
reduced capacity to repair DNA damage. A similar situation is, of

course, generally known to be true with regard to the susceptibility to cancer of humans that are homozygous for mutations causing various definite or presumed repair-deficiency syndromes. But more importantly from the standpoint of genetic risk, there is also good evidence which indicates that humans, heterozygous for certain repair-deficiency syndromes, also have increased risk of dying from cancer [12, 13]. Although at present there are only nine or so proven or presumed repair-deficiency syndromes in humans, it is almost certain that the total number of loci that are related to DNA repair processes is considerably larger. This statement is based upon what we already know in Drosophila and fungi. At present there are about 30 and 100 loci in Drosophila and yeast, respectively, known or presumed to be involved with DNA repair processes [7, 11]. These numbers are expected to increase as the considerable increase in interest in this area of research provides new data. The present data in these lower eukaryotes suggest that it is likely that in the human genome there are also numerous loci where mutations that lead to reduction in repair capacity can occur.

From the point of view of hazard evaluation, the two points mentioned above — large number of repair-related loci and possible expression of the mutations in these loci in the heterozygote state — add considerable significance to mutations induced in the germ line. There is a tendency for us to worry about cancer as a consequence of mutations in somatic cells a great deal more than we worry about cancer being the consequence of germinal mutations. Cancer as a direct effect of environmental chemicals is, of course, a very important health problem; but the impact of induced germinal mutations on the etiology of human cancer has been generally ignored. The presumably large number of repair-related loci where mutation can potentially occur and the possible expression of these mutations in the heterozygous state obviously suggest that there may be an important association between mutation induction in germ cells and human carcinogenesis. Furthermore, if the increased susceptibility of these heterozygotes to cancer is indeed attributable to their reduced ability to repair DNA damage, then it is possible that their germ cells might also be at higher risk with respect to mutation induction.

From the foregoing, the usefulness of a repair-deficient laboratory mammal in fundamental as well as practical research is obvious. There is a breakthrough in this regard as described below.

That certain repair processes exist in specific germ cell stages in male and female mice has been demonstrated in various studies (see separate reviews by Russell [9], Pedersen [8], and Sega [10], this volume). However, the relationship between repair processes and induction of mutations in mammalian germ cells has not been studied to any significant extent until recently, when we discovered the existence of a genetically controlled repair system in the fertilized eggs

of mice [3]. This repair system is described in the present report
as it is related to the formation of dominant-lethal mutations and
heritable translocations following treatment of postmeiotic male
germ cells.

EVIDENCE FOR REPAIR IN FERTILIZED EGGS

Although the subject of this paper is repair in fertilized eggs,
it is appropriate to describe a dominant-lethal study we did several
years ago on maturing dictyate oocytes [4]. In this study (SEC ×
C57BL)F_1, T-stock, and (101 × C3H)F_1 females were treated with isopropyl methanesulfonate (IMS) and mated to untreated (SEC × C57BL)F_1
males. It was found that the frequencies of presumed dominant-
lethal mutations induced in T-stock and (SEC × C57BL)F_1 females were
considerably higher than that induced in (101 × C3H)F_1 females.
However, because the females themselves received the treatment, the
basis for the large differences observed between these stocks was not
clear at that time, although differences in the repair of genetic
damage was offered as one of the possible explanations. Today, evidence is strong indicating that the differences between stocks are
attributable to differences in the ability of the oocytes to carry
out repair of IMS-induced premutational lesions. What is the evidence for repair?

To demonstrate the existence and magnitude of repair in fertilized eggs and to separate the effects of this process from other
factors, we used a simple procedure whereby males from one stock,
(101 × C3H)F_1, were treated with IMS and then mated to females from
four stocks [random-bred T-stock, (C3H × C57BL)F_1, (C3H × 101)F_1,
and (SEC × C57BL)F_1] at selected periods after treatment [3]. In
all cases the times after treatment when males were mated corresponded to postmeiotic germ cell stages. Afterwards, the yield of
dominant-lethal mutations in each of the four stocks of females was
determined.

The initial study was performed at a dose of 65 mg/kg to maturing spermatozoa (matings that occurred within the first few days
after treatment). Dominant-lethal data are summarized in Fig. 1.
A marginal effect of 9% dominant-lethal mutations was observed for
(C3H × C57BL)F_1 females, and a low, but clear-cut, dominant-lethal
effect of 18% was observed for (C3H × 101)F_1 females. In marked
contrast to these two stocks, (SEC × C57BL)F_1 and T-stock females
had much higher dominant-lethal frequencies (50 and 81%, respectively). Thus, the maximum difference between stocks is about one
order of magnitude.

The large maximum difference between stocks of females in their
yield of dominant-lethal mutations induced by IMS in sperm is truly

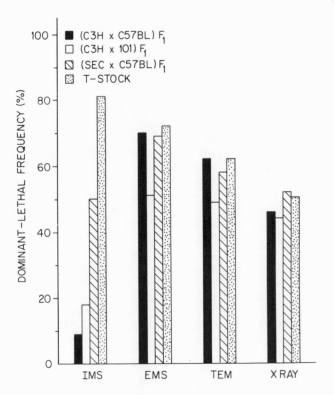

Fig. 1.   Differences in the capacity of eggs to repair genetic
lesions induced in spermatozoa and spermatids.   (The graph was constructed from data in ref. [3]).   Experimental males were mated at
the following intervals after treatment: IMS (65 mg/kg) or x-rays
(550 R), 0.5-3.5 days;   EMS (200 mg/kg), 6.5-9.5 days;   TEM (0.2
mg/kg), 4.5-7.5 days.

remarkable.   Because only one stock of males was exposed to IMS and
because the different stocks of females were not treated, the large
differences observed between stocks of females strongly suggest that
there are differences in the capabilities of the egg to repair the
premutational lesions that were induced in the male genome.   However,
it was essential to rule out one other possible explanation — i.e.,
that there might be differential survival of affected embryos in
different maternal environments.   To rule out this possibility, a
cytological study of first-cleavage metaphases was carried out [3].
The relative incidence of chromosome aberrations clearly paralleled
that of dominant-lethal mutations, thus confirming the repair-capa-
bility hypothesis.

How do other mutagens compare with IMS with respect to the magnitude of differences between stocks of females? Experiments similar to that done for IMS were also performed with the alkylating compounds ethyl methanesulfonate (EMS) and triethylenemelamine (TEM) and with x-rays [3]. These dominant-lethal data are also shown in Fig. 1. It was concluded that differences in the yields of dominant-lethal mutations between (C3H × 101)F_1 stock on one hand and T-stock, (SEC × C57BL)F_1, and (C3H × C57BL)F_1 stocks on the other exist for EMS or TEM treatments. However, it is important to emphasize that these differences are markedly smaller than the maximum difference found for IMS. No significant differences between stocks were observed in the case of x-rays.

The differences by which the four stocks of females responded to the four mutagens described above appear consistent with the concept that a number of different repair systems exist. For example, in cases in which repair differences were demonstrable, T-stock responded in the same relative order for each of the chemicals studied, whereas the other stocks did not. These results suggest that the mutagens differ in the types of lesions produced, each type requiring a corresponding repair process.

RELATIONSHIP BETWEEN REPAIR IN FERTILIZED EGGS AND ABERRATION FORMATION IN TREATED MALE POSTMEIOTIC GERM CELLS

The series of events that takes place from the time the premutational lesion occurs in the chromosome of male postmeiotic germ cells until the resulting aberration is transmitted to progeny is still not well understood. What happens to this premutational lesion during postmeiotic germ cell maturation and after the sperm has entered the egg? To what extent does the egg influence the conversion of the premutational lesion into aberrations? These are complicated questions that will not be easy to answer for at least two reasons. First, it is expected that the processes differ to a small or large extent depending upon the mutagens involved. Even within the class of alkylating chemicals, certain of these processes should be expected to vary depending upon the nature of the important premutational lesion produced. Second, most of these processes are not subject to direct study. Thus, in order to develop concepts regarding basic mechanisms, we need to rely upon indirect evidence that seems to explain the observation. In this context, formulation of a concept for the formation of chromosomal aberrations induced by alkylating chemicals in male postmeiotic germ cells was attempted [5]. This concept was based upon the dominant-lethal and heritable translocation data for IMS, EMS, TEM, and x-rays as well as the data on repair in fertilized eggs involving these mutagens.

The information on repair was discussed in the preceding section. The important point is that IMS differed markedly from EMS and TEM in the degree to which genetic lesions carried in postmeiotic male germ cells are repaired in the egg. Large repair differences between stocks of females were found in the case of IMS, but much smaller differences were found in the case of EMS and TEM.

Another remarkable difference that exists between IMS on one hand and EMS and TEM on the other lies in the relative rates at which dominant-lethal mutations and heritable translocations are produced. Over the years a close association between the production of dominant-lethal mutations and the production of heritable trans-locations in male postmeiotic stages has become somewhat of a dogma. This association certainly holds true for x-rays and for all of the alkylating compounds that were reported in the literature — e.g., EMS, TEM, cyclophosphamide, methyl methanesulfonate, etc. When dose-effect relationships were studied, there was a good positive correlation between the rates of induction of dominant-lethal muta-tions and heritable translocations [2, 6]. Our recent data on dominant-lethal mutations and heritable translocations prove that this dogma is not correct [5]. Data on relative inducibility of dominant-lethal mutations and heritable translocations are shown in Table 1. In the case of spermatids and spermatozoa treated before mating, the frequencies of heritable translocations observed at levels of dominant-lethal mutations that are more than 50% are in the neighborhood of 30% for EMS, TEM, and x-rays; in contrast, the frequencies produced by IMS are at least one order of magnitude lower for similar conditions. In the case of inseminated spermatozoa, x-rays produced a clear-cut increase in the frequency of heritable translocations even when the level of dominant-lethal mutation was marginal. IMS, on the other hand, did not produce a single case of heritable translocation in this germ cell stage even though the level of dominant lethals produced by the dose used was clearly higher than that in the x-ray study. The following conclusions may be drawn from the observations. EMS and TEM, but not IMS, are similar to x-rays with respect to the effective production of heritable translocations relative to the production of dominant-lethal mutations. IMS pro-duces mainly dominant-lethal mutations accompanied by a negligible frequency of heritable translocations.

To repeat, two striking differences exist between IMS on one hand and EMS and TEM on the other: first, in the relative rates at which dominant-lethal mutations and heritable translocations are produced; second, in the degree to which genetic lesions carried in postmeiotic male germ cells are repaired in the egg. The obvious question is what do these differences mean in terms of basic mech-anisms? We have explained these differences as a function of the types of chromosomal lesion present at the time of repair activity and whether or not chromosomal aberrations are already fixed at the time of postfertilization pronuclear DNA synthesis [5].

TABLE 1

RELATIVE INDUCIBILITY OF DOMINANT-LETHAL MUTATIONS AND
HERITABLE TRANSLOCATIONS IN MALE POSTMEIOTIC GERM CELLS[a]

Mutagen	Dose	Germ cell stage	Estimated dominant-lethal frequency (%)	Heritable translocation frequency (%)
EMS	200 mg/kg	Early spermatozoa	70	32.1
TEM	0.2 mg/kg	Middle spermatids	75	28.9
x-ray	700 R	Maturing spermatozoa and spermatids	67	27.2
	100 R	Inseminated spermatozoa	9	2.8
IMS	50 mg/kg	Inseminated spermatozoa	24	0
	75 mg/kg	Maturing spermatozoa	82	2.7
	75 mg/kg	Early spermatids	58	0.4

[a]This table was constructed from data published in refs. [2, 5, 6].

Because of the large repair differences between stocks of females, it was assumed that the unrepaired IMS-induced premutational
lesions in treated spermatozoa and spermatids persisted up to the
time of pronuclear DNA synthesis, whereupon they were converted
primarily into chromatid and isochromatid deletions which eventually
led to dominant lethality. The cytological analysis of first-cleavage metaphase has, in fact, yielded evidence for the production of
these deletions [3]. Consistent with this explanation is the finding
that although IMS effectively induced dominant-lethal mutations, it
induced only a negligible level of heritable translocations. Thus,
it was concluded that the majority of the important premutational
lesions induced by IMS in spermatozoa and spermatids were converted
into aberrations as a consequence of pronuclear DNA synthesis.

Conversely, since, like x-rays, EMS and TEM induced high levels
of heritable translocations relative to dominant-lethal mutations,

it was concluded that a significant proportion of the premutational lesions induced by these chemicals were converted into chromosome-type aberrations (i.e., the exchanges were already fixed prior to pronuclear DNA synthesis). In support of this conclusion is the cytological result of Bürki and Sheridan [1] on the first-cleavage division in which male postmeiotic germ cells of mice were treated with TEM. They found only chromosome-type aberrations — no chromatid fragments or chromatid-type exchanges were observed. It is not clear whether the small repair differences between stocks of females observed for EMS or TEM treatments mean that the induced premutational lesions were already converted to aberrations or to some intermediate form prior to the time of repair activity in the fertilized eggs.

On the basis of repair, heritable translocation, and dominant-lethal mutation data described above, a hypothesis concerning the mechanisms by which alkylating chemicals induce dominant-lethal mutations and heritable translocations can be postulated [5] — that the relative rates at which dominant-lethal mutations and heritable translocations are produced from treatment of postmeiotic male germ cells depend upon the longevity of important premutational lesions. Heritable translocations are produced at a high rate relative to dominant-lethal mutations by alkylating chemicals that induce primarily premutational lesions which are converted to breaks and interchanges prior to pronuclear DNA synthesis. Conversely, alkylating chemicals that induce primarily premutational lesions that persist up to the time of pronuclear DNA synthesis produce mainly the types of aberrations which lead to dominant lethality. This hypothesis does not state that the production of chromosome-type aberrations and the production of chromatid-type aberrations are mutually exclusive. On the contrary, it allows that both types of aberration are produced at rates that may differ from one mutagen to another depending upon the types of premutational lesions produced. It does require that the production of heritable translocations must result from exchanges that were already fixed prior to pronuclear chromosome replication.

CONCLUSION

The usefulness of repair-deficient laboratory mammals in fundamental as well as practical research in mutagenesis and in carcinogenesis and teratogenesis should be obvious. The results described in this report represent a significant advance not only in the study of repair processes in laboratory mammals but also in understanding the relationship between these processes and formation of chemically induced chromosomal aberrations. These results also demonstrate the effectiveness of the genetic approach in our efforts to discover repair deficiency in laboratory mammals.

Where do we go from here? One obvious question that needs to be answered is whether or not the large differences in the capacities of fertilized eggs of different stocks of female mice to repair IMS-induced genetic lesions in male germ cells are also present in somatic cells. We need to obtain information on the genetics of repair processes in the mouse. It is essential to extend the studies described in this report to determine the repairability of the ge-netic lesions produced by a wide variety of chemical mutagens. In addition to dominant-lethal mutations and heritable translocations it is necessary to determine how other genetic end points, such as point mutations and sex chromosome loss, are affected by the repair processes. From a practical standpoint, we need to classify existing stocks for their competence in repairing genetic lesions produced by various classes of chemical mutagens and ultimately develop tester stocks of females for use in practical screening of chemical muta-gens. Finally, it should be obvious that the area of research described in this report is still in its primordial stage. Consid-ering the fundamental as well as practical significance of this area of research and the leads provided by the results presented, obtaining the information described above appears essential.

ACKNOWLEDGEMENT

This research was sponsored by the Office of Health and Environmental Research, U.S. Department of Energy, under contract W-7405-eng-26 with the Union Carbide Corporation.

REFERENCES

1. Bürki, K., and W. Sheridan, Expression of TEM-induced damage to postmeiotic stages of spermatogenesis of the mouse during early embryogenesis. II. Cytological investiga-tions, Mutat. Res., 52 (1978) 107-115.
2. Generoso, W. M., K. T. Cain, S. W. Huff, and D. G. Gosslee, Inducibility by chemical mutagens of heritable transloca-tions in male and female germ cells of mice, In: Advances in Modern Toxicology, Vol. 5, W. G. Flamm and M. A. Mehlman, Eds., Hemisphere Publishing Co., Washington, D.C., 1978, pp. 109-129.
3. Generoso, W. M., K. T. Cain, M. Krishna, and S. W. Huff, Repair in the egg of chemically induced genetic lesions in sperma-tozoa and spermatids of mice, Proc. Natl. Acad. Sci. (U.S.), 56 (1979) 435-437.
4. Generoso, W. M., S. W. Huff, and S. K. Stout, Chemically induced dominant-lethal mutations and cell killing in mouse oocytes in the advanced stages of follicular development, Mutat. Res., 11 (1971) 411-420.

5. Generoso, W. M., S. W. Huff, and K. T. Cain, Relative rates at which dominant-lethal mutations and heritable translocations were induced by alkylating chemicals in postmeiotic male germ cells of mice, Genetics, 93 (1979) 163-171.

6. Generoso, W. M., W. L. Russell, S. W. Huff, S. K. Stout, and D. G. Gosslee, Effects of dose on the induction of dominant-lethal mutants and heritable translocations with ethyl methanesulfonate in male mice, Genetics, 77 (1974) 741-752.

7. Lemontt, J., Genetic and physiological factors affecting repair and mutagenesis in yeast, This volume, p. 85.

8. Pedersen, R. A., and B. Brandriff, Radiation and drug-induced DNA repair in mammalian oocytes and embryos, This volume, p. 389.

9. Russell, W. L., Radiation and chemical mutagenesis and repair in mice, In: Molecules and Cellular Processes, R. F. Beers, Jr., R. M. Herriott and R. C. Tilghman, Eds., John Hopkins University Press, Baltimore, 1972, pp. 239-247.

10. Sega, G. A., Relationship between unscheduled DNA synthesis and mutation induction in male mice, This volume, p. 373.

11. Smith, P. D., R. D. Snyder, and R. L. Dusenbery, Isolation and characterization of repair-deficient mutants of Drosophila melanogaster, This volume, p. 175.

12. Swift, M., and C. Chase, Cancer in families with xeroderma pigmentosum, J. Natl. Cancer Inst., 62 (1979) 1415-1421.

13. Swift, M., L. Sholman, M. Perry, and C. Chase, Malignant neoplasms in the families of patients with ataxia-telangiectasia, Cancer Res., 36 (1976) 209-215.

CHAPTER 29

REPAIR AND MUTATION INDUCTION IN MOUSE GERM CELLS: A SUMMARY

AND SOME THOUGHTS

LIANE B. RUSSELL

Biology Division, Oak Ridge National Laboratory
Oak Ridge, Tenn. 37830 (U.S.A.)

Evidence for repair of premutational lesions induced in
mammalian germ cells has come from several directions, and some of
it has been around for quite some time. Yet it is only as a result
of relatively recent work that we now have the opportunity, with
experimental mammals, to penetrate into areas of research that have
already yielded rich rewards in yeast and Drosophila, namely, the
genetics of repair capacity. This opportunity is particularly
welcome in view of the fact that experimental mammals, which obviously could provide animal models for human genetic disease, have
lagged behind man in the study of repair-deficiency states. Several
such states are known in humans; in the mouse, we are only now on
the threshold of discovering some.

The various lines of evidence for repair of premutational
damage in mouse germ cells were presented at this symposium. The
first indication of repair came, over 20 years ago, from the radiation dose-rate effect on mutations induced in both spermatogonia
and oocytes [15, 16]. W. L. Russell reviewed results from a
variety of specific-locus experiments, involving protracted or
fractionated doses, that point strongly to the existence of a
repair process. He believes that some premutational lesions - most
of which result from single-track events - can be repaired at low
doses and dose rates in certain germ-cell stages; but that, at
high doses and dose rates, the repair system is either damaged or
saturated [14]. Some others have interpreted Russell's data on the
basis of a linear-quadratic function, which assumes that a large proportion of the mutations found after irradiation at high dose rates
are two-track events [1]. W. L. Russell's talk at this symposium
demonstrated with detailed mathematical models what he has stated
earlier [12] that curve fitting alone can give few clues as to the
nature of the induced mutations: thus, models involving a single-

track hypothesis fit the data as well as (actually better than) does
the linear-quadratic model. In his view, the most cogent evidence
comes from an analysis of the nature of the mutations. Such studies
as deficiency and complementation mapping have indicated that the
bulk of the specific-locus mutations induced in spermatogonia are
either intragenic or deficiencies so small as to be almost certainly
one-track in origin [8, 10].

More evidence for repair comes from the finding of unscheduled
DNA synthesis (UDS) in mouse germ cells. UDS was discussed for the
male by Sega [17] and for the female by Pedersen [7].

In the female, UDS has now been demonstrated for all stages of
oocyte development following UV irradiation. If, as Pedersen
believes, UDS is a reflection of excision repair, such repair capacity appears to be highest in the growing oocyte; and, though lower,
still quite sizeable in the neighboring stages, i.e., the earlier
resting oocyte and the later germinal-vesicle stage (mature oocyte).
Unfortunately, no female mutation-rate data are available for any
agent that, like UV, induces long-patch repair, and it is therefore
not yet possible to relate oocyte long-patch repair capacity to
mutational endpoints. Only x-ray mutagenesis has been extensively
studied. This gives evidence for some sort of repair (dose-rate
effect for specific-locus mutations) in mature and maturing oocytes.
It also suggests that there might exist a highly efficient repair
mechanism in resting oocytes, since the mutation rate, even after
irradiation at high dose rates, drops to control levels during
post-irradiation intervals of more than 6 weeks, when such oocytes
are being utilized [11]. If this phenomenon is, in fact, due to
repair rather than to other possible causes (which Russell has
enumerated), then the resting oocyte could have the greatest capacity
for short-patch repair. The maturing oocyte presumably also pos-
sesses considerable short-patch repair capabilities, as indicated
by the major dose-rate effect on transmitted mutations (low dose
rates yielding no increase over control levels [13]). In addition,
UDS reveals the maturing oocyte to have the greatest capacity for
long-patch repair.

It is somewhat troublesome that Pedersen finds the lowest levels
of UDS in the very stage for which we now have some of the most
intriguing evidence for repair of premutational damage, namely, the
fertilized egg (see below). However, though low at that stage, UDS
is still clearly detectable. Further, we do not yet know whether
any of the agents for which genetic differences in repair capacity
of the fertilized egg have been demonstrated in fact induce long-
patch repair of the type presumably revealed by UV-stimulated UDS.

Sega's work with mouse males raises some basic questions about
the interpretations to be placed on UDS endpoints in chemical mutagenesis. How is UDS in mammalian germ cells related to removal of

DNA lesions? And how are these lesions related to transmitted
genetic damages of various types? There are, for example, very
marked differences in UDS between mature sperm and late spermatids
on the one hand, and earlier postleptotene germ-cell stages on the
other, whereas the initial levels of DNA alkylation are roughly the
same for both sets of stages. Sega finds that the rate of loss of
alkylated bases varies in the same direction as does UDS, i.e.,
both endpoints are much lower in mature sperm and late spermatids
than in earlier germ cells. On the basis of this stage correspondence, he suggests that excision of bases is associated with the UDS
response, and that low response of the stages that have condensed
chromosomes is the result either of nonproduction of repair enzymes
or of inaccessibility of lesions to the enzymes.

Stage correspondence is the main argument for another one of
Sega's conclusions: that UDS may not have a significant effect
on the lesions that lead to chromosome breakage. He believes that,
in the case of EMS, the primary target for such lesions is not DNA,
but protamine, since, with respect to stage of EMS treatment, the
ethylation curve for protamine matches the dominant-lethal curve,
while the ethylation curve for DNA does not. Similar relations will
have to be shown for a variety of agents before such a conclusion
can be broadened, especially since, for a number of chemicals, dominant lethals are readily inducible in germ-cell stages that have
chromatin devoid of protamine [2, 3].

If UDS, is, in fact, not related to chromosome breakage-derived
genetic endpoints, such as dominant lethals, is it related to point
mutations, as measured in the specific-locus test? Sega's conclusion - that it is not - is based on a comparison of specific-locus
mutation frequencies for irradiated postspermatogonial stages with
relative UDS levels for these same stages: the latter increase
during weeks 3 and 4 after treatment, while the former not only do
not decrease, but increase slightly. Sega's conclusion thus rests
on the assumption that UDS indicates restoration of a predamage
condition; if, in fact, UDS were related to error-prone repair
processes, the observed results would not be out of line. The standard specific-locus test is capable of detecting a wide array of
changes involving the loci - from intragenic alterations not associated with absence of material to deletions long enough to involve
neighboring markers [8, 10]. Even with radiation, a sizeable proportion of the mutations induced (though not necessarily at the
germ-cell stages at which UDS is induced) is the result of intragenic changes; UDS will have to be compared with specific-locus
mutations resulting from chemicals known to produce primarily
"subtle" changes before any conclusions can be drawn about its
relation to the specific-locus endpoint.

The challenge of building the bridge between initial lesion and
genetic endpoint is being approached in two ways. UDS observed in

male or female germ cell stages is presumably an indication of events that affect the initial lesion. However, the relation between UDS and measurable genetic endpoints still requires considerable exploration. Another study of repair in mammalian germ cells [4] takes the opposite direction, i.e., it starts with genetic endpoints and attempts to trace back to events affecting the initial lesions. This is the approach coming out of Generoso's finding that the genetic constitution of the female can strongly affect the level of dominant lethals induced by exposure of the male to various mutagens, but especially to isopropyl methanesulfonate (IMS, an agent that produces a high ratio of O-6 to N-7 alkylation of guanine). Possible alternative explanations for this phenomenon have been eliminated [5], leaving only the interpretation that the penetrated oocytes of certain strains are repair competent, while those of others are repair deficient. A similar condition has already been shown to exist in Drosophila [19], and I had early indications that paternal sex-chromosome loss might be affected by the strain of the female [9]. Generoso's work, however, provides the first well-documented evidence for an association between repair and induction of genetic damage in mammalian germ cells.

Much remains to be done, as Generoso himself points out: different genetic endpoints and different mutagens must be studied. However, the advantages of having gained a genetic handle on repair processes are maniford. The study of repair-deficiency states will now be possible in a laboratory mammal, and these states may provide experimental models for human genetic diseases. To elucidate the genetics of repair processes, it will be necessary to develop tests by which individuals can be classified as deficient or competent; presently, only population parameters are available (e.g., dominant-lethal frequencies). Explant tissue cultures may be made to serve this purpose if the genetic differences demonstrable in fertilized eggs also apply to somatic cells. The mammalian work must also attempt to discover whether there is an association between mutagen sensitivity and repair deficiency as in Drosophila, and such experiments have been initiated by Generoso. Another avenue of attack (which is also in progress at Oak Ridge) is to compare the effect of known repair inhibitors on the fertilized egg of repair-competent and -deficient strains.

Generoso proposes an hypothesis to account for the finding that the agent, IMS, that gives the greatest strain differences in repair capacity is also the one that gives the lowest frequency of translocations for a given level of dominant lethals. He suggests that lesions produced by IMS persist until the time of pronuclear DNA synthesis, at which time they are converted into chromatid or isochromatid deletions, whereas lesions induced by some other agents (e.g., EMS, TEM, x-rays) are converted to breaks and interchanges prior to pronuclear DNA synthesis [4].

Although it will be important to see how many other agents fit this pattern, the hypothesis already suggests testable cross references to Sega's UDS work. For example, by Generoso's hypothesis, lesions induced in sperm or late spermatids by EMS (and perhaps MMS?) might become "fixed" even before sperm entry into the oocyte, as indicated by the almost negligible differences between stocks of females in repair capacity for EMS-induced damage. On the other hand, such lesions could be available for possible repair for a short period between sperm entry into the oocyte and sometime prior to pronuclear DNA synthesis (which begins about 6 hr after sperm entry [6]). By Sega's evidence, probably no repair of these lesions occurs prior to sperm entry. Would this brief period of reparability of the male genome in the oocyte be detectable by UDS? That lesions induced in the male genome by EMS or MMS are, in principle, detectable by UDS is known from the treatment of postleptotene spermatocytes and early spermatids. However, UDS studies of eggs fertilized with MMS-treated sperm were negative [18]. It would seem important to do similar work with IMS-treated sperm, since Generoso's hypothesis predicts that lesions in such cells should be available for repair during the entire period between sperm entry and pronuclear DNA synthesis. This should result in UDS.

Other experiments, too, would provide cross references between UDS and genetic indicators. For example, UDS determinations in various oocyte stages, such as were summarized by Pedersen for UV treatment, should be done following IMS treatment of strains identified by Generoso as repair-competent or -deficient, respectively. In the male (early spermatid), Sega has identified high- and low-UDS strains following MMS exposure, and he suggests that the differences may be related to the relative efficiencies with which these strains remove the alkylation product. It will be of interest to check UDS in early spermatids exposed to IMS, specifically comparing those strains whose females (penetrated eggs) have shown high or low repair capacity in Generoso's experiments.

One important implication of the probable existence of genetic repair deficiency that has been pointed out by Generoso is a new relation between mutagenicity and carcinogenicity. No longer is mutagenicity of an agent merely an indication that such an agent also has a good probability of being an initiator of cancer. Mutagenicity per se achieves an added dimension of importance in that a presumably large number of loci in the germline could mutate to repair-deficiency alleles which, even in the heterozygous state (i.e., F_1) could increase susceptibility to carcinogenic agents. In addition, there is the possibility that a "self-feeding" process could be initiated with respect to mutagenicity. Thus, existing genetic differences (i.e., repair competency versus deficiency) apparently determine the level of probability at which new genetic differences (induced mutations) come about, and some of these new genetic states, in turn, could affect future mutability.

ACKNOWLEDGEMENT

This research was sponsored by the Office of Health and Environmental Research, U.S. Department of Energy, under contract W-7405-
eng-26 with the Union Carbide Corporation.

REFERENCES

1. Abrahamson, S., and S. Wolff, Re-analysis of radiation-induced
        specific locus mutations in the mouse, Nature, 264 (1976)
        715-719.
2. Ehling, U. H., Comparison of radiation- and chemically-induced
        dominant lethal mutations in male mice, Mutat. Res., 11
        (1971) 35-44.
3. Ehling, U. H., D. G. Doherty, and E. V. Malling, Differential
        spermatogenic response of mice to the induction of dominant-
        lethal mutations by n-propyl methane sulfonate and isopropyl
        methane sulfonate, Mutat. Res., 15 (1972) 175-184.
4. Generoso, W. M., Repair in fertilized eggs of mice and its role
        in the production of chromosomal aberrations, This volume.
        p. 411.
5. Generoso, W. M., K. T. Cain, M. Krishna, and S. W. Huff,
        Genetic lesions induced by chemicals in spermatozoa and
        spermatids of mice are repaired in the egg, Proc. Natl.
        Acad. Sci. (U.S.), 76 (1979) 435-437.
6. Krishna, M. and W. M. Generoso, Timing of sperm penetration,
        pronuclear formation, pronuclear DNA synthesis, and first
        cleavage in naturally ovulated mouse eggs, J. Exptl. Zool.,
        202 (1977) 245-252.
7. Pedersen, R. A., and B. Brandriff, Radiation- and drug-induced
        DNA repair in mammalian oocytes and embryos, This volume.
        p. 389.
8. Russell, L. B., Definition of functional units in a small
        chromosomal segment of the mouse and its use in interpreting
        the nature of radiation-induced mutations, Mutat. Res., 11
        (1971) 107-123.
9. Russell, L. B., Numerical sex-chromosome anomalies in mammals:
        their spontaneous occurrence and use in mutagenesis studies,
        in: Chemical Mutagens-Principles and Methods for Their
        Detection, Vol. 4, A. Hollaender (Ed.), Plenum Press,
        New York, 1976, pp. 55-91.
10. Russell, L. B., W. L. Russell, and E. M. Kelly, Analysis of the
        albino-locus region of the mouse. I. Origin and viability,
        Genetics, 91 (1979) 127-139.
11. Russell, W. L., The genetic effects of radiation, In: Peaceful
        Uses of Atomic Energy, Vol. 13. IAEA, Vienna, 1972,
        pp. 487-500.

12. Russell, W. L., Discussion, In: Biological and Environmental
       Effects of Low-Level Radiation, Vol. I, IAEA, Vienna, 1976,
       p. 17.
13. Russell, W. L., Mutation frequencies in female mice and the
       estimation of genetic hazards of radiation in women, Proc.
       Natl. Acad. Sci. (U.S.), 74 (1977) 3523-3527.
14. Russell, W. L., Radiation and chemical mutagenesis and repair
       in mice, In: Molecular and Cellular Repair Processes, R. F.
       Beers, Jr., R. M. Herriott, and R. C. Tilghman, Eds., The
       Johns Hopkins University Press, Baltimore, 1972, pp. 239-
       247.
15. Russell, W. L., L. B. Russell, and M. B. Cupp, Dependence of
       mutation frequency on radiation dose rate in female mice,
       Proc. Natl. Acad. Sci. (U.S.), 45 (1959) 18-23.
16. Russell, W. L., L. B. Russell, and E. M. Kelly, Radiation dose
       rate and mutation frequency, Science, 128 (1958) 1546-1550.
17. Sega, G. A., Relationship between unscheduled DNA synthesis
       and mutation induction in male mice, This volume, p. 373.
18. Sega, G. A., R. E. Sotomayor, and J. G. Owens, A study of
       unscheduled DNA synthesis induced by x-rays in the germ
       cells of male mice, Mutat. Res., 49 (1978) 239-257.
19. Würgler, F. E., and U. Graf, Mutation induction in repair-
       deficient strains of Drosophila, This volume, p. 223.

CHAPTER 30

CHROMOSOME-BREAKAGE SYNDROMES: DIFFERENT GENES, DIFFERENT

TREATMENTS, DIFFERENT CANCERS

JAMES GERMAN

The New York Blood Center, 310 East 67th Street
New York, New York   10021

SUMMARY

Comparison of the strikingly different distributions of types
of cancer that occur in the genetic disorders that feature chromosome instability raises several interesting points. (a) Bloom's
syndrome: the distribution suggests that many of the cancers that
occur with regularity in the general population just occur more
commonly and at an earlier age. (b) Ataxia telangiectasia: cancers
of many types are increased in frequency, but lymphoreticular
cancers are exceptionally common, the case also in several other
genetically determined immunodeficiency disorders. Both Bloom's
syndrome and ataxia telangiectasia share defective immunity as a
major clinical feature, but the respective roles, if any, of it and
of chromosome instability in producing the cancer predispositions
are unknown. (c) Fanconi's anemia: cancer apparently has become
common only recently. The types and distribution which occur are
unusual. Fanconi's anemia cells have been shown to be hypertrans-
formable by oncogenic virus and to be defective in handling certain
types of DNA damage (as well as to manifest chromosome instability)
so that the recent increase in cancer incidence is both surprising
and unexplained. The degree of cancer proneness of Fanconi's
anemia per se, untreated by modern methods, must at present be
considered unknown. (d) Xeroderma pigmentosum: the cancer predisposition apparently extends only to cells which receive solar
damage, i.e., to skin and eye. This would not have been predicted
in view of the fact that the cellular mechanism is defective for
repairing DNA damage produced not just by sunlight but also by
certain classes of chemical carcinogens.

INTRODUCTION

The disorders referred to as chromosome–breakage syndromes [11]
are four: Bloom's syndrome (BS), Fanconi's anemia (FA), ataxia
telangiectasia (AT), and xeroderma pigmentosum (XP). Clinical and
cytological aspects of these four rare, genetically–determined
disorders have been presented elsewhere [12, 13], and several
summaries have been published also concerning their hypersensitivity
to environmental mutagens and carcinogens and defectiveness in
repairing damaged DNA [2, 14, 22]. An important clinical feature
these four syndromes share is cancer proneness, and by definition
they all exhibit excessive chromosome instability, either spontaneously or under certain conditions. (The data in the tables are
documented elsewhere [17].) In BS and AT, tabulation of the cancers
was facilitated because of the existence of two central repositories
of information concerning them, the Bloom's Syndrome Registry [15,
16] and the Immunodeficiency-Cancer Registry [30]. For FA and XP,
with the exception of a tabulation made 20 years ago of cancer in
relatives of persons with FA [18], this had not been attempted
previously, and published case reports were my main source of
information.

BLOOM'S SYNDROME

The Bloom's Syndrome Registry, which is a repository of
information concerning persons throughout the world known to have
BS, provides the list of 19 cancers and 2 precancerous conditions
shown in Table 1. This registry provides not just the distribution
of types but also a reasonable estimate of the frequency of cancer
in BS: at present, approximately one cancer has occurred for every
four persons to have been diagnosed BS since the syndrome was
described 25 years ago. As to distribution of type, acute leukemia
is by far the commonest neoplasm: half of these are acute lympho-
cytic leukemia (ALL). However, a relatively large number of
carcinomata have occurred at sites commonly affected in other people,
large in view of the fact that those alive with BS constitute a
young group (average age of those alive in 1979 = 16.4 years).
Based on the information presently accumulated, therefore, distinguishing BS from the general population with respect to cancer
occurrence is a greater than normal incidence of some type of acute
leukemia during childhood and a premature onset of some type of
carcinoma thereafter.

FANCONI'S ANEMIA

FA was described in 1927, and something over 200 affected
individuals with what is widely considered a single clinical entity
have been reported or mentioned in the medical literature [1]. The
31 entries in Table 2 appear sufficient to permit the conclusion

TABLE 1

CANCERS KNOWN TO HAVE OCCURRED IN BLOOM'S SYNDROME

Type, site	Age at diagnosis
Leukemia, acute nonlymphocytic	4
Leukemia, acute nonlymphocytic	4
Lymphosarcoma, abdominal	4
Leukemia, acute lymphocytic	9
Lymphosarcoma, cervical	12
Leukemia, acute nonlymphocytic	13
Lymphoma	13
Leukemia, acute lymphocytic	15
Leukemia, acute lymphocytic	15
Leukemia, acute nonlymphocytic	23
Refractory anemia with excess blasts[a]	23
Leukemia, acute nonlymphocytic	25
Carcinoma, squamous cell, base of tongue	30
{ Carcinoma, squamous cell, epiglottis[b]	30
{ Lymphoma	30
Lymphoma, diffuse histiocytic	31
{ Carcinoma, adeno-, sigmoid colon[b]	39
{ Carcinoma, squamous cell, esophagus	39
{ Carcinoma, adeno-, sigmoid colon[b]	37
{ Polyps, colon[a,b]	38
{ Carcinoma, squamous cell, gastroesophageal junction	44

[a]Premalignant condition.

[b]Multiple primaries in one person shown by brace.

that cancer occurs more commonly in FA than in the general population of children and young adults. It must be admitted that the number of persons who have been affected with FA in whom these 31 cancers emerged is unknown; although FA is a rare condition, little reason exists any longer to report typical cases of it, whereas the ones with cancer very possibly would be reported, thus a bias of ascertainment of cancer in FA.

Although many authors have written during the last dozen or so years that FA is a cancer-predisposing condition, for four decades following 1927, little attention was paid to cancer. Reviews of the FA literature made in 1955 [7] and 1959 [18] disclosed only one possible report of cancer, a child reported to have a leukemoid reaction [29]. Cancer had been reported also in four relatives of individuals

TABLE 2

NEOPLASMS REPORTED IN PERSONS WITH FANCONI'S ANEMIA

Type	Age
Leukemia, acute nonlymphocytic - 10 cases	7-29
Carcinoma, squamous cell, gingiva	20
Neoplasm, liver, primary - 9 cases	12-38
{ Carcinoma, squamous cell, gingiva[a]	21
Carcinom , squamous cell, tongue	22
{ Leukemia, acute myelomonocytic	21
Hepatoma	21
Carcinoma, squamous cell, esophagus	26
{ Carcinoma, squamous cell, anus[a]	31
Carcinoma-in-situ (Bowen's disease), vulva	31
{ Carcinoma, squamous cell, anus[a]	37
Carcinoma-in-situ, labium minus	38
{ Carcinoma, squamous cell, tongue[a]	38
Carcinoma, hepatocellular	38

[a]Two primaries in one person shown by brace.

with FA [18]: leukemia in two cousins, an uncle, and a brother.   (The
brother [7], although he had no hematological symptoms prior to
onset of leukemia at 27, had some features associated with FA:
shortness (150 cm), unusually small genitalia, and dermal hyper-
pigmentation as well as "very short first metacarpals and wasting of
the thenar eminence.")   When Fanconi reviewed FA in 1967 [10], 40
years after he had described it [9], he did not emphasize predisposition to cancer as a prominent feature of the syndrome.   FA has
been known as a clinical entity for over half a century; why have
30 of the 31 cancers that have ever been reported in persons with it
been reported just in the last 14 years?   Is cancer in FA a result
of the underlying molecular defect, as is generally assumed, perhaps
via an increased mutation rate in somatic cells on the basis of
defective DNA repair?   Could it not just be secondary to the medical
management in vogue since 1959, androgen administration [27, 28]?
Table 2 shows that the distribution of types of solid tumors which
have been reported is strikingly different from that which occurs in
the general population.   The several acute leukemias include not a
single example of ALL, the commonest leukemia of childhood.   Also,
the occurrence of so many hepatic cancers is puzzling; in America
and Europe primary cancer of the liver is rare, usually emerging only
in a cirrhotic liver, but in certain parts of the world it is one
of the commonest cancers, apparently on the basis of some

environmental factor. In this regard, it is noteworthy that both
leukemia and hepatocellular carcinoma have been reported in persons
with conditions other than FA who have received androgen therapy.
A third possibility is that the management enhances an underlying
genetic propensity to cancer. And, a fourth possibility is that
cancer predisposition is a feature of the syndrome, the medical
management simply delaying death from marrow failure, permitting
time for the predisposition to be expressed as neoplasia; it is my
impression that this is the generally accepted explanation.

ATAXIA TELANGIECTASIA

For AT, the incidence of cancer is generally acknowledged to be
high, but just how high is unknown. However, the distribution of
cancer type and site affected is known from a study of 101 entries
currently in the Immunodeficiency-Cancer Registry (Table 3). [AT
contributes more cancers by far to the Registry than any other single
genetically determined immunodeficiency (GDID)]. Cancer occurs with
increased frequency in most if not all immunodeficiency states,
whether genetic or therapeutically induced. It is noteworthy that
although chromosome instability and sensitivity to ionizing radiation
are prominent findings in AT but not in most other GDID, the
distributions of type cancer in AT and in immunodeficiency generally
are approximately the same. The distribution in AT differs however
from that in the general population of immunocompetent children, and
from that among children who have received excessive ionizing
radiation [20].

It is noteworthy that, of the four conditions being discussed
in the present paper because they share chromosome instability, not
just one but two of them must be classed GDIDs. BS probably was
described only 25 years ago because very few affected persons
survived early life before antibiotics were in general use; a defect
in immune function is a major feature of BS [19]. AT, although
described the year before FA [35] and again fifteen years later [21],
was not generally known until after the report of Boder and Sedgwick
[3] which was in the period when antibiotics had come into widespread
use. Chromosome instability is not a recognized feature of most
GDIDs (Bruton's agammaglobulinemia, severe combined immunodeficiency,
the Wiskott-Aldrich syndrome, et cetera). This raises the question
of what the relative roles of chromosome breakage and of immune
dysfunction are in the conversion of normal cells to neoplastic, and
of the progression of neoplastic clones. Do they both contribute
significantly to the cancer proneness? (Defective immunity is not
recognized as a feature of FA and XP.)

TABLE 3

CANCER OCCURRENCE IN THE ATAXIA-TELANGIECTASIA SYNDROME[a]

Histological type	Number of cases	
Mesenchymal		
Lymphoreticular	69	
Lymphocytic lymphoma		17
Histiocytic lymphoma		13
Malignant reticuloendotheliosis		1
"Lymphoid" leukemia		20
Other		18
Hodgkin's disease	10	
Myeloid leukemia	0	
Other mesenchymal tumor	5	
Epithelial		
All sites excluding nervous system	14	
Nervous system	3	
Total	101	

[a]Median age at diagnosis of malignancy 9 years (range 2-31).

XERODERMA PIGMENTOSUM

Skin cancers of multiple types occur with great frequency in most persons with XP. (Information is not available as to the relative incidence by complementation group.) Skin and eye cancers in XP may be assumed to be a consequence of the defective repair of solar damage. Increased cancer of internal tissues, with unusually early onset, also could have been predicted in view of the fact that XP cells are defective at the repair not just of UV-induced but also of chemical carcinogen-induced DNA damage. Table 4 does not support this prediction, however, and permits the tentative conclusion that cancer in areas other than the body surface is not unusually common in XP. The explanation for the unexpected paucity of internal cancers may be interesting and important, although a trivial matter, underreporting of the occurrence of nonskin cancer in XP, could be a contributory factor. (In the future, I shall attempt to learn more of the occurrence of nonskin cancer in XP and will make a more significant report than is possible at present if published and unpublished information about its occurrence is communicated directly to me.)

TABLE 4

NON-SKIN, NON-EYE CANCERS IN REPORTED CASES OF XERODERMA PIGMENTOSUM

Type	Age
Leukemia, acute lymphocytic[a]	3
"Neoplasm of the tongue"	Unstated
Carcinoma, squamous cell, tip of tongue	11
{ Carcinoma, squamous cell, tip of tongue[b]	11
Carcinoma, squamous cell, tip of tongue	1
Sarcoma, testis[c]	12
Glioblastoma multiforme, brain	15
Leukemia, myelogenous	32

[a]This child's sib, also with XP, is thought also to have developed leukemia, but is unreported.

[b]Two primaries in one person shown by brace.

[c]Unconfirmed death-certificate data; details of case unreported.

HETEROZYGOTES

Tables 1-4 pertain to cancer in persons homozygous for one of these rare genes, i.e., with the clinical disorders. Surveys concerning cancer proneness in relatives of persons with FA, with AT, and with XP have been made, and evidence interpreted as significant of an increased propensity has been reported for all three groups [31-34]. The question as to whether persons heterozygous for the genes determining these rare conditions are themselves at in increased risk of developing cancer is without doubt an important one to have answered [13], and further studies aimed at confirming those reports are needed. However, for several reasons, reliable information is difficult to obtain. Persons heterozygous for each of these rare genes can be recognized with certainty only by becoming the parent of an affected homozygote, and affected homozygotes are rare. In FA, the matter is complicated because of the variability in the clinical syndrome itself and by the existence of several disorders that are easily confused with it [1], some as yet themselves defined only vaguely or not at all as clinical entities. Even the genetic analysis of FA is made difficult for these same reasons. To obtain firm information pertaining to cancer incidence in carriers of the FA gene, careful ascertainment of index cases and the analysis of a sizeable but "pure" sample of families seem

highly desirable, certainly at the outset. (The same can be said
for the genetic analysis of FA. I am not convinced that it should
be classed a recessive disorder in the usual sense.) AT also may
be genetically heterogeneous; it certainly is so clinically. The
study of cancer in carriers of the AT gene may eventually be facilitated by the fact that carriers may demonstrate chromosome
instability [6] or sensitivity to γ-radiation [23, 24]. It seems
quite possible that the cancer risk for carriers of these several
genes will await reliable and easy methods for carrier detection.
In my opinion, judgement on the matter should, for the present, be
withheld.

In our species, the genes for BS, FA, AT, and XP are essentially
the only "mutants" known to be responsible for DNA-repair defectiveness, mutagen-carcinogen hypersensitivity, and chromosome
instability. This paucity contrasts to the wealth of repair
defective mutants being generated in nonhuman eukaryotic species.
A few recessive mutations which affect chromosome behavior in human
meiosis have been detected, but in somatic cells of the few affected
persons studied so far [4, 5], repair and chromosome behavior seem
normal. It cannot be assumed, however, that the genes for BS, FA,
AT, and XP and for the few other recessively transmitted disorders
known to be associated with cancer are the only recessive genes
segregating in the human population which may, in single dose, be
important in determining a person's risk of cancer - if in fact these
have this importance. All of the conditions these few known genes
produce when homozygous seriously interfere with a normal postnatal
life and lead to early death (with the exception of the meiotic
mutants just mentioned). It is possible that other recessive genes
exist, homozygosity for which is lethal to the embryo, so that they
could never be responsible for entities to be observed in clinical
medicine. For the detection of such hypothetical genes, the use of
laboratory methods by which repair defectiveness or hypersensitivity
of a person's cells to some known mutagen-carcinogen can be revealed
seems a plausible approach [e.g., 22, 24, 25]. Such testing
well might yield more "mutants' than a search among clinical disorders, though this latter approach, already proven, should also be
continued.

ACKNOWLEDGEMENTS

I acknowledge the valuable advice of Dr. Blanche P. Alter of
Boston and Dr. Kenneth H. Kraemer of Bethesda in preparing Tables
3 and 4. This work is supported partially by research grants from
N.I.H. (HD 04134, HL 09011) and the American Cancer Society.

REFERENCES

1. Alter, B. P., R. Parkman, and J. M. Rappeport, Bone marrow
   failure syndromes. In: Hematology of Infancy and
   Childhood, D. G. Nathan and F. A. Oski, Eds., 2nd ed.,
   W. B. Saunders, Philadelphia, 1979, (in press).
2. Arlett, C. F., and A. R. Lehmann, Human disorders showing
   increased sensitivity to the induction of genetic damage,
   Ann. Rev. Genet., 12 (1978) 95-115.
3. Boder, E., and R. P. Sedgwick, Ataxia-telangiectasia, Univ.
   of Calif. Med. Bull., Spring (1957) 15-27, 51.
4. Chaganti, R. S. K., and J. German, Human male infertility,
   probably genetically determined, due to defective meiosis
   and spermatogenic arrest, Am. J. Hum. Genet., in press.
5. Chaganti, R. S. K., Familial azospermia in human male infertility, Am. J. Hum. Genet., in press.
6. Cohen, M. M., M. Sagi, Z. Ben-Zur, T. Schaap, R. Voss, G. Kohn,
   and H. Ben-Bassat, Ataxia telangiectasia: chromosomal
   stability in continuous lymphoblastoid cell lines.
   Cytogenet. Cell Genet., 23 (1979) 44-52.
7. Cowdell, R. H., P. J. R. Phizackerley, and D. A. Pyke,
   Constitutional anemia (Fanconi's syndrome) and leukemia in
   two brothers, Blood, 10 (1955) 788-801.
8. Day, R. S. III, and C. H. J. Ziolkowski, Human brain tumour
   cell strains with deficient host-cell reactivation of N-
   methyl-N'-nitro-N-nitrosoguanidine-damaged adenovirus 5,
   Nature, 279 (1979) 797-799.
9. Fanconi, G., Familiäre infantile perniziosartige Anämie
   (perniziöses Blutbild und Konstitution), Jahrb. Kinderheilk,
   117 (1927) 257-280.
10. Fanconi, G., Familial constitutional panmyelocytopathy,
    Fanconi's anemia (F.A.), Seminars in Hematology, 4 (1967)
    233-240.
11. German, J., Chromosomal breakage syndromes, Birth Defects:
    Original Article Series 5 (1969) (5) 117-131.
12. German, J., Oncogenic implication of chromosomal instability,
    In: Medical Genetics, V. A. McKusick and R. Clairborne,
    Eds., HP Publishing Co., New York, 1973, 39-50.
13. German, J., Genetic disorders associated with chromosomal
    instability and cancer, J. Invest. Dermatol., 60 (1973)
    427-434.
14. German, J., The association of chromosome instability,
    defective DNA repair, and cancer in some rare human genetic
    diseases. In: Human Genetics, Proc. the Fifth Intern.
    Congress of Human Genetics (1976), S. Armendares and
    R. Lisker, Eds., Excerpta Medica International Congress
    Series No. 411, 1977, pp. 64-68.
15. German, J., D. Bloom, and E. Passarge, Bloom's syndrome:
    V. Surveillance for cancer in affected families, Clin.
    Genet., 12 (1977) 162-168.

16. German, J., D. Bloom, and E. Passarge, Bloom's syndrome:
     VII. Progress report for 1978, Clin. Genet., 15 (1979)
     361–367.
17. German, J., The cancers in the chromosome-breakage syndromes.
     Proc. Sixth Internatl. Congress of Radiation Research,
     Tokyo, 1979 (in press).
18. Garriga, S., and W. H. Crosby, The incidence of leukemia in
     families of patients with hypoplasia of the marrow, Blood,
     14 (1959) 1008–1014.
19. Hütteroth, T. H., S. D. Litwin, and J. German, Abnormal immune
     responses of Bloom's syndrome lymphocytes in vitro, J.
     Clin. Invest., 56 (1975) 1–7.
20. Kraemer, K. H., Progressive degenerative diseases associated
     with defective DNA repair: xeroderma pigmentosum and ataxia
     telangiectasia. In: DNA Repair Processes, W. W. Nichols
     and D. G. Murphy, Eds., Symposia Specialists, Miami (1977)
     37–71.
21. Louis-Bar, Mme.: Sur un syndrome progressif comprenant des
     télangiectasies capillaire cutanées et conjonetivales
     symmetriques, à disposition naevoide et des troubles
     cérébelleux, Confin. Neurol. (Basel), 4 (1941) 32–42.
22. Paterson, M. C., Environmental carcinogenesis and imperfect
     repair of damaged DNA in Homo sapiens: causal relation
     revealed by rare hereditary disorders. In: Carcinogens:
     Identification and Mechanism of Action, A. C. Griffin and
     C. R. Shaw, Eds., Raven Press, New York, 1979, pp. 251–276.
23. Paterson, M. C., A. K. Anderson, B. P. Smith, and P. J. Smith,
     Enhanced radiosensitivity of cultured fibroblasts from
     ataxia telangiectasia heterozygotes manifested by defective
     colony forming ability and reduced DNA repair replication
     after hypoxic γ-irradiation, Cancer Res., 39 (1979)
     3725–3734.
24. Paterson, M. C., and P. J. Smith, Ataxia telangiectasia: An
     inherited human disorder involving hypersensitivity to
     ionizing radiation and related DNA-damaging chemicals,
     Ann. Rev. Genet., 13 (1979) 291–318.
25. Rainbow, A. J., Production of viral structural antigens by
     irradiated adenovirus as an assay for DNA repair in human
     fibroblasts. In: DNA Repair Mechanisms, P. C. Hanawalt,
     E. C. Friedberg, and C. F. Fox, Eds., Academic Press, New
     York, 1978, pp. 541–545.
26. Schroeder, T. M., and J. German, Bloom's syndrome and Fanconi's
     anemia: Demonstration of two distinctive patterns of
     chromosome disruption and rearrangement, Humangenetik, 25
     (1974) 299–306.
27. Shahidi, N. T., and L. K. Diamond, Testosterone-induced remission
     in aplastic anemia, Amer. J. Dis. Child, 98 (1959) 293–302.

28. Shahidi, N.T., and L. K. Diamond, Testosterone-induced
    remission in aplastic anemia of both acquired and congenital
    types. Further observations in 24 cases. New Engl. J. Med.,
    264 (1961) 953-967.
29. Silver, H. K., W. C. Blair, and C. H. Kempe, Fanconi syndrome;
    multiple congenital anomalies with hypoplastic anemia.
    A.M.A. Am. J. Dis. Child, 83 (1952) 14-25.
30. Spector, G. D., G. S. Perry III, and J. H. Kersey, Genetically
    determined immunodeficiency diseases (GDID) and malignancy:
    Report from the Immunodeficiency-Cancer Registry. Clin.
    Immunol. Immunopath., 11 (1978) 12-29.
31. Swift, M., Fanconi's anaemia in the genetics of neoplasia.
    Nature, 230 (1971) 370-373.
32. Swift, M., L. Sholman, M. Perry, and C. Chase, Malignant
    neoplasma in the families of patients with ataxia-
    telangiectasia. Cancer Res., 36 (1976) 209-215.
33. Swift, M., Malignant disease in heterozygous carriers.
    Birth Defects: Orign. Art. Series, 12 (1976) (1) 133-144.
34. Swift, M., and C. Chase, Cancer in xeroderma pigmentosum
    families. Am. J. Hum. Genet., 29 (1977) 105A.
35. Syllaba, L., and K. Henner, Contributions a l'independance de
    l'athétose double idiopathique et congénitale. Rev.
    Neurol., 1 (1926) 541-562.

CHAPTER 31

SUMMARY AND PERSPECTIVE:

RELEVANCE TO HUMAN HEALTH HAZARD ASSESSMENT

CHARLES H. LANGLEY

National Institute of Environmental Health Sciences
Research Triangle Park, North Carolina 27709 (U.S.A.)

In this session Drs. German, Paterson, and Swift presented
their thoughts and research results on human genetic variation that
is known or suspected to involve DNA repair and/or mutagen sensitivity. Their discussion brought out some of the salient issues in
this area: (1) the difficulties in identifying mutant phenotypes
that might involve disturbances in the function of the genetic
machinery, (2) relationships between cellular and molecular phenomena
and possible associations with phenotypes and environmental interactions, and (3) the possibility of increased cancer risk in heterozygotes.

The two dominant features of research in this area are dependence upon a small number of rare syndromes for material and
dependence upon the large body of nonmammalian information for ideas.
Many of the difficult problems have their source in the probable in-
adequacies of quantity and qualities of the mutants available and
in lack of concordance between DNA metabolism in humans and organisms
that serve as models.

Dr. German presented tabulations [1] of cancer occurrence in
the four most widely studied syndromes: Bloom's syndrome (BS),
ataxia telangiectasia (AT), Fanconi's anemia (FA), and xeroderma
pigmentosum (XP). Dr. German noted the association of BS and AT
with severe immunodeficiency and questions whether the cancer proneness of these syndromes might not be associated with immunodeficiency rather than increased somatic mutation. He also suggested
that the increased cancer incidence in FA might be attributable to
the androgen therapy rather than somatic mutations. Finally, Dr.
German pointed out the apparent lack of increased cancer in tissues
other than those exposed to sunlight among XP individuals. Although

data are still meager, it is remarkable that XP individuals do not
show increased incidences of other tumors thought to be largely
environmental in origin. This is especially puzzling, in light of
growing vidence for increased sensitivity of cultured XP cells to
a bro. range of chemical mutagens/carcinogens. Dr. German's
discus ion clearly indicates the difficulties in identifying and
characterizing human variation in DNA metabolism which might affect
mutation and/or cancer incidence.

     Dr. Paterson discussed results from experiments with
cultured fibroblast cells from individuals with AT and other
possibly interesting diseases. The details of these experiments
and their analyses can be found in the literature cited in the review
of Paterson and Smith [2]. Using plating efficiency as a measure of
sensitivity to various mutagenic agents (primarily ionizing radiation), Dr. Paterson and his colleagues demonstrated sensitivity to
hypoxic γ-irradiation of some presumed AT heterozygotes to be intermediate between the AT homozygotes and the normal homozygotes. This
finding is significant, in that it supports the indication of increased cancer risk in heterozygotes. It also suggests the feasi-
bility of identifying AT heterozygotes and other high risk individuals in the population. Dr. Paterson also presented data indicating
variation in sensitivity to several varied mutagens among cells from
different AT patients. This points toward a significant heterogeneity in this syndrome. This heterogeneity makes characterization
more difficult and has serious implications for the risk considerations in the general population. Dr. Paterson showed data indicating
the Rothmund-Thomson syndrome (RTS) cells are more sensitive to UV
light and γ-irradiation. These findings must be confirmed on cells
from other patients, but suggest shared repair pathways of UV and
ionizing irradiation damage in man. Dr. Paterson has surveyed
several other syndromes predisposing to cancer. There is a suggestion of increased sensitivity to ionizing irradiation in FA and
tuberous sclerosis as measured to reduction in plating efficiency.
Most interesting was the investigation of cells from members of a
family with clustered acute myelogenous leukemia. There was a
strong suggestion of association between sensitivity to γ-irradiation
and occurrence of cancer in individuals in this family. These
results demonstrate the complex phenomena being characterized in
the study of rare and heterogeneous syndromes and the associated
statistical problems.

     The rarity and heterogeneity of these recessively inherited
autosomal diseases indicate that the frequencies of heterozygotes
are certain to be much higher than the homozygotes. Dr. Swift
spoke of his investigation of cancer risk among family members of
patients with AT [5]. Comparing cancer incidence before the age of
45 years among blood relatives of AT patients, he estimated a fivefold increase in fatal cancer. He pointed out that AT heterozygotes
may make up 1% or more of the general population. With this

frequency and the fivefold increased risk, cancer in this unidenti-
fied high risk subgroup may account for as much as 5% of the cancer
in the general population. Dr. Swift has also investigated cancer
risk in relatives of patients with XP and FA and found some evidence
for increased risk [4].

There is good reason to suspect that genetic variation in
DNA repair or other aspects of the genetic machinery may play a
large role in the susceptibility to cancer and germinal mutations.
As mentioned above identified mutations may account for much, but
there is every reason to expect the known variation to be just "the
tip of the iceberg." The number of genetically distinct genes contributing to these known diseases may be grossly underestimated,
since complementation is likely to be tested only among the most
frequent alleles/loci. More important, we can expect many mutants
at most loci to be selected so strongly in the heterozygote (and
perhaps lethal in the homozygote) that identification of these
mutations in the population would be completely improbable, although
their cumulative impact over loci would be substantial [3].

Dr. German suggests that in vitro identification of heterozygotes of DNA metabolism mutants holds the most promise in the
study of human genetic variation in DNA metabolism. Dr. Paterson's
efforts are clearly headed in that direction. The facile elucidation of the complexities of the already-identified syndromes (considered above), as well as the evaluation of human genetic variation
in DNA metabolism in general, will have to rely on in vitro detection
of individuals with relevant phenotypes.

REFERENCES

1. German, J., Chromosome-breakage syndromes: different genes,
        different treatments, different cancers, This volume, p. 429.
2. Paterson, M. C., and P. J. Smith, Ataxia telangiectasia: an
        inherited human disorder involving hypersensitivity to
        ionizing radiation and related DNA-damaging chemicals,
        Ann. Rev. Genetics, 13 (1979) 291-318.
3. Simmons, J., and J. C. Crow, Mutations affecting fitness in
        Drosophila populations, Ann. Rev. Genetics, 11 (1978) 49-78.
4. Swift, M., Fanconi's anemia in the genetics of neoplasia,
        Nature, 230 (1971) 370-373.
5. Swift, M., L. Sholman, M. Perry, and C. Chase, Malignant
        neoplasms in families of patients with ataxia-telangiectasia,
        Cancer Res., 36 (1976) 209-215.

CONTRIBUTORS

Carmen Attolini, Laboratorio CNR di Genetica Biochimica ed
    Evoluzionistica and Instituto di Genetica dell'Universita'
    di Pavia, 27100 Pavia, Italy

K. N. Ayres, Department of Microbiology, The University of Chicago,
    Chicago, Illinois 60637, U.S.A.

Bruce S. Baker, Biology Department, Universify of California,
    San Diego, La Jolla, California 92093, U.S.A.

Michael A. Bender, Medical Department, Brookhaven National
    Laboratory, Upton, New York 11973, U.S.A.

Umberto Bertazzoni, Laboratorio CNR di Genetica Biochimica ed
    Evoluzionistica and Instituto di Genetica dell'Universita'
    di Pavia, 21700 Pavia, Italy

K. Bose, Department of Microbiology, The University of Chicago,
    Chicago, Illinois 60637, U.S.A.

James B. Boyd, Department of Genetics, University of California,
    Davis, California 95616, U.S.A.

Brigitte Brandriff, Laboratory of Radiobiology and Department of
    Anatomy, University of California at San Francisco,
    San Francisco, California 94143, U.S.A.

Herman E. Brockman, Department of Biological Sciences, Illinois
    State University, Normal, Illinois 61761, U.S.A.

Adelaide T. C. Carpenter, Biology Department, University of
    California, San Diego, La Jolla, California 92093, U.S.A.

C. C. Chang, Department of Human Development, College of Human
    Medicine, Michigan State University, East Lansing, Michigan
    48824, U.S.A.

T. Y.-K. Chow, Departments of Biochemistry and Biology, McGill
     University, Montreal, Quebec, Canada, H3G 1Y6

Frederick J. de Serres, Office of the Director, National Institute
     of Environmental Health Sciences, Research Triangle Park,
     North Carolina 27709, U.S.A.

Ruth L. Dusenbery, Department of Biology, Emory University,
     Atlanta, Georgia 30322, U.S.A.

A. J. Fornace, Jr., Department of Physiology, Laboratory of
     Radiobiology, Harvard School of Public Health, Boston,
     Massachusetts 02115, U.S.A.

M. J. Fraser, Departments of Biochemistry and Biology, McGill
     University, Montreal, Quebec, Canada, H3G 1Y6

Errol C. Friedberg, Laboratory of Experimental Oncology, Department
     of Pathology, Stanford University, Stanford, California
     94305, U.S.A.

Maurizio Gatti, Instituto de Geneticà, Faculta di Scienze, Citta
     Universitaria 00185, Roma, Italy

Walderico M. Generoso, Biology Division, Oak Ridge National
     Laboratory, Oak Ridge, Tennessee 37830, U.S.A.

James German, The New York Blood Center, 310 East 67th Street,
     New York, New York 10021, U.S.A.

Tom Glover, Department of Human Development, College of Human
     Medicine, Michigan State University, East Lansing, Michigan
     48824, U.S.A.

U. Graf, Institute of Toxicology, Swiss Federal Institute of
     Technology and University of Zürich, CH-8603 Schwerzenbach,
     Switzerland

M. M. Green, Department of Genetics, University of California,
     Davis, California 95616, U.S.A.

Paul V. Harris, Department of Genetics, University of California,
     Davis, California 95616, U.S.A.

P. J. Hastings, Department of Genetics, The University of Alberta,
     Edmonton, Alberta, Canada, T6G 2E9

E. Käfer, Departments of Biochemistry and Biology, McGill
     University, Montreal, Quebec, Canada, H3G 1Y6

R. F. Kimball, Biology Division, Oak Ridge National Laboratory,
     Oak Ridge, Tennessee 37830, U.S.A.

Charles Langley, National Institute of Environmental Health Sciences,
     Research Triangle Park, North Carolina 27709, U.S.A.

Jeffrey F. Lemontt, Biology Division, Oak Ridge National Laboratory,
     Oak Ridge, Tennessee 37830, U.S.A.

J. B. Little, Department of Physiology, Laboratory of Radiobiology,
     Harvard School of Public Health, Boston, Massachusetts 02115,
     U.S.A.

Veronica M. Maher, Department of Microbiology and Department of
     Biochemistry, Carcinogenesis Laboratory, Michigan State
     University, East Lansing, Michigan 48824, U.S.A.

J. Justin McCormick, Department of Microbiology and Department of
     Biochemistry, Carcinogenesis Laboratory, Michigan State
     University, East Lansing, Michigan 48824, U.S.A.

P. Moore, Department of Microbiology, The University of Chicago,
     Chicago, Illinois 60637, U.S.A.

H. Nagasawa, Department of Physiology, Laboratory of Radiobiology,
     Harvard School of Public Health, Boston, Massachusetts 02115,
     U.S.A.

Loree D. Olson, Program in Genetics, Washington State University,
     Pullman, Washington 99164, U.S.A.

Christopher J. Osgood, Department of Genetics, University of
     California, Davis, California 95616, U.S.A.

Roger A. Pedersen, Laboratory of Radiobiology and Department of
     Anatomy, University of California at San Francisco, San
     Francisco, California 94143, U.S.A.

Sergio Pimpinelli, Instituto de Geneticà, Faculta di Scienze, Citta
     Universitaria 00185, Roma, Italy

Louise Prakash, Department of Radiation Biology and Biophysics,
     School of Medicine, University of Rochester, Rochester,
     New York 14627, U.S.A.

Satya Prakash, Department of Biology, University of Rochester,
     Rochester, New York 14627, U.S.A.

Richard J. Reynolds, Laboratory of Experimental Oncology, Department
        of Pathology, Stanford University, Stanford, California 94305,
        U.S.A.

Liane B. Russell, Biology Division, Oak Ridge National Laboratory,
        Oak Ridge, Tennessee 37830, U.S.A.

Masao S. Sasaki, Radiation Biology Center, Kyoto University,
        Sakyo-ku, Kyoto 606, Japan

Koki Sato, Division of Genetics, National Institute of Radiological
        Sciences, 9-1, Anagawa 4, Chiba 260, Japan

Alice L. Schroeder, Program in Genetics, Washington State University,
        Pullman, Washington 99164, U.S.A.

Roger S. Schultz, Department of Human Development, College of
        Human Medicine, Michigan State University, East Lansing,
        Michigan 48824, U.S.A.

Gary A. Sega, Biology Division, Oak Ridge National Laboratory,
        Oak Ridge, Tennessee 37830, U.S.A.

R. B. Setlow, Biology Department, Brookhaven National Laboratory,
        Upton, New York 11973, U.S.A.

R. Sklar, Department of Microbiology, The University of Chicago,
        Chicago, Illinois 60637, U.S.A.

David A. Smith, Biology Department, University of California,
        San Diego, La Jolla, California 92093, U.S.A.

Karen E. Smith, Department of Genetics, University of California,
        Davis, California 95616, U.S.A.

P. Dennis Smith, Department of Biology, Emory University, Atlanta,
        Georgia 30322, U.S.A.

Ronald D. Snyder, Biology Division, Oak Ridge National Laboratory,
        Oak Ridge, Tennessee 37830, U.S.A.

Miria Stefanini, Laboratorio CNR di Genetica Biochimica ed
        Evoluzionistica and Instituto di Genetica dell'Universita'
        di Pavia, 21700 Pavia, Italy

B. Strauss, Department of Microbiology, The University of Chicago,
        Chicago, Illinois 60637, U.S.A.

K. Tatsumi, Department of Microbiology, The University of Chicago,
        Chicago, Illinois 60637, U.S.A.

James E. Trosko, Department of Human Development, College of Human
      Medicine, Michigan State University, East Lansing, Michigan
      48824, U.S.A.

R. C. von Borstel, Department of Genetics, The University of
      Alberta, Edmonton, Alberta, Canada, T6G 2E9

Raymond Waters, Genetics Department, University College, Singleton
      Park, Swansea SA2 8PP, U.K.

Sheldon Wolff, Laboratory of Radiobiology and Department of Anatomy,
      University of California at San Francisco, San Francisco,
      California 94143, U.S.A.

F. E. Würgler, Institute of Toxicology, Swiss Federal Institute of
      Technology and University of Zurich, CH-8603 Schwerzenbach,
      Switzerland

INDEX

451